Reversing Heart Disease and Preventing Diabetes

D1555083

Apply Science to Lower Cholesterol 100 Points;
Reduce Arterial Plaque 50% in 25 months;
and Improve Heart Rhythm and Valves

Kent R. Rieske, BS/ME

Reversing Heart Disease and Preventing Diabetes

Library of Congress Cataloging-in Publication Data
Kent R. Rieske, Reversing Heart Disease and Preventing Diabetes

Library of Congress Control Number: 2011943818

| ISBN-10: | 0-9828485-4-4 | (Paperback) |
| ISBN-13: | 978-0-9828485-4-8 | (Paperback) |

Subject 1:	Medical: Cardiology
Subject 2:	Medical: Diet Therapy
Subject 3:	Health & Fitness: Disease - Diabetes

Third printing June 2015
Printed in the United States of America, United Kingdom, and Australia
Exalt Publishing®

Contents

Dedication

To my wife, Marti; son, Matthew; and daughter, Michelle.

To God who has said, "Which things also we speak, not in the words which man's wisdom teacheth, but which the Holy Ghost teacheth; comparing spiritual things with spiritual. But the natural man receiveth not the things of the Spirit of God: for they are foolishness unto him: neither can he know them, because they are spiritually discerned." 1 Corinthians 2:13–14

Acknowledgement

I am very grateful to my wife, Marti, for her excellent editing of this book. Her medical secretarial degree from Concordia College, Bronxville, NY; extensive experience as a medical transcriptionist; previous book editing; and natural command of the English language have given her the unique ability to edit the scientific content of this book.

Thank you, Marti, for your wonderful help and continued support.

Medical Disclaimer

Autobiography

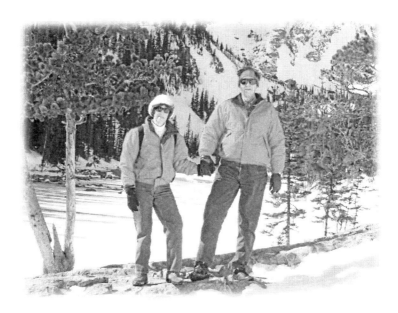

Kent and Marti Rieske
Hallet Peak and Emerald Lake on February 14, 2011
Rocky Mountain National Park, Colorado

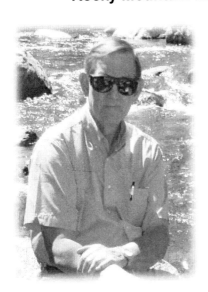

I was born at home on a small farm in Provo, Utah, in 1939. We grew potatoes, carrots, onions, beans, strawberries, raspberries, and corn in abundance, along with the apples from a large orchard. We had one lonely pear tree and three sour pie cherry trees.

We had one milk cow that produced a calf each year and a chicken coop with two dozen chickens. Milk, butter, and eggs were plentiful in addition to the meat from slaughtered chickens and the cow or her grown male offspring. My mother prepared meals from this abundance, and my father loved honey on the cornbread made from home-grown, home-ground corn. She bought honey in a large bulk container, and we used a spoon to scoop it out when it crystallized. Mother was addicted to carbohydrates because her grandfather was a beekeeper.

My maternal great grandfather, Christian Jensen Peterson, was a child when his mother remarried. They lived in Utah before it was a state, and President Brigham Young of the LDS Church instructed the family to move from Salt Lake City to Castle Valley, Utah, in 1880 as one of several families who founded the present town of Price. Their initial home along the Price River was a single room dug into the hillside and enclosed in the front by logs. These common dwellings for the pioneers were called *dugouts.* The soil was a good insulator in summer and winter.

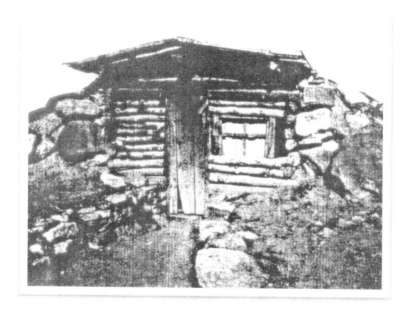

Christian later married and provided for his family by farming, hunting, and keeping bees. The honey created an addiction to carbohydrates that did the family no good. In those days, fruits were limited to their seasons because canning wasn't done, but honey was available throughout the year.

When I was about 10 years old, I enjoyed shooting my father's .22 Winchester® pump rifle around the farm and hunting birds and small game in the nearby woods. My father shot a mule deer nearly every year, and so did I after I reached the legal hunting age of fourteen.

When I was in college, I bought a Browning® 12-gage, 5-shot automatic shotgun that was awesome for hunting ducks and pheasants. I successfully hunted pheasants in the nearby field and woods as well as other areas of Utah. This is the same gun that I used in Otis, Colorado, about ten years ago to shoot three cock pheasants within two seconds when they all flew up at once. Bang-bang-bang! It happened as fast as you can say it. Instead of the smaller No. 4 shot usually recommended, I used No. 2 shot, 3" magnum shells that left the pheasants dead on impact as they fell in the weeds. I had finally matched the record set by my brother-in-law while he was hunting in our cornfield many years before.

When I was a teenager, I caught trout with my hands in Spring Creek that ran along our farm property, and I often cooked them over an open fire. We took our 16-foot (5 meter) aluminum fishing boat to Yellowstone National Park every summer, where we easily caught our daily limit of three cutthroat trout per person.

Those were the good ol' days when we had fun playing with the bears. My friend and I were about 14 years old when he went with us to Yellowstone. We had fun with a half-grown, golden-colored bear who was more concerned about us than we were about him. We chased him from the cabin area into the forest, but when he was out of sight and very quiet in the thick trees, we began to worry about where he was. We panicked and ran back to the cabin as fast as we could.

One big male bear wasn't as much fun. He got agitated at the kids running around in all directions and yelling. He was on the other side of a parked car when I heard a low, rumbling growl and noticed the hair standing up on the back of his shoulders. Yikes! I ran around several cabins and into our cabin, slamming the door to make sure it was latched. I hadn't taken one second to look back, and have no I idea if he chased me or not. I suspect that he didn't bother with me once I was out of his sight.

I gathered morels in the woods by the Provo River and brought them home, using my shirt as a carry bag. They ranged in color from black to brown, and my mother was thrilled because some of them were 4" (100 mm) high. Morels are the most delicious food on earth and fit for a king as were the quail that I shot. Mother fried the morels in fresh butter that I helped her make with a hand churn. The flavor was so delicious it is indescribable. Small, half-dehydrated morels cost $50 per pound today if you can find them. Morels won't grow in captivity or in a mushroom barn, so they are rare and expensive.

You may be wondering what all this history has to do with reversing heart disease. Actually, it has everything to do with my ability to reverse my heart disease, and I think you will grasp the connection when you study my current diet in the following chapters. Reversing heart disease depends on the amount of protein, fat, and carbohydrates in the diet. It is not as you may have been taught.

The modern food shopper would be astonished at the amount of food that we threw away or let rot. Most of the farm products were naturally organic, but we sprayed the apples and beans with insecticides several times each season. Worm-free organic apples are impossible to grow, and those sold in the supermarkets are frauds. In the years when the spring frost didn't freeze the blossoms, every farmer had more apples than he could sell, and at least half of them fell on the ground to rot.

When I was a child, my mother bottled all kinds of fruits and made sugar-rich jams and jellies. When she went to the store, I helped her by carrying the 10-pound (4.5 kg) bags of sugar and flour to the truck and into the house.

We had cow that provided plenty of raw milk, cream and butter, but my mother got duped into buying factory margarine made from pure white hydrogenated corn oil. It came in a flexible plastic bag (a new invention) with a bubble of orange dye inside that easily ruptured when we squeezed it. I thought it was fun to massage the bag until the dye turned the white fake fat into something that looked a lot like butter. We ate this instead of the real butter that I had previously helped my mother make by cranking the cream separator and the butter churn.

When I was growing up, our diet was a precursor of the *USDA Food Guide Pyramid*. My mother died from cancer at age 50, and my father from heart disease at age 56 as a result of this high-carbohydrate diet of whole grains, potatoes, fruit, honey, and refined sugar. You may think that white sugar is not recommended on the pyramid, but as you will see in the following chapters, fruit juice and white sugar have exactly the same sugar molecules. The body doesn't know the difference.

Life on the farm had health risks from pathogens, such as bacteria, viruses, fungi, protozoa, and parasites, because of the close proximity of farm animals, fecal matter that was spread as fertilizer for the row crops, and contact with the soil itself. We were not germ freaks in those days, but perhaps we should have been.

The apple orchard presented a health risk because all apple orchards must be sprayed heavily with insecticides to prevent worms from boring into the center of the apples to lay their eggs. As a teenager on a farm, I was literally drenched in four insecticides: DDT®, Malathion®, and two others. My father put these four insecticides into the tank of a heavy-duty sprayer that I pulled with the tractor. The sprayer had a 1" (25 mm) diameter hose and a pump discharge pressure of 400 pounds per square inch (27.6 bars) that would literally drench a full-grown apple tree in seconds. This was not like a garden hose. The high-pressure, high-volume spray created a cloudy mist of overspray that dried on contact to form a pure white coating of insecticides that remained on my arms, neck, and face as a visible residue for several hours until spraying was completed. I could taste the chemicals as I breathed the misty air. I received more insecticide from each spraying than the average person receives in a lifetime. My mother would tell me to go wash off the spray with the garden hose, but like most kids, I did a sloppy cleaning job with the icy cold water. I never even considered using soap.

We sprayed several times each year for many years, but my severe overdose of four insecticides has not affected my health in any way that I can discern—even though DDT® and Malathion® have been banned by government regulations. Maybe the insecticides prevent the cancer, diabetes, inflammatory bowel disease, and more than four dozen autoimmune diseases that I have avoided.

Eating organic apples may be a larger cancer risk than eating the insecticides instead of the apples. I will give the scientific proof that fructose sugar as found in apples and other fruits can cause fatty liver disease that in turn causes liver cancer. Fruit also increases the diabetes risk, and 25% of diabetics die from cancer. Fructose and glucose found in fruit, and glucose from whole grains causes systemic candida yeast and systemic fungal infections that I believe are the cause of deaths resulting from tumors incorrectly diagnosed as cancerous. Lung cancer is probably caused by fungus in many cases, but it can also be caused by radiation and free radical chemical damage to the cells.

One of the greatest health risks on the farm was exposure to bacteria and viruses from breathing the pathogen-ladened air during the annual spring cleaning of the chicken coop. The chickens slept on a wooden frame about 12" (305 mm) off the concrete floor that was covered with chicken wire screen. This area was about 10% of the size of the chicken coop. They walked on 2" x 2" (50 mm x 50 mm) horizontal wooden strips placed over the screen and parallel to the front of the platform on 12" (305 mm) centers. By natural instinct, the chickens jumped onto the platform as nighttime approached and slept on the strips in rows. Most of their fecal droppings accumulated on the concrete floor under the wire screen. The floor was covered with wood chips after cleaning, but the floor later became a mixture of fecal droppings, feathers, and wood chips. Everything was scooped up, tossed into the pickup truck, and taken to the field where it was thrown in order to spread it evenly.

Cleaning the chicken coop was a dreaded chore. The chickens would fly and scatter from the activities, and the pathogen-laden dust filled the air. My sisters and I were just naïve children and attacked our assignment with vigor. We inhaled the pathogen-laden air and never thought about wearing any protective clothing or breathing masks. This was my first introduction to organic farming.

Work in the fields was also high risk. Cuts and scrapes were common and became infected most of the time. Our favorite topical antiseptics for the cuts were mercurochrome and Merthiolate®, both mercury-based products that have since been banned for general public use. (Many people are outraged that Merthiolate® is still used as a vaccine preservative.) However, these antiseptics appeared to be more effective than those available for general public use today.

Injuries commonly became red and swollen with puss. My mother always gave me instructions to tell her immediately if I saw a "red line running up my arm." I knew she was serious, but I didn't know her warning was about a deadly systemic infection that could have flashed throughout my body. I watched for the red line but it never appeared.

By age ten or earlier, I became fairly knowledgeable and effective at treating myself. I found from experience that the best treatment was to rip the scab off an infected injury and scrub it with the fiber hand brush and very soapy water. I am now sure the brush was a mass of bacteria too, but I didn't know it at the time. I found that hard scrubbing until the injury was bloody, red flesh was more effective than being gentle. I just had to endure the pain and get the job done. One of our mercury-based antiseptics was applied generously after cleaning, and the injury was covered with a band aid, which didn't stay on very long as I work or played around the farm. I repeated the whole procedure when the injury was in a location that could not be easily protected.

I also dreaded picking sweet corn. My father had severe hay fever that kept him inside the house, sneezing and wiping his nose. He didn't even approach the cornfield when the pollen was flying. I had to respond whenever anyone came to buy a few dozen ears of corn. The dust and pollen from the corn left me a filthy mess. It was in my hair, down my shirt, and was itchy. I tried to ignore the slices on my arms and neck from the razor sharp edges of the corn leaves.

Harvesting the onions was another hazard. The large Golden Spanish onions were harvested in the fall when the tops began to fall over. We grasped several tops in one hand and pulled the onions out of the ground. By harvest time, they had pushed themselves above the soil and the roots pulled out easily. A very large, sharp paring knife in the other hand was used to cut the tops, and the onions dropped into the irrigation furrow between every other row where they remained for several days to dry. The index finger on the hand holding the onion tops took the slice several times each season. My sisters and I found that onion juice was a very good disinfectant. It also seemed to stop the bleeding. I pried the cut open as I squeezed a few drops of onion juice onto the injury. It stung but not badly. We forgot the band aid, ignored the blood, and just kept "topping onions." I can still see the scars on my index finger.

We harvested the carrots in the late fall before a hard frost. Our carrots were mainly used as food for the cow, and she loved them. They turned the milk slightly orange, but the flavor was not affected. My father cut the tops off with a very sharp round-nose shovel while they were still in the ground. The walk-behind tractor had two staggered blade plows that simply lifted the large carrots out of the ground. They were about twice the size of the average large potato, unlike those in the supermarkets today. Because the weather was generally cold and our hands became numb, we held them in the tractor's engine exhaust to keep them warm. The carrots were stored in a pit cellar that had a dirt-covered roof.

Our neighbor down the lane was quoted as saying, "Max Rieske is killing those kids." He and his obese wife lived on a small lot with two overweight girls. They didn't farm and had the only lawn in our neighborhood and a sidewalk to the lane. I guess we were blue collar rednecks and they were proper. His prophesy was wrong. Their entire family has since passed away, but my two sisters and I continue to celebrate our birthdays.

Our gravel road was about a mile long from our house to the highway on which I rode my bike daily to and from school or just for fun. One day when I was about 12 years old, I crashed hard on the gravel and ripped a silver dollar-sized hole in my knee. I scrubbed the injury as hard as I could with the fiber hand brush to get the sand and dirt out of the flesh, but since the pain prevented me from doing a thorough cleaning, it got infected. It might have been a blessing when I fell again and tore off the scab. The second treatment was followed by increased caution to allow the injury to heal. I also learned to allow a scab to fall off naturally and not to pick at it.

As children, we seemed to be sick with a cold or bronchial infection half of the time. I had both of my ear drums lanced to help drain and heal the infections. That was one approach doctors used. I was very thankful for penicillin even though it caused a rash on my chest that we largely ignored.

I received the standard vaccinations in school until I was in the third grade and one of the shots made me severely ill. I knew the shot had made me sick, and I threw an absolute fit when anyone suggested giving me another vaccination. My mother relented and I had very few vaccinations after that. I did get a tetanus shot when I was 12 years old after I stepped on a nail while helping to build our new house. The carpenter was amazed that I could cut a board square without drawing a line to follow.

One day I fell out of an apple tree and landed on the barbed wire fence. To my amazement, I didn't get badly hurt or cut. When I was in college, my father asked me to cut down the apple orchard of about 100 old mature trees. It was a bigger job than simply cutting the tree off near the ground. I cut off all of the small limbs, dragged them to one spot, and threw them in a large pile to be burned. I cut the bigger limbs off the main trunk, cut them into 6' (2 meters) lengths, and placed them in a pile. Later my father hired a man with a large mobile circular saw to cut them into smaller pieces for the fireplace. The job went on day after day for weeks until the new chainsaw came close to expiring. Luckily I never got hurt, but in one careless split second, the whirring chain came too close to my thigh. The blade ripped into my Levis® and cut a 6" (153 mm) jagged tear. I shuddered before looking. Surprise—not a scratch on me! I threw the Levis® in the trash because in those days we wouldn't be caught dead in jeans with a hole in the knee. Those were the days of the iron-on knee patches. I always hated to see a hole worn in the knee, and I still prefer dark blue jeans that are not faded. You may be wondering what work, injury, and exposure to pathogens have to do with heart disease. Actually, they are very relevant as I hope to explain in the following chapters.

I received a Bachelor of Science degree in Mechanical Engineering in 1962 and became a registered Professional Engineer in several states. My career included positions as Chief Mechanical Engineer and Director of Engineering. In 1985 I started a home-based consulting engineering firm, developed and marketed engineering software worldwide, and created a non-denominational Christian website based on dispensational theology. The website also includes a scientific approach to health and nutrition.

I believe bacterial and viral infections are risk factors for heart disease as I will discuss in more detail in Chapter 3. When I suddenly developed high blood pressure of 150/100 in 1983 at age 44, I went to the Arizona Heart Institute in Phoenix where we were living. At the time, treatment was limited, and I was advised to exercise more even though I was already very active. Many years later, I tried several blood pressure medications but rejected each one because of the side effects. My blood pressure fluctuated but generally remained in 150/90 range for 24 years before my heart attack in September 2007 at age 68.

By random chance, I was treated by an excellent cardiologist. He placed a stent (expanded metal screen device that holds the artery open) in one of my major heart arteries and left two other small areas of plaque (a restrictive deposit in the artery) with 40% and 50% occlusions untreated. It came as no surprise when the report from the radiologist who interpreted my emergency room X-rays noted scar tissue on my bronchial tubes from previous infections. I have had many bronchial infections as an adult and during my childhood.

I developed the diet, supplement, and drug regimen within a few months after placement of the stent, and my cardiologist agreed with my approach. In October 2009, he performed another angiogram because my blood pressure became erratic. He chose an angiogram because it is the most accurate method available for diagnosing the health of the heart arteries and valves, and he could insert another stent at the same time if necessary. We were both thrilled that the two small areas of plaque had been reduced to half the size in only 25 months. His advised me to, "Stay on your program and see me again in one year."

I will not divulge the name of my cardiologist, but I will say that he goes by the science, is an excellent surgeon, and has placed two thousand stents in patients' arteries. His bedside manner is relaxed and calm, not rushed in order to get to the next patient. Best of all, he completely agrees with my method for reversing my heart disease and doesn't push the low-fat dogma. In fact, he didn't recommend any diet after my heart attack except to say, "Stay on your diet" when I told him I was eating low-carb. This was before I started my cholesterol-lowering regimen and before seeing the angiogram that proved I had reduced my two small areas of heart artery plaque by 50% in only 25 months.

Yes, I have proved that heart artery plaque can be removed. I have reversed my heart disease.

Everyone seems to like him. I referred a friend to him when her cardiologist was out of the office. She immediately wanted to switch after the first visit but decided not to do so because she didn't want to hurt her cardiologist's feelings. My cardiologist is so busy that I must call six weeks in advance to get an appointment. He doesn't need me to promote his business.

Credits

William Banting (1797–1878) was a formerly obese and sickly undertaker in London, England, who wrote the 22-page booklet, *Letter on Corpulence,* in 1859 to explain how a fairly low-carbohydrate diet greatly restored his failing health in a very short time. His success was based on his persistence in trying every diet suggested to him by several doctors until he stumbled upon the absolute truth regarding the connection between diet and health. To his dismay, the majority of physicians and citizens instantly rejected the information.

Vilhjalmur Stefansson, BA, ethnologist (1879–1962), and **Rudolph Martin (Karsten) Anderson**, PhD, zoologist (1876-1961), were Arctic explorers who ventured to northern Canada beyond the Arctic Circle during 1906–1912 to bring back the secrets of the Eskimos' all-meat diet. Mr. Stefansson was shocked that the public and doctors rejected his reports and insisted that man cannot live without eating vegetables. Mr. Stefansson wrote several books about his adventures.

Weston A. Price, DDS, dentist and nutritionist (1870–1948), traveled around the world with his wife, Florence, in the 1920s and 1930s. He visited many primitive villages in order to assess the connection between diet and their excellent health. He authored the popular book, *Nutrition and Physical Degeneration.*

Robert C. Atkins, MD, cardiologist and nutritionist (1930–2003), authored the best-selling low-carbohydrate book, *Dr. Atkins' Diet Revolution,* and several others.

Michael R. Eades, MD, and **Mary Dan Eades**, MD, doctors and nutritionists who authored the very popular low-carbohydrate book, *Protein Power,* and several others.

Reversing Heart Disease and Preventing Diabetes

Introduction

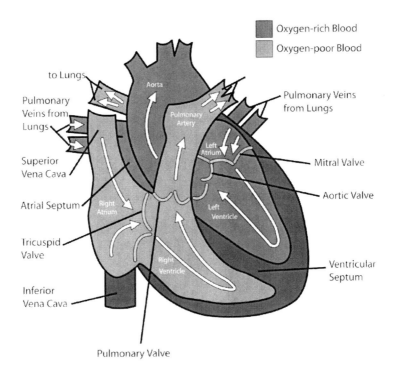

Diagram of the Human Heart

This is a science book. You may think this declaration is unnecessary because books, articles, and studies about health, nutrition, and disease are not expected to be fiction. This book is based on scientific facts that will reveal why many books and references about health and nutrition are pure fiction. I used science to develop the diet therapy; vitamin, mineral, and supplement program; and the selection of pharmaceuticals to formulate the regimen that reduced my two areas of heart artery plaque by 50% in only 25 months. Consult your physician before you proceed with any diet therapy suggested in this book.

Millions of people have been diagnosed with coronary artery disease and have had one or more stents inserted to open the plaque-plugged arteries. The patients are told to follow the government's official low-fat dietary guidelines afterward but are consistently disappointed when they discover their conditions have worsened, not improved as the medical authorities promised. The result is a very high-risk and painful open heart operation and quadruple heart artery bypass procedure that they must undergo in the hope of saving their lives. After surviving the ordeal, the frightened patients follow the official government guidelines even closer. The result is another major disappointment when they are told the replacement arteries are filling up with plaque as well. The more they comply with the guidelines, the faster their disease progresses.

Remember. This is a science book.

Patients generally expect that the dietary guidelines and drugs prescribed for them will reverse their heart disease and prevent them from having future heart attacks. Professional medical societies and government health departments tell them the treatment has been scientifically tested and proven to be effective. The patient will read books and pamphlets that give scientific studies by people and organizations with advanced credentials. Could most of this information be false? Yes! It is scientifically false! Most of it is only false conjecture and political correctness that are opposite to scientific facts. The obsessive compulsive controlling élite have an agenda that is not in your best interest.

Yes, most of the information given to patients for the prevention and reversal of heart disease is scientifically false. Patients become so discouraged that they don't know whom to trust or what to believe. These patients may have a hard time believing that my awesome success is real because they have been tricked many times. Well, it is real, and I am overjoyed that I have reversed my heart disease.

The word *science* is automatically interpreted to mean that the topic and information are true. Deceived or unscrupulous individuals throw the word around loosely in order to give the false impression that their claims are valid. Organizations get away with deceiving society because they are the highest authorities both inside and outside of government. They have no one who can challenge them because they blast their agendas across the major media with billions of dollars of government funding.

Don't be brainwashed by the obsessive compulsive controlling élite with agendas.

After a person receives a devastating health diagnosis, he begins to question the previous dietary advice he received from government health authorities. The public is having a health concern meltdown as test results often reveal several deadly diseases or symptoms of diseases, such as plugged arteries, leaky heart valves, terrible EKG charts, irregular heart rhythms, fatty liver disease, cancer, diabetes, hypertension, and dreadful blood chemistry readings. They should be concerned. The rates of heart disease, cancer, diabetes, and obesity continue to increase despite the public's attempts to adhere to official dietary recommendations.

They rush to the supermarket and load their carts with organic whole grain cereals and breads; potatoes and yams; soy or rice milk; ten different kinds of fruits; and a dozen boxes of frozen low-fat, zero-cholesterol frozen meals. Now they feel more at ease about becoming stronger and healthier. They grumble out loud as they hurry past the dairy and meat departments, "It must have been that egg and piece of meat I ate at the fast food restaurant."

Are there areas of science that are based on pure conjecture without any real scientific foundation? Yes! Biology is a good example. Biology is classified as a *natural science* (the study of living organisms), but biology has degenerated into a field of study that is rarely based on scientific truth. Biology references, studies, and textbooks are based primarily on conjecture and theories that have little basis in scientific truth. Because biology as taught in the schools and universities can't be confirmed by repeatable measurements and observations, it is not classified as a *pure science*—nor should it be.

Music is more of a science than biology, yet music is classified as an art. The musical scale is based on physics, a pure science, and the instruments are made by highly precise scientific calculations. The Middle C musical note has the same frequency in all countries, languages, and societies at 261.625565 hertz. Indeed, it is a strange, uneven number. Biologists would claim that Middle C was once 200 hertz and is in the process of evolving toward 300 hertz. No! Middle C has always been the same frequency.

Sciences are classified as being *fundamental, basic,* or *pure* when they are based on proven fundamental laws that can be repeatedly confirmed, measured, and verified by carefully controlled experiments and observations. We call the results of these experiments and observations *scientific laws* because they can be confirmed at any time by anyone using repeatable experiments. Middle C is a scientific law of music. As a mechanical engineer, I work daily with scientific laws that can be used repeatedly without fear that the results may be different than expected. A load placed on a beam in a building, bridge, or piece of equipment will produce a deflection that can be determined by scientific formulas and confirmed by actual load tests. Another example is the pressure in a vessel that will produce a stress in the wall of the vessel that can be accurately determined by scientific formulas and confirmed by actual tests. Electrical engineers know the formulas they used will give the same dependable answers as when their fathers were in college. Engineers don't need to run these tests over and over in order to assure themselves that the results of the scientific formulas are accurate, true, and have not evolved to produce different results. All engineers get the same answers regardless of the language they speak or country in which they live. Diet and health guidelines that government health departments, medical associations, and medical departments in universities give to the public are pure propaganda controlled by these groups with an agenda.

Many diet-health reports and studies are pure propaganda controlled by groups with an agenda.

Introduction

We read studies concerning health, nutrition, and disease that appear in the mass media on a daily basis. The news report usually begins with the statement, "In a new scientific study..." and continues to give the results of the study. However, many of these studies contradict each other, are not repeatable, and appear to violate other observations. These are not scientific studies that the lead-ins claim or that most people assume. They are often formulated and structured in such a manner that the researcher knows in advance what his report will conclude in accordance with his predetermined agenda or motive. For these reasons, studies should always be viewed with a great deal of skepticism. A report delivered today by an organization with the highest credentials can be expected to be proved false tomorrow. This leaves the general public in a state of confusion, not knowing what information is true and what is false. Many people write to me and complain that they are extremely frustrated by the contradictory information they read. They are frustrated because they tend to be susceptible to propaganda and are not skeptical enough when the information is first presented. The trick used in many reports and studies is to present one foundational statement at the beginning that is treated as a given; however, that statement has not been proven as the reader assumes and is actually false. The public gets taken in by the false assumption without realizing that the conclusion of the study is also false. The mass media are a lot like magicians. They present the lead-in material in a way that appears to be true only to trick the observer into believing a result that is actually false.

In order to separate fact from fiction, one must have a broad, comprehensive knowledge in many areas of study and apply this knowledge to the information being presented. When a scientific truth cannot be validated by each and every test and observation, it ceases to be scientific or true. A theory does not need an overwhelming amount of evidence against it to be proved false. Only one test or observation needs to fail in order to prove that the theory cannot be trusted. We wouldn't want to risk our lives on a formula for the design of airplanes that was right some of the time but occasionally wrong.

I will go back to the very basics of science, nutrition, and human physiology to arrive at conclusions, recommendations, and remarks that you will find differ greatly from those propagated by the major media, university textbooks, individuals with high credentials, health and nutrition associations, government departments of health and nutrition, and religious groups. You will find many of the statements in this book to be harshly contrary to other references. I make no apology for the differences.

The controlling government élite are not innovative entrepreneurs.

I have been criticized for the lack of references to support my statements and claims. The general public has been brainwashed to believe that original thought is nonexistent. People want a long list of references to support each and every statement. I will give many references, but much of my analysis of the effect of diet on human physiology is original. Thomas Edison did not have any references for his incandescent electric light bulb, and the Wright brothers did not have any references for the design of their airplane. If you would rather be brainwashed, gather all the references available and believe the majority opinion.

The media, individuals, and organizations use brainwashing to protect their agendas. For example, the United States Department of Agriculture's *USDA Food Guide Pyramid* and the new *2010 USDA My Plate* are diet programs that claim a healthy diet must contain 50–60% carbohydrates in order to supply the body with the daily energy it needs. Scientifically, this claim is false. The amount of carbohydrates essential for good health is zero. The body does not require dietary carbohydrates for energy.

The scientific requirement for carbohydrates in the diet is zero.

The body's essential requirements for sustaining life are protein and fats, not carbohydrates. Carbohydrates are not one of 57 or more scientifically essential nutrients required for humans. Numerous references say you must eat carbohydrates because they are the energy source for the brain and heart. Again, this statement is false. We have all been brainwashed to some degree by the obsessive compulsive controlling élite to believe we must eat some carbohydrates or we will contract a disease.

For example, on October 13, 1972, an airplane carrying a team of rugby players, along with other family members, crashed in the Andes Mountains in Uruguay near the Chilean border. Some of the 45 passengers in the plane survived. After many days of starvation, these survivors decided to save their own lives by consuming the flesh of their dead companions, and they began with the body of the pilot whose faulty judgment caused the crash. (The survivors wanted a little justice as well.) Several days after the crash, an avalanche buried the remaining section of the airplane's fuselage and filled it with snow, killing more of the survivors. Sixteen people survived this tragedy for a period of 72 days before they were rescued. They didn't suffer brain or heart damage even though carbohydrates were totally absent from their diet for the entire 72 days.

Introduction

Let me paint an alternate scenario that is totally fictitious. Imagine an airplane on its way to Australia for the fictitious International Conference of Vegetarians. Imagine that the plane is identical to the one that crashed in the Andes. Far out over the South Pacific Ocean, the plane develops electrical and mechanical problems that force it down. The pilot is relieved to see an island immediately to his right, turns toward it, and gently glides the plane to a soft landing. The passengers are elated that they landed without difficulty, and they are amazed at the beautiful scenery as they look out of the windows of the plane. "This looks like paradise," one of the passengers says as the others nod in agreement. The island is covered with ground plants, fruit trees, and fruit vines loaded with mangos, apples, oranges, peaches, apricots, grapes, blackberries, raspberries, pineapples, cherries, plums, pears, bananas, kiwis, dates, and nectarines that are randomly ripening. There are also numerous vegetable plants, including broccoli, beets, rhubarb, celery, cabbage, lettuce, onions, garlic, spinach, and tomatoes. Best of all, herbs are growing everywhere to flavor the fruit and vegetable salads. The naturally organic fruits and vegetables are not bothered by insects, rodents, birds, or other animals because there are none of these pests on the island.

We have all been brainwashed to some degree by the obsessive compulsive controlling élite.

The daily rain shower provides ample water for the plants and survivors, and the soft sea breeze is as pure as one could imagine. The stranded passengers cannot reach the ocean because waves are crashing against the rocks on all sides, but that doesn't bother them since they are vegetarians who don't want to eat the fish anyway.

Introduction

They have one major problem. The airplane's communication radio has been destroyed by the electrical problem that brought down the craft. Even so, the survivors are not concerned because they have plenty of food, water, and shelter in the perfect climate, and they expect to be rescued shortly. This is better than *Gilligan's Island* except they don't have a doctor and are confident they don't need one. However, as the days pass, they begin to feel weak and sick even though they are getting all the calories they need from the food on the island.

One year later, an airplane spotted the downed craft on the little island and sent a radio message to alert authorities, who had assumed the plane ditched in the ocean with a total loss of lives. Upon arrival, the authorities were shocked to discover that the plane landed without damage, but the passengers were all dead. The bodies showed no signs of trauma, but they had obvious signs of emaciation. The investigation that followed revealed that the passengers had a generous supply of fruits and vegetables to provide all the calories and most of the vitamins and minerals they needed, but they died because their diets were almost devoid of essential amino acids and essential fatty acids. If you were starving to death on an island with fields of tomatoes, you would still starve to death.

You can thrive on meat alone, but you can't survive on only fruits and vegetables.

These people would not have died if the island had been covered with animals such as pigs, cows, seals, or sheep instead of all the fruits and vegetables and the passengers had been willing to kill and eat animals. Fruits and vegetables are not essential scientific requirements for human nutrition even though health authorities and school lunch nutritionists are pushing this agenda as if it were the optimal diet. The calories from fruits and vegetables are classified primarily as carbohydrates. Once they are digested, all carbohydrates are reduced to individual sugar molecules. The most common dietary sugars are:

- Sucrose   - common in table sugar and honey
- Glucose   - common in table sugar, honey, and grains
- Fructose   - primarily in fruit, table sugar, and honey
- Xylitol   - sugar alcohol in fruits and vegetables
- Sorbitol   - sugar alcohol in fruit
- Mannitol   - sugar alcohol in plants
- Trehalose   - in plants, mushrooms, and sunflower seeds
- Galactose   - in milk and sugar beets
- Maltose   - sugar from brewing grains
- Lactose   - common sugar in milk

Some sugars are combinations of two sugar molecules. A sugar molecule composed of two smaller sugar molecules is called a *disaccharide.* Table sugar (sucrose), composed of one molecule of fructose and one molecule of glucose, is the best example.

A molecule composed of three sugar molecules is called a *trisaccharide.* Trisaccharides can have different physical and chemical properties depending upon the configuration of the bond and the types of sugar molecules within the bond.

A molecule composed of various sugars bonded in a group of three to ten sugars is called an *oligosaccharide,* which is found in many vegetables.

Carbohydrates are comprised of sugar molecules.

Starches and glycogen are examples of storage carbohydrates called *polysaccharides,* which are composed of a large number of branched chain glucose molecules. The calories in potatoes are primarily starches, and the body produces glycogen to store energy in the liver and muscles.

Sugar alcohols are hydrogenated forms of carbohydrates that are used as sweeteners in place of table sugar (sucrose), high-fructose corn syrup (fructose sugar), and artificial sweeteners. Some diet candy bars were labeled, "low-carbohydrate" or "only 2 grams of carbohydrate," and the U.S. Food and Drug Administration forced their manufacturers to change the ingredient label because sugar alcohols can be metabolized as carbohydrates. I found that a great weight-loss program would be immediately sabotaged by eating these bars. Sugar alcohols cause weight gain just like any other carbohydrate. Do not buy foods that contain the following additives:

- Arabitol
- Dulcitol
- Erythritol
- Glycerol
- Glycol
- Iditol
- Isomalt
- Lactitol
- Maltitol
- Mannitol
- Polyglycitol
- Ribitol
- Sorbitol
- Threitol
- Xylitol

What are the scientific facts concerning human anatomy and physiology? Does the human body function well on a high-carbohydrate diet with unlimited fruits and vegetables as some commercial "pay-to-lose weight" programs suggest? No! The high-carbohydrate diet causes many diseases.

Introduction

Perpetual Deception of Humanity

The study of humanity's susceptibility to mass deception is worthy of a voluminous book in itself, but I will only summarize the history to see where we have been and where we are now. Looking back in history, we see mankind's continual struggle—a little progress followed by a major setback. The ancient achievements of the Greeks, Romans, and Egyptians are good examples. Each had advanced developments in the written languages, mathematics, science, surgery, metal refining, construction, architecture, shipbuilding, and warfare. These advancements parallel our current achievements in the industrial revolution, scientific equipment, communications technology, aircraft, electronics, engineering, metallurgy, pharmaceuticals, surgery, spacecraft, shipbuilding, and warfare.

Despite all their achievements, Europe crashed into the misery of the Dark Ages after the fall of the Greek, Roman, and Egyptian empires. This wretched condition of the masses lasted for the outrageous period of 500 years. Human existence was so deplorable that people could not even read the existing manuscripts or write a simple letter to a friend. It appeared as if ignorance engulfed everyone.

Nutritional brainwashing is off the charts and so is the obesity rate.

Today most people would say that we have progressed greatly in the areas of nutrition, health, and medicine, but a closer look reveals the actual shocking results. Yes, we have great medical equipment that was invented and manufactured by members of the pure sciences. These engineers and scientists invent and design the equipment and teach the physicians how to use them.

Introduction

The heart artery stent is a great example of a scientific invention that a skilled physician used to save my life in 2007. Diabetics are grateful as well for the discovery and manufacture of synthetic insulin as a lifesaver, but the incidence of diabetes continues to soar. It should not be this way because the diet I present in this book will prevent Type 2 Adult-Onset Diabetes 100% of the time. Many societies in past centuries lived totally free from diabetes because they ate a diet identical to that which I present.

A cure for cancer was promised to be on the horizon 50 years ago if universities were simply given a little more money to study the disease. Chemotherapy, radiation, and surgery have been a dismal failure, and cancer prevention using pharmaceuticals is practically nonexistent. The latest statistics show the death rate from cancer has surpassed heart disease, and the life span of citizens in all English-speaking countries is expected to decline in coming years, not increase as has been the trend for the last 100 years. Surprisingly, heart disease is still the leading cause of death in women, yet women tend to be very fearful of cancer and almost nonchalant about heart disease. Men tend to fear heart disease and for the most part dismiss cancer, especially if they have never smoked or used tobacco.

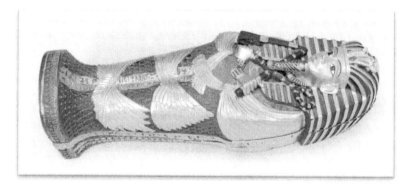

Replica of Pharaoh Tuthankamen's Tomb
Ruler of Egypt 1333 BC – 1323 BC

Introduction

Ask a Mummy if Fruits and Vegetables Are Healthy Foods

The ancient Egyptians suffered in a manner similar to our present society because they ate a diet almost identical to that eaten by the masses today. The Nile River Delta was a lush, well watered, sunny garden where the people could grow organic fruits, vegetables, and grains in abundance with little effort. They had domestic animals for milk and meat as well as fish from the Nile River and the Mediterranean Sea. This was the epitome of a balanced diet. The area was thought to be a paradise, and they were envied by neighboring countries which often suffered famines. Because the ancient Egyptians had an abundance of food, they had the free time they needed to construct the gigantic pyramids that were monuments to their rulers.

Mummies reveal Egyptians' poor health.

The Egyptians had a unique process for mummifying the dead. The very dry climate, chemicals used to dehydrate the body, and other preparations allowed the corpse to remain almost unchanged for thousands of years. The bodies have been so well preserved that even the skin remains. In the 1800s and early 1900s, visitors to Egypt could buy one of the more than 100,000 mummies to take home and display in their personal libraries, offices, or homes. These mummies are a scientific gold mine for studying the health of the people who ate the balanced diet that was in perfect agreement with the present-day *USDA Food Guide Pyramid*.

The Egyptian mummies clearly show signs of rheumatoid arthritis in the joints. This reveals that they suffered from autoimmune diseases as a result of leaky gut syndrome, most likely caused by the organic whole grains. Therefore, it is highly probable that they had many of the more than four dozen other autoimmune diseases that I describe in my book, *Absolute Truth Exposed - Volume 1*. They had very poor dental and bone health unlike the excellent dental and bone health seen in skeletons of the Inuit (Eskimos), who ate a 100% meat diet. The Egyptians' writings described health afflictions that clearly show they suffered from heart disease, myocardial infarctions, and other ailments that have been confirmed by scientific examinations of the mummies. Many were obese, diabetic, and more than likely had high blood pressure.

Proof heart disease is an ancient problem: Autopsy finds 3,500-year-old Egyptian princess had clogged arteries
Daily Mail, May 18, 2011
http://www.dailymail.co.uk/sciencetech/article-1388244/Egyptian-princess-3-500-years-ago-clogged-arteries-proving-heart-disease-modern-condition.html#ixzz1MiMexcFd

"An Egyptian princess who lived more than 3,500 years ago is the oldest known person to have had clogged arteries, dispelling the myth that heart disease is a product of modern society, a new study says.

To determine how common heart disease was in ancient Egypt, scientists performed computer scans on 52 mummies in Cairo and the United States.

Among those that still had heart tissue, 44 had chunks of calcium stuck to their arteries - indicating clogging.

44 out of 52 mummies examined had clogged arteries."

Introduction

Ancients 'had heart disease too'
BBC News – November 18, 2009
http://news.bbc.co.uk/2/hi/8363200.stm

"Hardening of the arteries has been found in Egyptian mummies - suggesting that the risk factors for heart disease may be ancient, researchers say.

The team of US and Egyptian scientists carried out medical scans on 22 mummies from Cairo's Museum of Antiquities.

They found evidence of hardened arteries in three of them and possible heart disease in three more.

All the mummies were of high socio-economic status and would have had a rich diet.

Details of the study by the University of California, the Mid America Heart Institute, Wisconsin Heart Hospital and Al Azhar Medical School in Cairo appear in the Journal of the American Medical Association.

The team said the subjects' bodies had been preserved by mummification because they were serving in the court of the Pharaoh or were priests or priestesses.

The X-rays were checked by five experienced cardiovascular imaging physicians on the team.

They showed that 16 of the 22 mummies had identifiable arteries or hearts left in their bodies after the mummification process.

Nine of these had calcified deposits in the wall of the artery leading to the heart or in the path where the artery should have been.

Some mummies had calcification in up to six different arteries.

Introduction

Definite hardened arteries or atherosclerosis, in other words a build-up of fat, cholesterol, calcium and other substances in the blood vessels, was present in three.

Of the mummies who had died when they were older than 45, seven out of eight had calcification whereas only two out of eight of the younger mummies did.

There were no differences in calcification between men and women."

'No hunter-gatherers'

The researchers said that while ancient Egyptians did not smoke tobacco, eat processed food or lead sedentary lives, they were not hunter-gatherers.

Agriculture was well-established and meat consumption appears to have been common among those of high social status.

Dr Gregory Thomas, from the University of California, said: "While we do not know whether atherosclerosis caused the demise of any of the mummies in the study, we can confirm that the disease was present in many.

"So humans in ancient times had the genetic predisposition and environment to promote the development of heart disease.

"The findings suggest that we may have to look beyond modern risk factors to fully understand the disease."

- The most ancient mummy diagnosed with atherosclerosis was Lady Raj.
- She lived for 30 to 40 years around 1530 BC.
- She was nursemaid to Queen Ahmose Nefertari.
- She predated Moses by 300 years and King Tutankhamun by 200.

Introduction

The ancient Egyptians ate a balanced diet just like the one recommended by government health agencies in all English-speaking countries. Their diet is now called the *Mediterranean diet* that many professional nutritionists today support as the ideal, optimal, healthy diet. They used olive oil in abundance, ate only organic foods, drank raw goats' milk, made whole grain breads, and ate some meat and fish to make it the perfect *balanced diet*. The air and water were not polluted with industrial or natural wastes or toxic chemicals, and they were not exposed to man-made radiation. They did not smoke dried plant leaves like tobacco.

So why did the ancient Egyptians suffer from poor health exactly like our present societies? The answer is clear when analyzed in a scientific manner, but as usual, the researchers in the above studies simply could not figure it out and blamed it on their affluence. They had a preprogrammed *healthy diet* bias that prevented them from doing a clear scientific analysis as I have done. The ancient Egyptians developed the same deadly diseases as our present societies because they ate the same levels of deadly carbohydrates. The less affluent in our societies have higher rates of obesity, diabetes, cancer, heart disease, and autoimmune diseases for the same reason. They eat more of the less expensive grain products and less of the more expensive meat and fish. The commoners in ancient Egypt probably suffered ill health more than the affluent because they also ate more whole grains and less of the more costly meat and fish. As expected, the researchers arrived at the answer backward and blamed the heart disease in the mummies on their affluence. The fact remains that the commoners' relatives could not afford the expensive mummifying technique and burial locations that preserved the corpses of the affluent.

Introduction

> "All the mummies were of high socio-economic status and would have had a rich diet."

What is a "rich diet?" The researchers could have given a clear prognosis but instead gave an undefined, garbled explanation that is scientifically wrong. They had a predetermined bias as to the components of a rich diet and tried to point the finger at meat in a very subtle statement about their "high socio-economic status," even though they present no evidence that the mummies had a higher incidence of heart disease than the commoners or slaves. Their conclusions are pure conjecture.

> "Agriculture was well-established and meat consumption appears to have been common among those of high social status."

Certainly those of high social status ate meat because they had no religious law that prohibited it, but the researchers did not have mummies from the commoners or slaves for comparison. The commoners and slaves most likely had shorter life spans than the affluent. The diet, health, and environmental factors in ancient Egypt did not produce a healthy society. I will analyze these factors and compare them to the diet philosophy of today's professional nutritionists, government health departments, prestigious medical schools, popular world-renown medical clinics, diet gurus, and universities.

Egyptian Environmental Factors

- The Egyptians did not have toxic industrial emissions in the air, water, or on the land.
- The Egyptians, crops, and livestock were not exposed to insecticides, herbicides, factory chemicals, synthetic hormones, or inorganic fertilizers.

- The Egyptians' food did not contain preservatives, thickeners, flavor-enhancing chemicals, refined sugars, processed white flour, or refined fats.
- The Egyptians had no means of refrigeration, and the hot climate led to easy spoilage of food products. Therefore, the food went from the field to the table.
- Food storage consisted of grains for food and wines for refreshment. Since the exceedingly dry climate was perfect for long-term grain storage, grains were the primary off-season food source. Uh-oh! Now we see what killed them—an abundance of whole grains.
- Canals from the Nile River were the source of irrigation for the fruits and vegetables, and the spring floods enriched the soils in the Delta. The Nile was known for fertility and must have been rich in minerals.

Egyptian Economic Factors Concerning Diet

- The Egyptians grew an abundance of organic grains that were affordable for everyone.
- The Egyptians grew a large variety of organic fruits that also provided juices.
- The Egyptians grew an abundance of citrus fruits and had an abundance of citrus juices.
- The Egyptians grew an abundance of grapes for juice and fermented wine.
- The Egyptians grew a large variety of vegetables but did not grow potatoes, which were unknown in that area. Potatoes came from South America. They may have had yams but not sweet potatoes.
- The Egyptians grew date palms from which they harvested the sugary fruit.
- The Egyptians colonized honey bees and collected the honey.

- The Egyptians had cattle, goats, and birds, but these were not abundant because the majority of the land was used for farming fruits and vegetables. The fish from the Nile River and Mediterranean Sea were plentiful for those living near the water with a boat and fishing skills, but fish were not available for those living just a short distance from the water because they could not be preserved.
- The Egyptians were basically farmers, and the majority did not hunt or fish.

Egyptian Health Based on the Above Factors

- With the exception of a few modern diseases like HIV, the Egyptians suffered at an early age from every disease in our modern medical dictionary.
- Heart disease was rampant in the Egyptians.
- The Egyptians had severely decayed teeth at an early age.
- They had weak bones, degenerative disc disease, rheumatoid arthritis, and other autoimmune diseases.
- They certainly suffered from diabetes and cancer.
- They had other autoimmune disease as a result of inflammatory bowel diseases that caused the arthritis.
- Life expectancy of the Egyptians was short for everyone independent of their status in society.

Ancient Egyptian Diet and Health Compared to That of All English-Speaking Countries Today

- The Egyptians' all-organic, 100% natural diet was almost identical to that of people today who comply with the *USDA Food Guide Pyramid*.
- They ate an abundance of organic whole grain foods, identical to the base of the *USDA Food Guide Pyramid*.

- They ate an abundance of organic fruits and vegetables, which is identical to the second level of the *USDA Food Guide Pyramid.*
- Their limited amount of animal fats, butter, and no saturated coconut oil is identical to the top point of the *USDA Food Guide Pyramid.*
- They did not have coconut oil, since coconut palms were not growing in Egypt at that time. They were grown in Polynesia, South Asia, and South America.
- They grew date palms that produced the sugary fruit and had honey exactly like we have available in today's supermarkets.
- The Egyptians suffered from a multitude of diseases common in all English-speaking countries today because these two civilizations ate nearly identical foods—the ultra high-carbohydrate diet.

The ancient Egyptians have already proved that an organic diet rich in fruits and vegetables is very unhealthy. Just ask a mummy.

Egyptian mummies prove that organic fruits, vegetables, and whole grains are unhealthy.

When professional nutritionists and health organizations can't make the physical evidence agree with their paradigm, they immediately point the finger at the guaranteed scapegoat— genetics. They often state that the Eskimos and North American Plains Indians did not suffer from obesity, diabetes, cancer, or heart disease because they adapted to the 100% meat and animal fat diet over many centuries. However, they can't explain why the ancient Egyptians never adapted to the balanced diet after living on the Nile River Delta since the dawn of civilization.

> "So humans in ancient times had the genetic predisposition and environment to promote the development of heart disease."

The researchers end the article by admitting that they don't have a clue as to why the mummies had heart disease.

> "The findings suggest that we may have to look beyond modern risk factors to fully understand the disease."

We can always count on the professional medical and nutritional élite and government organizations to get the answer backward. This is why they can't prevent or reverse heart disease as I have done.

Government organizations and the medical and nutritional élite always get nutritional recommendations backward—guaranteed.

The escalating rates of Type 2 diabetes and morbid obesity prove that the health recommendations from the American Medical Association (AMA), American Heart Association® (AHA), and others are wrong. They claim that heart artery plaque can be prevented by eating a balanced diet according to the *USDA Food Guide Pyramid* and exercising vigorously. Professional government health organizations claim that the low-fat, anti red-meat diet, and exercise will eliminate obesity, heart disease, cancer, diabetes, fatty liver disease, and make people skinny. Oh, really? It hasn't done so!

Introduction

While shopping in a health-food supermarket, I noticed that most of the advertisements and packages contained the modern dogma and buzzwords to attract the shoppers:

- Low-cholesterol
- Zero-cholesterol
- Low-fat
- No saturated fats
- Whole grains

- Vegetarian
- 100% vegan
- All natural
- Organic

The supermarket was crowded, and I began to observe the shoppers and the contents of their carts. I do this every time I shop. You should try it. Most shoppers were women, many between the ages 20–50. It is a shock (but no surprise) that many of the younger women are getting plump, if not fat. Are their shopping carts full of fatty red meat, eggs, and cheese? Absolutely not! The carts looked just like the diet in the *USDA Food Guide Pyramid* that the women are told to eat.

The following are some of the typical products I saw in the carts of the chubby women:

- Boxes of organic whole grain cereals
- Bags of potato chips and corn chips
- Small half-dozen packages of cage-free eggs, if any
- Bags and boxes of pasta of every imaginable shape
- Cartons of soy or rice milk
- Specialty nutrition snack bars
- Nuts or trail mix with nuts and dried fruits
- Potatoes
- Yams
- Lettuce and carrots
- Fruit, fruit, fruit, fruit, and more fruit

Introduction

Meanwhile, new reports are telling us that cancer has zoomed past heart disease as the number one cause of death. How could this be? I did not see one package or carton of cigarettes. We were told that lung cancer would be eliminated if everyone would simply stop smoking and if shoppers would buy organic fruits and vegetables. Fifty years ago we were promised that the cure for cancer was just around the corner if we would only give researchers more money. Society gave more money and got more cancers.

Women were told that breast cancer and osteoporosis would be eliminated if the middle-aged women would simply pop that little hormone pill in their mouths every day. Well, the health and medical experts were wrong. The hormone replacement pills proved to cause breast cancer and osteoporosis after millions of women suffered and died. Lung cancer among women who have never smoked has increased, not decreased as promised. Women were also told that an annual mammogram would end breast cancer, but the death rate has increased.

The cure for cancer is promised year after year.

Cancer is blamed on the bad pollutants in the air, but this is false as well because the air is much cleaner than in past years. Are you beginning to get the strange feeling that the entire diet and health program recommended by the professionals is headed in the wrong direction?

Introduction

Understanding Your Doctor

Doctors use the Latin or Greek languages for many of the medical terms as do other professionals in the sciences. Latin was the language of Ancient Rome and became the source for the French and Spanish languages. Latin is often considered to be a dead language because it is no longer the primary spoken language in any country or by any group of people.

Greek was a highly respected language in the sciences and medicine, and it was studied and spoken by professional people and scholars. Early medicine developed in Europe and used Greek or Latin medical terms to enable physicians in other countries to communicate with each other without the need to translate. Latin and Greek were universal languages for medicine and other sciences.

Ask your physician to please explain in common English words.

Written communications were generally in the Latin alphanumeric characters with 26 Latin letters A-Z plus 10 Arabic numbers: 1, 2, 3, 4, 5, 6, 7, 8, 9 and 0 for a total of 36, or 62 if case-sensitivity is considered. The Greek language was written with characters composed of a set of 24 that has been in use since the 8th century BC and is still used today. Examples are: β, θ, T, λ, etc., but I will not attempt to explain the Greek alphabet. Greek words used by physicians and scientists are generally translated into the Latin alphanumeric characters as is the case with the word *hepatic* in Greek that means *liver* in English.

Conditions, diseases, and parts of the anatomy are often described only with a Latin or Greek word, and the general public must learned to understand the meaning of these words.

Introduction

Other Latin words have an English equivalent that is easier to understand. If your doctor uses words that you don't understand, ask him to explain them in common everyday English.

I present the material in common English wherever possible along with the Latin or Greek when appropriate. This material will be easier to understand than the information in a professional medical book or reference because this book is written for the general public, not physicians.

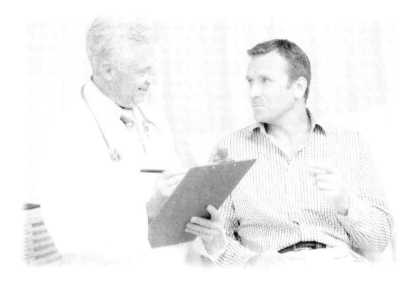

Doctors vary on diet recommendations.
Select a doctor who agrees with your approach.

Reversing Heart Disease and Preventing Diabetes

Chapter 1

Cardiovascular Disease Overview

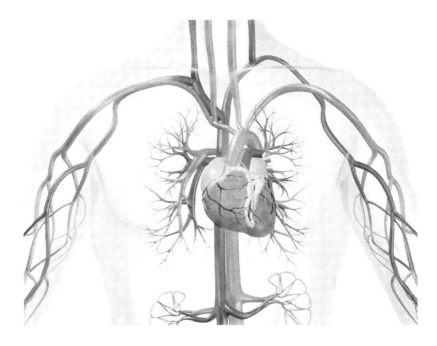

C ardiovascular disease is generally referred to as *heart disease* but actually involves the veins and arteries throughout the body as well as the heart, including the heart muscles, valves, arteries, veins, and nerves. Death can result from a wide range of malfunctions, diseases, infections, mineral abnormalities, or cardiac arrest when the heart simply stops beating. The various diagnoses can be divided into several categories as listed below. First I will describe a heart attack, the symptoms, and what you or bystanders should do immediately to prevent the victim from dying and to minimize damage to the heart and brain.

Heart Attack Symptoms and Emergency Treatment

A cardiologist will describe a heart attack as a *myocardial infarction* when a portion of the heart muscle is deprived of oxygen due to the interruption of the blood flow, which results in the death of muscle cells. The disruption of blood flow is usually brought about by the accumulation of arterial plaque or a blood clot called a *thrombus*. The common symptoms of a heart attack are pain in the center of the chest, left side of the chest, or radiating to the left arm. The pain can easily be dismissed as acid reflux, and women often have less noticeable symptoms than men. Abnormal sweating in combination with the pain is a more positive indicator. The heartbeat can become irregular (palpitations), and the pulse rate may be elevated or abnormally low. Weakness, shortness of breath, indigestion, nausea, or vomiting is common.

The immediate reaction should be the cessation of activity. Sit down in a relaxing position, summon emergency assistance, chew one full-strength (325 mg) aspirin tablet slowly, seek help from someone nearby with knowledge of cardiopulmonary resuscitation (CPR) in case the victim loses consciousness, and seek an oxygen supply. (Caution: Do not take aspirin for symptoms of a stroke.) The victim has a much greater chance of minimal heart muscle damage when these actions are taken. The aspirin works faster if the first tablet is chewed before swallowing with water. A small person should only take one tablet. Mineral water may be a better choice than tap water, but any liquid is acceptable including a soft drink, coffee, or tea.

Cardiac arrest is caused by a disruption of the nerve impulses to the muscle, a mineral imbalance, the blockage of a major coronary artery by plaque or a blood clot, or blockage of a heart valve by a blood clot. The symptom is immediate lapse into unconsciousness that may be accompanied by a cessation of breathing. Immediate action is imperative since brain death will occur within five minutes and brain damage in a much shorter time.

CPR is the immediate course of action when the heart has stopped, and emergency assistance must be summoned. Medical personnel will administer CPR, supplemental oxygen, and defibrillation (a strong, direct-current shock to the chest) in an attempt to regain a pulse.

Save a life by learning CPR.

Because the heart is surrounded by a semi-rigid rib cage, pressure at the center of the rib cage over the heart will compress the heart and thereby pump the blood. This manual manipulation (CPR) is an emergency procedure often used on people who become unconscious and are suspected to have cardiac arrest, myocardial infarction (heart damage from a blockage of the heart artery), or ventricular fibrillation (heart fluttering instead of beating). An observer's first action should be to check the victim's pulse in either the neck or wrist. Placing the ear against the chest is another way to detect if the heart is beating normally. A stroke can render a person unconscious while the heart is beating normally. If you don't know how to find a pulse or if none is observed, begin CPR immediately. Don't waste time. Start CPR within 10 seconds at the most.

In cases like a high impact automobile crash, CPR may not be the right thing to do. Princess Diana's death in Paris is a good example. The emergency personnel who arrived on the scene attempted to stabilize her before taking her to the hospital, but this was a very bad decision. The high impact tore the aorta near the heart, which caused her to bleed to death internally. If they had given her multiple blood transfusions on the way to the hospital, she might have been saved in surgery. I saw a similar case on a television program that was filmed live in a hospital emergency room. The patient arrived from the scene of a motorcycle accident with a fairly reasonable pulse rate and blood pressure, but his blood pressure kept dropping lower and lower. I was screaming at the television, "Take him into surgery quickly because he has internal bleeding!" I groaned as the hospital emergency personnel decided to perform a scan. He died from internal bleeding before the scan was finished because his liver had been ruptured. CPR would not have helped him either. He needed immediate surgery to stop the bleeding from a ruptured liver. People who have suffered severe trauma and have a pulse should not be given CPR. They should be treated for possible internal injuries that could cause them to bleed to death.

CPR is generally given after the heart has been restarted by defibrillation in an intensive care facility. Older training videos and CPR classes often taught that the pressure applied to the chest must be done at a rate of about one compression per second, or 60 per minute. These instructions have now been found to be erroneous. The CPR rate should be more than 100 compressions per minute, or nearly double the frequency previously taught. One training program used the song *Staying*

Alive by the Bee Gees as background music to force the students to increase the CPR rate to 104 compressions per minute. The slower rate used in the past has resulted in the death of many patients who could have been saved had the rate been increased. CPR videos that show a substandard rate may still be around. If you are ever in a situation where you must administer CPR, pick up the pace with fast, heavy, and deep compressions. Soft little pushes on the chest are not going to accomplish anything and the person may die. The chest must be noticeably compressed in order to compress the heart and aid in pumping the blood. It is better to break a rib and save a life than simply let the person lie there and die.

Recent studies have also indicated that chest compression is much more important for saving the life of the victim than is blowing air into the victim's mouth and lungs. In the past, these were given equal importance, but that has been shown to be incorrect. Major attention should be given to the new hands-only CPR procedure because it will also help to ventilate the lungs that are in the chest cavity on either side of the heart. It's more important to get the blood circulating to the brain than to inflate the lungs.

If the hands-and-mouth method is used, it should be done by giving 10 compressions before blowing into the victim's mouth and lungs. Don't stop the CPR procedure simply because the victim remains unconscious. Many lives have been saved because rescue personnel failed to give up on the victim. It may take a long time before the heart begins to beat on its own. Don't expect the victim to regain consciousness easily even after the heart begins to respond.

Several years ago, my wife, Marti, and I were driving home on a four-lane divided highway at about 10:00 PM. We approached a car and a pickup truck that were stopped in the middle of the two lanes with the headlights of the truck shining on the car. It didn't appear to be an accident, and we thought the problem was a stalled vehicle. As we slowly drove past, we could see three young adult men in the car. They were sitting up but slumped backward and not moving. The car looked like it had no damage at all. I said to Marti, "The people look like they're dead." She agreed. We drove past the car and truck, and vehicles behind us did the same. We did not see a reason to stop because the car and truck showed no signs of having had a collision. The person in the pickup truck was there and appeared to be uninjured.

The next day we heard about the accident in which three people had died. We later drove past the scene on the way to town, and I noticed two marks through the grass across the highway median. The marks were spaced at a greater width than those of the tires on a car, and I realized they represented the wheelbase of the car (not the tread width) as the car slid sideways across the grass, up the slope, and onto the roadway on the other side. The median sloped downward at about a 5° angle as it approached the other side and then turned up at an angle of about 20°. The tires left a heavier mark in the soil as they dug into the upslope because the car slid sideways. Later in a radio newscast, the father of one of the young men who died was describing the accident. The driver had been traveling at a high rate of speed and lost control of the car, causing it to slide sideways across the median, impact the upslope, and stop in the middle of the two lanes on the other side. The young men all died from the rupture of the major arteries or veins near the heart. The sudden upward change in the direction of the car as it impacted the slope caused the heavy hearts to drop in the chest cavity and tear the veins and arteries. The young men had lost consciousness before they could even attempt to get out of their seats and no doubt died within minutes.

In another auto accident, a young woman in a small car slammed head-on into the side of a large car, hitting it in the engine area. She was not wearing a seat belt, and the impact left her beneath the steering wheel and compressed between the pedals and the seat. She was semiconscious as another man and I lifted her up onto the seat and out of the car to the pavement. Many of the people at the scene would have left her there to be extracted by rescue personal. I heard someone say, "Don't move her" as the other man and I both ignored the incorrect advice. If we had not moved her, she would have died from suffocation. Accident victims must be quickly moved from a slumped-forward position to a supine position (lying flat on the back) to enable them to breathe easily. A person left unconscious while slumped forward will quickly suffocate.

When I was about 12 years old, a neighbor girl one year younger was wearing a small chain around her neck while swinging on her swing set. I was told that her chain caught on a clothesline at the back of her neck and pulled her out of the swing. She was left hanging with her feet barely touching the ground and the clothesline very taut. By the time her parents saw her, she was unconscious. Her father released her from the clothesline and called the fire department. CPR was not a general procedure at that time, and I doubt that anything was done to attempt to revive her until the firemen arrived to begin giving her oxygen with a face mask. She was not responding after a considerable amount of time, so her father suggested that they leave her alone because "she was dead," but the firemen refused. She finally responded because the firemen would not give up, and she later recovered with very little permanent damage.

Chapter 1

General Description of the Cardiovascular System

Cardio refers to the heart and *vascular* refers to the arteries and veins that carry blood throughout the body. The arteries carry nutrient and oxygen-rich blood and branch to become smaller and smaller in diameter until they are classified as *capillaries.* The blood then returns through the convergent veins until it reaches the heart. The arteries go to every organ, muscle, and tissue in the body, including some of the major bones. The blood collects carbon dioxide, waste products, and heat and returns to the heart. The lungs remove a considerable amount of this body heat by evaporative cooling and thermal conduction as we breathe. Dogs must remove body heat through the lungs, because they do not sweat in the same manner as humans; therefore, dogs pant to cool themselves. On the other hand, pigs or swine do not sweat or pant, and they will overheat and die when forced to overexert or if they are placed in a hot location.

The heart of the average man at rest will pump about 5 quarts (4.7 liters) of blood per minute and the rate can be increased to 20 quarts (18.9 liters) per minute during fairly heavy physical activity as the pulse rate and the pressure both increase. You can visualize from these numbers that the heart is doing a lot of work and pumps a considerable amount of blood every day.

The brain is very sensitive to the amount of oxygen in the blood that it receives. When the supply of oxygenated blood to the brain is interrupted, a person quickly lapses into unconsciousness, and brain damage can occur within a few minutes at normal room temperature. Brain damage occurs at a slower rate at lower temperatures as occurs when someone falls through the ice into very cold water. Other organs, muscles, and tissues of the body are less sensitive to oxygen deprivation, and cell death may not occur for some period of time after the blood supply has been cut off. These examples are seen when someone accidentally severs a finger. The finger can be retrieved and the veins, arteries, ligaments, and tendons reattached without the finger dying. The major problem with severed extremities is the inability to reconnect the nerves, which prevents full use and function of the member.

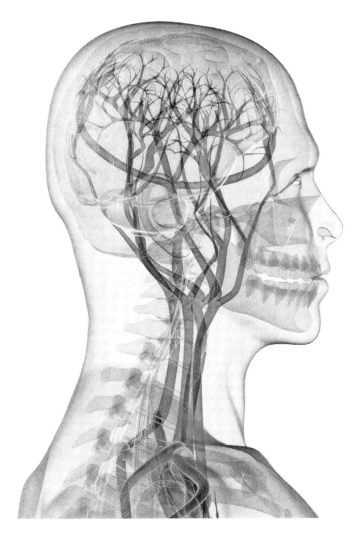

Vascular System of the Brain

Geometry of the Heart

The heart functions like a two-stage pump with two minor chambers, two major chambers, and four valves. Each pair of chambers consists of an atrium (upper minor chamber) and a ventricle (lower major chamber) that are separated by an atrioventricular valve. The right atrium at the top of the heart receives oxygen-depleted blood via two major veins as the blood returns to the heart. The upper vein, called the *superior vena cava*, delivers blood to the right atrium from the head and upper body extremities. The lower vein, called the *inferior vena cava*, also delivers blood to the right atrium from the body and lower extremities. The word *atrium* means *court, entrance, or foyer* to the heart.

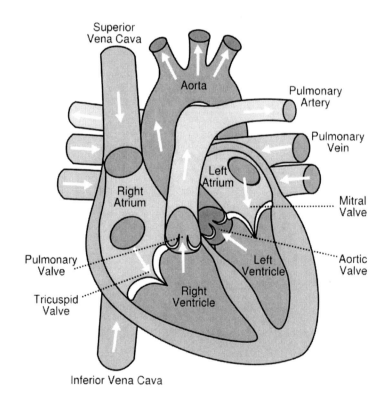

The lower right chamber is called the *right ventricle,* and the tricuspid (atrioventricular) valve is between the two chambers. Blood enters the right ventricle from the atrium through the tricuspid and is discharged from the ventricle through the pulmonary semilunar valve into the pulmonary artery that leads to the lungs. Blood comes from the head, body, and extremities and flows into the right side of the heart. From there it is pumped to both lungs. The blood leaves the lungs and returns to the left side of the heart through the pulmonary vein.

The two chambers on the left side of the heart are the left atrium and the left ventricle separated by the bicuspid or mitral (atrioventricular) valve. The left atrium at the top of the heart receives oxygenated blood from the lungs via the four pulmonary veins as it returns to the heart. Blood flows from the left atrium down through the bicuspid valve into the left ventricle. Blood is discharged from the left ventricle through the aortic semilunar valve to the aorta, which is the main artery delivering oxygenated blood to the entire body.

The two atria function as collection or surge chambers to even the flow in the veins during the opening and closing of the atrioventricular valves. Because the atrium has only one valve that is common with the ventricle, the atrium cannot produce any pressure. It is only a surge chamber that can increase or decrease in volume. The contraction of the heart muscles surrounding the ventricles closes the atrioventricular valves, which stops all of the blood flow from the atria. This action slams the atrioventricular valves closed like half-opened doors in a strong wind. The sound produced when the valves slam closed can easily be heard by the physician through his stethoscope. I will discuss this below in more detail. The atria begin to expand with blood after the atrioventricular valves close, allowing the flow in the veins to remain more constant. Some references may state that the atrium expands and contracts with the ventricle, but this is incorrect. The atrium and ventricle are out of phase with each other such that the atrium enlarges as the ventricle contracts. The atrium contracts as the ventricle enlarges with the intake of blood from the atrium.

Each ventricle functions as a pressure chamber that fills with blood when the heart muscles expand, and it pumps the blood out by the contraction of the muscle. Many references describe the ventricle filling process as a period of relaxation. I believe this is misleading. The muscles of the heart do not simply relax. They forcefully expand. The ventricle expands in order to draw blood in from the atrium because the atrium simply does not have the ability to produce pressure. The ventricle literally opens the door (atrioventricular valve) and sucks the blood in from the atrium. The heart is certainly not at rest during this part of the cycle. You can easily test my description by holding your breath and compressing your chest cavity with your diaphragm. If the heart were at rest during the filling of the ventricle, this test would stop the filling and cause cardiac arrest. We know this does not happen. The ventricle continues to expand and fill even though you are holding your breath and compressing your chest cavity with the diaphragm. The pulse remains strong and the blood flow continues to be adequate, although it may be slightly reduced. Don't perform this test. Take my word for it.

Functions of the Heart Valves

Each ventricle has two valves to control the flow—one to allow the flow of blood into the chamber and the other to allow the flow out of the chamber. The one-way valves each function as check valves that open easily in one direction to allow blood flow and close tightly in the other direction to block the blood flow. The design of the valves is exceedingly clever. The tricuspid valve is at the inlet to the right ventricle and is formed by three leaflets, flaps, cusps, or petals facing into the chamber. The cusps have stringy attachments called *chordae tendineae* extending to the opposite side of the ventricular chamber. The papillary muscles at the lower end of these stringy attachments contract to pull the valve open as the heart begins to fill. They relax somewhat to allow the valve to close, yet they provide continual support to the valve to prevent its collapse, inversion, or prolapse during the strong contraction of the heart. The papillary muscles in each ventricle are like a doorman at the hotel entrance who opens and closes the door to allow the guests to enter. The pressure in the veins is low, and the valve needs assistance in order to open for easier blood flow. Some references suggest that the chordae tendineae are slack when the valve is open, but these references neglect to understand that they aid in the opening of the valve. The chordae tendineae between the cusps of the valves and the papillary muscles perform three functions, not just one. They open the valve, hold it open, and prevent it from collapsing upon closing.

The atrioventricular valves are very large in order to allow blood flow with very little pressure difference across the valve. The bicuspid mitral valve that allows blood to flow into the left ventricle has a design similar to the tricuspid atrioventricular valve in the right ventricle, but the bicuspid has only two leaflets or cusps.

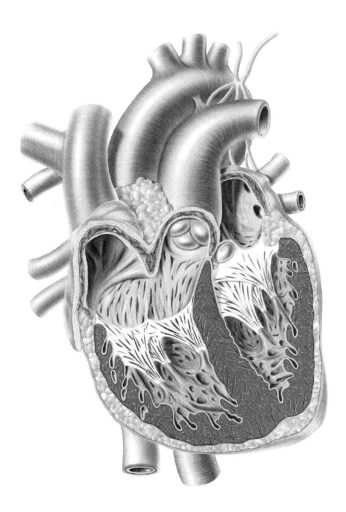

Another valve near the top of each ventricle allows the blood to exit during contraction of the heart muscles. These are called the *semilunar valves* and face in the opposite direction to the atrioventricular valves. The leaflets protrude outward from the heart into the corresponding artery without an atrial chamber. They are smaller in size and stout because the heart muscle has a great deal of power that is able to force the valves open during the contraction. The bicuspid aortic valve in the left ventricle has only two cusps or leaflets that allow blood flow to the aorta, and the pulmonary valve in the right ventricle that has three cusps or leaflets that allow blood flow to the pulmonary artery. We can see that the two valves in the right side of the heart each have three cusps, and the two valves in the left side each have only two cusps.

Defective, damaged, or malfunctioning valves often allow the blood flow to leak in the wrong direction. The sound made by this leakage is often referred to as a heart murmur and is called *regurgitation* or *prolapse* of the valve. The flow of blood through the valve can be easily seen during an angiogram, and the leakage or reverse flow is obvious to the physician. Mitral valve prolapse is a commonly diagnosed heart ailment, but the other valves can also have regurgitation disorders.

Since both chambers of the heart are within the same muscular structures, the pumping action occurs almost simultaneously in both chambers. The sound of the heart pumping that we hear is actually produced by the closing action of the valves, not by any sound of the contraction. Since the heart has four valves, we are actually listening to four different sounds as two pairs of sounds. The first sound usually identified as *lub* or *lu-ub* is produced by the closure of the two atrioventricular valves. These valves produce the louder sound because the contraction begins sharply and slams both of the valves closed. The pulmonary vein (from the lungs) connects to the left atrium. The mitral valve between left atrium and the left ventricle produces the loudest *lu* sound because the left ventricle produces a higher pressure at the exit to the aorta (primary artery to the body) through the aortic valve. The tricuspid valve between the right atrium of the superior vena cava (primary vein from the body) and the right ventricle produces the *ub* sound.

The second sound usually described as *dup* is that made by two valves. The aortic valve between the aorta and the left ventricle produces the *d* part of the sound as the aortic valve closes and is the louder of the two valves. The closing of the pulmonary valve in the right ventricle is the second part of the sound that is usually described as *up*. The sound produced by these two valves is not as loud as the first sound because the contraction ends slowly and tapers off, allowing the two valves time to close at a slower rate.

No sound is produced as the valves open to fill the chambers of the heart with fresh blood, creating a pause in the sound and leading many to believe the heart is at rest. Actually, the heart is expanding rather than contracting. The sound produced by the two cycles sounds like *lub-dup—pause—lub-dup*.

The sound of the heart pumping reminds me of a Harley Davidson® motorcycle with the older V-twin engine. The connecting rods from the two pistons were attached to the same crankshaft bearing journal with the cylinders at a 60° angle to each other. The design makes the two cylinders fire in an unequal manner or uneven spacing between two cylinder strokes. This design also makes the engine vibrate excessively at idle as can be seen when a rider is idling at a red light and the entire motorcycle is shaking, particularly the handlebars. The engine produces the rhythmic sound similar to the sound of the heart beating, boom-boom—pause—boom-boom. The Harley Davidson® engine may sound severely out of tune or in need of repair but actually it's just fine.

The aorta is the main artery from the heart, and it carries blood to every part of the body except the lungs. The arteries branch and bifurcate into smaller and smaller vessels as they progress throughout the body until they become so small they can't be seen with the human eye. When the blood crosses the smallest part of the capillary vessels, it enters the vascular system of veins that merge and enlarge as the veins progress back toward the heart. The design of the entire system is amazing.

Abnormalities of the Heart Valves

The valves of the heart undergo an unrelenting service demand. They must open and close approximately once every second throughout a person's lifetime. The valve must resist aging and disease in order to stay functional. Each of the four heart valves must allow easy flow in one direction and seal tightly against any leakage in the other direction. There are three primary problems that occur with heart valves.

- The valve does not open properly and the flow through the valve is limited. This is called *stenosis*, which means abnormal narrowing.

- The valve does not seal perfectly when closed and allows blood to leak or flow in the wrong direction. This condition is called *regurgitation*.

- The cusps or flaps of a valve can collapse or partially collapse and cause the valve to malfunction, allowing it to leak in the wrong direction. This is called *prolapse* of the valve.

What Is a Heart Murmur?

The physician can easily observe and diagnose all of these conditions by performing an angiogram. When leakage occurs, he can hear the sound emitted that has been called a *heart murmur.* This is also called *valve prolapse*—the failure to function properly. The cusps or leaflets of the valve can collapse or flop in the wrong direction, which is the result of weak cusp tissues. Two percent of adults have this condition to some degree.

The body must maintain the proper function of the valves while they are in constant use. Valves can be attacked by a disease such as rheumatic fever, and they must be healed while they continue to function. Rheumatic fever begins as a sore throat caused by the common Group A Streptococcus bacterium and may often lead to permanent heart damage. Contrary to popular belief, damaged heart valves can undergo a noticeable amount of repair when given the proper nutrition and supplements as will be discussed in greater detail in Chapter 6, but the low-fat, high-carbohydrate diet recommended by health authorities will not heal the heart valves. Physicians rarely prescribe strict nutritional guidelines and supplements for treating heart valve problems. Treatment is usually done by a highly skilled surgeon who can replace dysfunctional heart valves with either an animal heart valve or a manufactured synthetic heart valve. Pig heart valves are a common choice.

What Is the Heart Septum?

The left and right sides of the heart are divided by a muscular structure called the *septum.* The septum between the two ventricles of a fetus has a hole in it that closes naturally within a few days after birth. This hole can reopen later in life if the body enters a catabolic state caused by hyperinsulinemia (abnormally high blood insulin) and the resulting hypercortisolemia (abnormally high blood cortisol level). Surgery should be performed to plug the hole in the septum because leaving it untreated allows regurgitation of blood between the two adjoining chambers that can result in a blood clot forming that can pass throughout the body. A hole in the septum between the two atriums can also occur as a congenital (birth) defect.

Irregular Pulse and Blood Clots

An irregular pulse is a condition in which the ventricle does not have a regular, evenly-spaced cycle. One cycle is often skipped or the cycles may be unequally spaced. This condition can be temporary and produces no ill effects, but it can be life-threatening when the pooling blood circulating within the atrium and ventricle coagulates and forms a clot called a *thrombus*. The thrombus is passed to the aorta and can migrate to the brain, resulting in a stroke that may lead to brain damage or death. A thrombus in the right ventricle flows to the lungs and creates a pulmonary embolism (arterial blockage). The blood clots can be dissolved if fast action is taken by the patient, others near the patient, or medical staff. The clot-dissolving drug called *Tissue Plasminogen Activator (tPA)* is a thrombolytic agent that has the nickname *clot buster*. It must be administered within two hours after the onset of symptoms if brain damage is to be prevented. The severity of the stroke and resulting damage depend upon the size of the artery that is blocked, location, percentage of blockage, and length of time the blockage remains. The physician's challenge is to determine whether the stroke is caused by an arterial hemorrhage (bleeding through the wall of the artery) or blockage. The clot buster will make the problem worse if it's given to a patient who is having a hemorrhagic stroke.

Measuring Electrical Nerve Impulses of the Heart

The heart is regulated by electrical nerve impulses that can be measured by an instrument, and the recorded results are called an *electrocardiogram* (EKG or ECG). The first nerve impulse from the right atrium called the *P wave* or *sinoatrial node* as shown in the EKG, is the beginning of atrial contraction. Some references indicate the atrium forces blood into the ventricle. This concept is misleading because the atrium is a chamber completely open to the vein and therefore cannot produce any pressure. It cannot force blood into the ventricle.

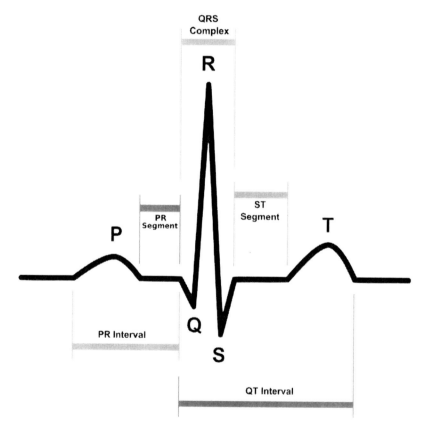

Sinus Heart Rhythm from an ECG Chart

Cardiovascular Disease Overview

The P wave signal begins at the right atrium, spreads to the left atrium, and starts the atrial contractions. The nerve impulse flows from the left atrium to the top of the septum and signals both ventricles to begin expanding in order to fill with a new surge of blood from the atria and veins. The next impulse called the *QRS complex* travels down the septum and spreads to the ventricular muscles to begin the contraction that pumps blood to the arteries. The QRS wave begins with a sharp spike at point R. The ventricles then continue the contraction to discharge the blood during the next wave called the *ST segment*. The final T wave ends the contractions. The atria are contracting as the ventricles are expanding and vice versa to allow an unvarying flow in the veins.

Atrial and Ventricular Fibrillation of the Heart

The atrium begins to expand, and blood accumulates when the ventricle closes the atrioventricular valve and begins the power stroke to pump blood to the arteries. If the sinoatrial node fails to produce a nerve impulse, the ventricular QRS node misfires and the heart begins to quiver. This failure to produce a heartbeat is known as *fibrillation*. Most references call this *atrial fibrillation* or *A-fib* and describe it as a condition in which the weak muscles of the atrium begin to quiver. This description is universal, but I believe it is misleading. Fibrillation is caused by failure of the ventricle to produce a contraction stroke, and because the ventricle is actually in a state of fibrillation called *ventricular fibrillation or V-fib,* the atrium is forced to do likewise. The large muscles and power of the heart are in the ventricles, not the atria. The nerve signal begins in the atrium, but the physical response and effectiveness of the heartbeat is determined by the ventricle.

21

As the ventricle contracts and creates an arterial pulse, the atrium must expand because the atrioventricular valve is closed. This is followed by the expansion of the ventricle in order to draw in the blood from the atrium and cause it to contract. References often state cause and effect incorrectly. For example, if the atrium did not exist, the ventricle could pump the blood and refill quite effectively, but the flow in the veins would be a start-and-stop pulsating situation that would be undesirable. The starting and stopping of blood in the major vein would cause the muscles of the ventricle to work harder. Atrial fibrillation or failure of the atrium to expand or contract is not a life-threatening situation, but the ventricle must pump the blood to keep us alive.

Ventricular fibrillation is a life-threatening condition that occurs when the heart fails to restart after skipping several beats. The major muscles of the heart fail to contract and expand in the normal pumping cycle and cause blood flow to the arteries to stop. The blood pressure drops drastically. Naturally, when the ventricle stops pumping blood, the atrium goes into fibrillation as well. It has no choice, but ventricular fibrillation is the causal factor. Ventricular fibrillation degenerates into a flat line called *asystole* on the EKG and sets off a sudden alarm when a patient is attached to a heart monitoring machine. The medical staff must begin emergency procedures immediately in order to prevent brain damage and death. These procedures start by giving the heart a strong electrical shock with a defibrillator, which has been given the nickname *paddles*, although stick-on patches are also used. The scene is very familiar in the movies where two large suction cups on the end of heavy electrical wires are first rubbed together to neutralize the charge. They are then placed on opposite sides of the patient's chest after which the command is given for the attendant to energize the paddles. The sharp high-voltage, direct-current electrical shock jolts the patient's heart muscles into a sharp contraction, and the heart is often restored to its normal rhythm. Several shocks may be required when the heart fails to restart immediately.

Patients at risk for ventricular fibrillation are often treated with a defibrillator implanted in the chest along with a heart pacemaker. The implanted defibrillator fires a sharp electrical shock in the hope of restarting the heart during ventricular fibrillation.

Accidental Electrical Shocks

A normal EKG produces a graph that shows the nerve impulse waves of the heart generally referred to as the *sinus rhythm*, meaning the impulse waves are sinusoidal (wavy oscillation) in nature. However, the heart impulses are very jagged, not smooth waves as seen in alternating electrical current that the power company distributes to your home. Nerve impulses control the heart at one cycle per second for a 60 beats-per-minute pulse rate compared to 60 cycles per second for the electricity in your home. An electrical shock by household current is very disturbing to the heart because the higher frequency throws the heart into fibrillation.

The first electrical power distribution systems in the United States were operated with direct current (DC) as proposed by Thomas Edison but opposed by George Westinghouse, who suggested the use of alternating current (AC). The AC current allows the voltage to be easily increased or decreased with a transformer. Changing the voltage on a DC system was essentially impossible at that time and is still very difficult today. The DC current is first changed to AC, the voltage is changed in a transfer, and the AC is then changed back to DC current at the new voltage. In an attempt to gain public support for the direct current system, Thomas Edison used the argument that the alternating current was very deadly. Alternating current was used in the electric chair to execute prisoners, and this gave a very vivid description of the hazard. Thomas Edison correctly stated that alternating current was more hazardous to anyone who received an electrical shock, but the disadvantage of not being able to adjust the voltage in DC systems eventually proved George Westinghouse to be the winner of the "war of currents."

What Is Heart Muscle Disease?

Cardiomyopathy is the term given to chronic heart muscle disease. For unknown reasons, the heart muscles can grow to an abnormal thickness called *hypertrophic cardiomyopathy*, but more than likely this is a genetic factor. The muscle mass in the left ventricle can grow to be larger or thicker than normal and cause an obstruction of blood flow because the mitral valve is compressed between the ventricular muscle and the septum. In other cases, the heart muscles become weak and too flexible to sustain a strong, normal heartbeat. This leads to an enlarged heart and congestive heart failure.

When the heart stops beating for no known reason, the condition is called *primary cardiomyopathy*. Mineral imbalances are a prime suspect. A regular heartbeat can also be interrupted by rapid palpitations or arrhythmias (irregular or non-uniform heartbeats) as will be discussed in Chapter 6.

What Is Coronary Artery Disease?

Coronary artery disease (CAD) is a condition in which the inside of a heart artery narrows as a result of a buildup of atheromatous plaque between the inside lining of the artery, called the *endothelial lining,* and the second layer called the *smooth muscle layer.* The smooth muscle layer is covered by a layer of connective tissue that provides structural containment and support for the two layers beneath. The narrowing of the artery by plaque beneath the endothelial lining is called *atherosclerotic heart disease* or *atherosclerosis.* The atheromatous plaque deposit is composed primarily of macrophage cells, cholesterol, glycated LDL cholesterol, glycated proteins, glycated hemoglobin A1c, oxidized polyunsaturated omega-6 triglycerides, calcium, and fibrous tissue.

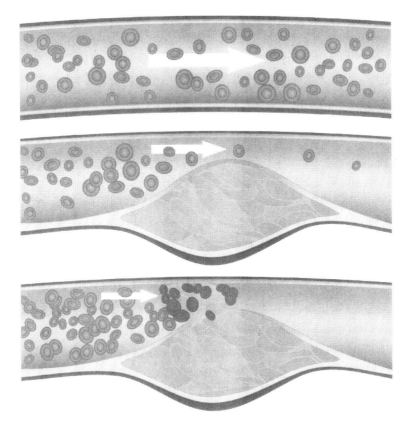

Atheromatous Plaque Deposit

The arteries of the heart can be very healthy except for only one atheroma, which can be treated by placement of a stent. In severe cases, several of the major arteries are lined with many atheromas, making treatment with stents less practical and requiring the replacement or bypass of a longer segment of the artery with a section of vein taken from the leg. This approach may be required for several arteries in a single surgery, and we often hear about someone who had a quadruple bypass.

Symptoms of Coronary Arterial Plaque

Symptoms of coronary artery disease do not generally appear until the plaque reduces the artery opening by 75%. People who do not engage in strenuous exercise may not notice symptoms of chest pain or tightness until the artery is 90% closed when the reduced blood flow deprives the heart muscle of oxygen. A heart attack (myocardial infarction) occurs when the blockage suddenly increases or when strenuous exercise is attempted.

Passing a treadmill test doesn't mean that the patient is not without risk. The plaque that restricts the heart artery is a ticking time bomb because of the threat of sudden rupture. The body attempts to repair a tiny rupture but in doing so, a life-threatening blood clot forms. Unfortunately, the blood clot can restrict the entire artery or break loose to flow down the artery and form a block where the artery becomes smaller. A very small plaque deposit is not without risk. Even though the plaque buildup may be small, the rupture in the endothelial lining can occur and form a blood clot that can cause a sudden, fatal heart attack. Autopsies have shown that many heart attack victims died because a small plaque deposit ruptured even though a much larger plaque deposit remained intact elsewhere in the heart arteries. This is the reason why a person can pass all the physician's tests without experiencing any symptoms and have a sudden, fatal heart attack.

Cardiovascular Examination Technologies

Physicians have several methods available to examine the blood flow in the arteries and veins throughout the body, and each has advantages, limitations, and risks. The following are the major methods physicians use to diagnose cardiovascular problems.

Catheter Angiography (Angiogram)

Catheter angiography, or angiogram, is the most definitive test for locating cardiovascular plaque and defective valves. It is a procedure in which a radio-opaque agent (impenetrable to X-rays) is injected into the blood. The agent appears as an area of dark contrast on the X-ray image and gives a sharp picture of the blood flow, size of arteries and veins, and the backflow or leakage in the heart valves. The result is a live video that clearly shows the blood flowing. If you have had an angiogram, ask your cardiologist for a copy of this very interesting video that you can view on your computer.

During the angiogram, the cardiologist should be prepared to place a stent in the site of arterial plaque or any artery restriction in order to restore full blood flow. The placement of the stent is restricted to arterial locations that are accessible, but a stent cannot be placed at the junction of an arterial branch. Physicians have to make the decision whether or not to place a stent in a small plaque deposit that creates a 50% or less restriction. It has been a difficult call because plaque deposits tend to grow, and even small deposits can rupture and result in a blood clot and heart attack. My regimen in this book makes that decision easier for those physicians who become aware that it can remove arterial plaque.

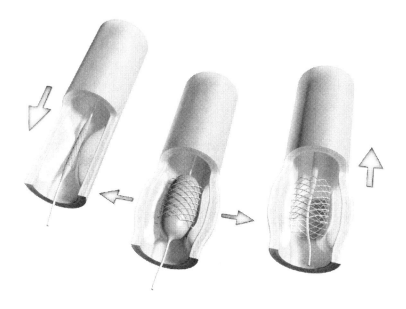

Stent Insertion in an Artery

Plaque and the placement of stents are not limited to the heart arteries. Plaque in the artery that supplies blood to the kidneys can result in total kidney failure. The diagnosis is difficult, and treatment is impossible without an angiogram in which a catheter is inserted in the peripheral femoral artery near the groin and a contrast agent is injected near the branch to the kidneys. The X-ray clearly shows the condition of the primary kidney (renal) arteries and the two branches leading to each kidney. The restricted artery can be opened by placing a stent at the location of the plaque in the same manner as is commonly done with restricted coronary arteries.

The nuclear isotopes used in the angiogram procedure have a fairly high radiation exposure rating of 20 millisieverts (2000 millirems). This compares to 0.36 millisieverts of exposure for a two-view mammogram, 3.0 millisieverts of exposure for

28

everyone from the annual atmospheric background radiation, and 50 millisieverts—the annual exposure limit—for a nuclear power plant worker. Since the nuclear isotopes have a very short half-life, the health risk is negligible.

Magnetic Resonance Angiography (MRA)

Magnetic resonance angiography is based on the magnetic resonance imaging (MRI) technology in which images of the arteries and veins are obtained and plaque restrictions are identified. MRA is noninvasive because no catheters are introduced into the arteries. For this reason, it is more frequently used for the neck and brain rather than the invasive catheter angiography procedure used for the heart and kidneys. MRA presents a much lower risk for stroke than the angiography.

The MRA is a good technique for diagnosing coronary artery disease and presents a lower risk than the angiography. The contrast dye is less toxic and allergenic than the ionizing radiation used in the catheter angiography. MRA is strictly diagnostic, and therefore a stent cannot be placed at the site of an artery plaque restriction as can be done with the angiography.

Computed Tomography Angiography (CTA)

Computed Tomography Angiography is a procedure used to visualize the blood flow in the arteries and veins throughout the body. A contrast ionizing radiation dye is injected into a vein in the arm, and a rotating X-ray beam is passed through the patient from many different angles to allow the computer to assemble a three-dimensional image of the subject area. CTA is often used to diagnose blood flow in the kidneys, lungs, arms, legs, neck, and brain.

CTA is diagnostic only and is used less frequently on the heart because the catheter angiography allows coronary artery stents to be inserted during the same procedure if necessary. Even though CTA is safer and less expensive than the catheter angiograph, it is not the preferred procedure.

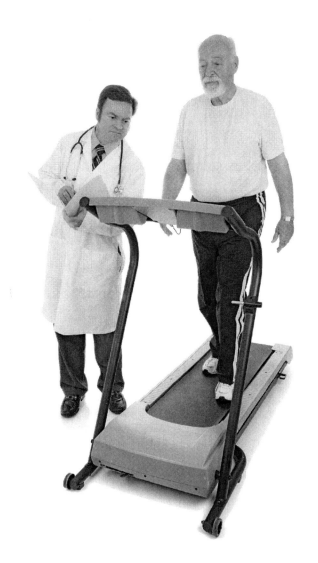

Doctor Monitoring a Senior Man on a Treadmill

Medical Treadmill Stress Tests Can Kill You

The Merck Manual® states that taking a treadmill or exercise stress test causes 1 person in 5000 to suffer a heart attack or death. This is said to be "a small risk" but in fact is an outrageous rate. If 1 person in 5000 had a heart attack or died while mowing the lawn, the daily death rate in the United States during the summer would be in the hundreds of thousands and lawn mowing would be outlawed. Keep in mind that a high percentage of those taking the treadmill stress test have mild or no heart disease and are not at risk whatsoever. For them it is simply a great, highly-intensive workout. The test proves they didn't have a heart attack at that energy level. Others who have an artery blockage severe enough to be detected by the test are at an extreme risk for heart attack or death on the treadmill or within 24 hours thereafter. The treadmill stress test for patients with hypertension (high blood pressure) is extremely risky. Giving patients a test that will kill them if they test positive is absolutely ridiculous. The doctor tells the family members of the deceased, "Yep, he had heart disease alright."

Hypertension and a treadmill stress test are a dangerous combination.

Relatives of those who died as a result of a treadmill stress test should file a massive class action lawsuit against the professional medical community. This would be similar to those brought against the tobacco and asbestos fiber industries for causing cancer in people exposed to those products. Taking a treadmill stress test presents a much higher risk for death than smoking, and the treadmill retribution is almost instantaneous.

31

Nearly everyone knows a friend, relative, or neighbor who went to the doctor for a routine examination that included a treadmill stress test only to die with 24 hours following the test. In many cases, the patient was aware of a heart condition and had been suffering from symptoms of heart disease. He didn't need a treadmill stress test to tell him he had heart disease. I have had about a dozen neighbors in my lifetime, and one died as the result of a treadmill stress test. That percentage is outrageous.

The standard medical procedure for the treadmill test is to stress the heart to the point of damage that is confirmed by electrocardiogram (ECG) or echocardiogram. The patient is then told he has a heart problem. The point of damage is actually a heart attack. A high percentage of patients have a very serious heart attack on the treadmill, collapse, and die soon afterward. More commonly, the patient goes home and suffers a serious heart attack within hours or days and often dies. His death, caused by the doctor's unnecessary and dangerous test, is easily dismissed because the patient had heart disease. This practice is not unlike the past medical practice of draining blood from the patient until he finally succumbed as was the case with United States President, George Washington.

A negative treadmill stress test is not proof that the arteries are free from plaque deposits.

A treadmill stress test does not rule out coronary artery disease because it does not measure the amount of plaque in the heart arteries. A patient can have as many as four heart arteries with 60% plaque restrictions and still pass the test. He can receive a good report from his doctor without either of them knowing that he has several arteries obstructed 60% by plaque. Treadmill stress tests are not definitive and they are dangerous.

Nuclear Isotope Treadmill Stress Tests Are Acceptable Under Certain Conditions

Radionuclide imaging (or radionuclide angiography) is safe from a physical basis only if a catheter angiography, magnetic resonance angiography (MRA), or computed tomography angiography (CTA) has found the arteries to be free from dangerous arterial plaque deposits. One or a combination of two nuclear isotopes is injected into a vein and allowed to circulate throughout the body. A detector outside of the body records the radiation emanating from the heart to form a 3-D image of the blood flow. Heart muscles that are receiving normal blood flow can easily be seen in contrast to those areas receiving less blood or none. The physician can effectively observe those areas of the heart where arterial flow is restricted or blocked.

The nuclear isotope treadmill stress test is moderately good, but it is not a precise method for measuring blood flow to all areas of the heart during rest and under stress. The radioactive isotope is injected into a vein in the arm while the patient is at rest. The patient then lies horizontally on the table while the detector rotates over the chest area. The arms are placed above the head in a position that becomes very uncomfortable during the 20-minute examination. The device takes a 20-second exposure before rotating in increments, for a total of 30 exposures. Radiation from the heart creates pictures of the blood flow in the heart arteries and muscle tissue that reveal which areas are being deprived of blood due to blockage from plaque, arterial fat, or other defects. They also show areas of the heart muscle that may have been damaged by an earlier heart attack and the extent of the resulting scar tissue.

The patient is then taken to the treadmill where ECG sensors are attached. The treadmill starts slowly and increases in both speed and slope until the patient achieves a pulse rate of 85% of maximum or greater. The patient is again injected with the radioactive isotope one minute before the treadmill is stopped. He is then taken immediately back to the radiology machines for another 20-minute session of 30 exposures. A radiologist then analyzes the resting and stress pictures and prepares the report.

This test is best used after placement of a stent or after arterial bypass surgery as a tool to determine the effectiveness of the treatment and the condition of the heart. It can also be used several years later for an ongoing evaluation of the patient's heart. It is an excellent tool to ensure that stents, bypass arteries, and other arteries are not becoming plugged with plaque or scar tissue. This test can see the inside condition of a stent where others may not. Stents can be subject to the growth of scar tissue in the inside and thereby restrict the blood flow in the artery. The problem can be resolved by placing and expanding another stent inside of an existing stent to relieve the restriction. As many as three stents, one inside of the other, can be inserted when required.

The nuclear isotopes used in the treadmill test have a fairly high radiation exposure rating of 9.4 millisieverts (940 millirems). This compares to 0.36 millisieverts of exposure for a two-view mammogram, 3.0 millisieverts of exposure for everyone from the annual atmospheric background radiation, and 50 millisieverts—the annual exposure limit—for a nuclear power plant worker. Since the nuclear isotopes have a very short half life, health authorities claim the risk is negligible.

The nuclear isotope treadmill stress test could cause a delayed surge in blood pressure to 160/95, which I noticed ten days after my first test and thirty days after the second. This undocumented hypertensive side effect could last two weeks or longer. The

Technetium TC 99M Sestamibi (Cardiolite) nuclear isotope appears to deplete potassium from the heart muscle, causing hypertension, elevated pulse, and an irregular heart rhythm. The combination can be life threatening. Take ¼ teaspoon of Morton's Salt Substitute® (610 mg of potassium chloride) in ½ cup of water. Test the blood pressure and pulse rate again after 60 minutes. Continue to supplement if an improvement is noted.

Artery Stent Limitations

Death is almost certain to occur when a main coronary becomes totally blocked with plaque and/or a blood clot. The resulting heart attack will certainly cause the patient to suffer severe heart damage with long-lasting implications. The smaller arteries of the heart present a different picture. When they become plugged, the patient will suffer a much milder heart attack, and the result is not likely to be life-threatening. Smaller arteries make blockage more difficult to correct by the placement of a stent, and in many cases nothing is done for the patient. The heart will form bypass arteries around the blockage and begin to heal even though the damage is not entirely corrected. The ability to remove or significantly reduce plaque deposits with my regimen is an awesome achievement that modern medicine can only dream about.

Stents have other limitations. They cannot be placed in areas where the artery has a sharp bend or where a branch occurs. Arterial plaque in these areas is much more difficult to handle than in straight sections of larger arteries. Plaque at a corner or branch can be life-threatening and must be treated by performing open-heart bypass surgery. My regimen can be used to reduce the size of the plaque deposit or possibly remove it completely if the artery is not totally blocked and the symptoms are mild enough to endure the waiting time.

Chapter 1

Artery Plaque Etiology and Pathology

The formation of arterial plaque can have several possible causes (etiologies) as will be discussed in Chapter 3. They are highly controversial, and this book will refute and counter several of the commonly accepted etiologies for the formation of arterial plaque. This is not a closed topic, and prevention of the disease is highly dependent upon our understanding of the true scientific etiology. The correct analysis that I present will allow the condition to be reversed, while the wrong analysis will result in a progression of the disease and death.

In the study and diagnosis (pathology) of arterial plaque, it is often described and pictured as a coating of fat and cholesterol that sticks to the inside wall of the artery, and the etiology is said to be a high-fat, high-cholesterol diet. Both of these descriptions are wrong. The plaque deposit is not on the inside wall of the artery but rather between the artery lining and the smooth muscle layer. The deposits contain low-density cholesterol and a small amount of fat in the form of triglycerides. Plaque is not caused by eating animal fats. Omega-6 fatty acids from vegetable oils, grains, seeds, and nuts are more common in arterial plaque than saturated fats that we have been told to avoid. I will present the scientific facts that health professionals, government health organizations, medical organizations, health books, physicians, and professional nutritionists often ignore. You should be prepared to read statements that are contrary to those presented by the mass media. Hopefully, the detailed scientific information I present will register in your mind and displace erroneous information.

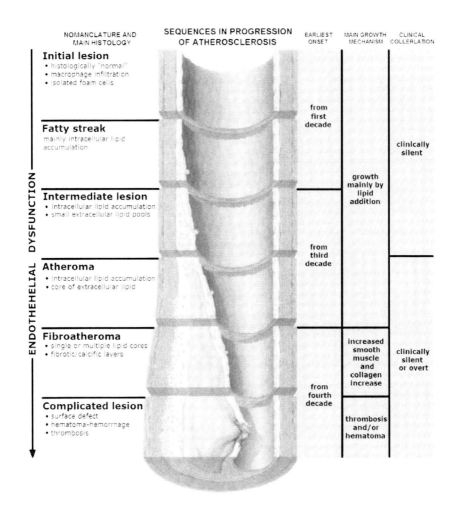

Sequences in the Progression of Atherosclerosis

Arterial plaque also contains white blood cells called *macrophages* that defend the immune system by attacking pathogens (disease-causing organisms such as viruses, bacteria, protozoa, parasites, and other undesirable creatures) and less harmful cellular debris. The macrophages neutralize pathogens by encasement, isolation, and digestion. Macrophages engulf and eat the pathogens. What? Are you surprised to hear the scientific truth that arterial plaque can be created by an immune system response to pathogens? Are you beginning to question the common rhetoric that heart disease is caused by eating meat, eggs, and cheese? If so, you are correct. Heart disease is not caused by eating meat, eggs, and cheese. The scientific facts are being ignored or suppressed by health authorities and others with high credentials and in many cases are being replaced by outright false statements, distortions, and lies. For more information on this topic, read the chapter about brainwashing in *Absolute Truth Exposed – Volume 1*. Books, reports, studies, dietary guidelines, and medical references are awash with statements from those who have been brainwashed or those who intend to brainwash you. Chapter 3 will explain in greater detail why arterial plaque contains macrophages.

Avoiding Blood Clots Caused by Plaque Rupture

The threat of sudden plaque rupture, blood clot formation, and heart attack can be greatly reduced or eliminated with drugs that keep the damaged lining of the artery from forming a clot when the artery lining ruptures. The body can then heal the damaged spot without the person ever being aware that anything happened. He does not suffer a heart attack in these cases, and he feels no pain because arteries do not contain nerve cells. He has avoided a heart attack without even changing his daily activity. This method will be discussed in more detail in Chapter 4.

What Is Arteriosclerotic Vascular Disease?

Arterial plaque can occur throughout the vascular system but is most common in the heart, legs, and neck. Other less common locations are the kidneys, intestines, and brain. It is seldom observed in the arms, liver, or lungs. Plaque in the arteries of the legs is a condition known as *peripheral artery disease.* This is not life-threatening, but it can be severely debilitating and painful. Because the muscles are deprived of blood and oxygen, damage and muscle cell death occur.

The two common carotid arteries with numerous branches are located on the sides of the neck and supply oxygenated blood to the neck and head. Arterial disease is common in this area where plaque deposits tend to form. Attention to symptoms and proper treatment are much more critical than similar conditions in the legs because the slightest restriction will deprive the brain of oxygen and result in cell death known as a *stroke*. Treatment is difficult because any blood clot or debris broken loose by medical procedures will travel to the brain and block the branches and very small artery branches (arterioles).

The liver receives oxygenated blood from a short arterial branch called the *common hepatic artery.* This branch also supplies blood to the pancreas, the first part of the small intestine called the *duodenum*, and a part of the stomach called the *pylorus.* Arterial disease in these branches is much less common but not impossible.

The lungs are less susceptible to arterial disease but highly susceptible to blood clots that can develop in the veins of the legs and travel through the body and into the heart before being pumped into the lungs. The clots are stopped as the branches become smaller and smaller in the transition toward the capillaries. The lungs act like filters that protect the brain and the rest of the body from being damaged by a blood clot in the peripheral veins. A blood clot in the lungs is much easier to treat, and damage is much less severe than a clot in the brain. However, a large blood clot can cause severe damage to one of the lungs, and a clot in both lungs is often fatal.

What Is Hemorrhagic Artery Disease?

Hemorrhagic artery disease is another life-threatening abnormality of the cardiovascular system in which an artery or vein develops a hole that allows blood to leak into the surrounding tissue. This condition in the brain is called a *hemorrhagic stroke* in which blood leaks out of an artery into the surrounding tissue of the brain or skull. It is often fatal or leaves the victim severely disabled.

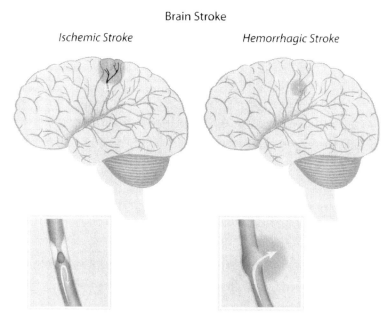

Brain Stroke

Ischemic Stroke   *Hemorrhagic Stroke*

Blockage of blood vessels; lack of blood flow to affected area   Rupture of blood vessels; leakage of blood

A bruise on the arm or leg is an example of hemorrhagic bleeding that is generally caused by trauma. The artery or vein is cut or torn and the blood leaks into the surrounding tissue. These bruises are generally of little consequence, and the blood is usually absorbed back into the system, unlike the dangerous effects of blood pooling that can occur within the brain.

Weak arteries are a side effect of a diet that is deficient in protein and essential fatty acids. For this reason, vegetarians are at a higher risk for hemorrhagic stroke than the general meat-eating population. Amino acids from the digestion of the protein found in red meat, fowl, fish, and seafood promote the growth and repair of healthy arteries and veins.

What Is Calcification or Hardening of the Arteries?

Arteriosclerosis is a general term used to describe the thickening or hardening disease of the larger arteries. In past years, hypertension was thought to be caused by a general hardening of the arteries throughout the body, but this concept may have been incorrect. Arteriosclerotic plaque can occur in small areas at many locations within the arteries, and these localized areas of plaque cause hypertension, not a general hardening. Smaller arteries and arterioles that lead to the capillaries can become diseased with plaque in a condition known as *arteriolosclerosis*. The reasons why people develop hypertension and suggested treatments will be discussed in great detail in Chapter 5.

Intracellular microcalcification causes deposits of calcium in the arteries between the vascular smooth muscle and the surrounding muscle layer adjacent to the atheromatous plaque. As a result, some of the cells die and calcification between the cells begins. This condition in the arteries leading to the brain may eventually cause a stroke, and a similar condition in the arteries of the legs produces peripheral artery disease. *Claudication* is a general term often used to describe these diseases.

The cervical section, nicknamed the *bulb,* is the lower part of the inner carotid artery and is very susceptible to the formation of calcified plaque that can be detected by a common X-ray examination. The bulb is a relatively straight section just above the bifurcation where the two carotid arteries begin. Since it is larger than what appears to be necessary, it is referred to as being *dilated.* LDL cholesterol and lipid deposits in this section may be due to the lower velocity of the blood flow that results in laminar flow—a condition in which the flow at the periphery of the artery is moving slowly and the velocity in the center is moving faster. Restricted blood flow in the bulb area as a result of plaque formation, plaque rupture, and the resulting blood clot can lead to an ischemic stroke. Surgical intervention called *carotid endarterectomy* in this area of the vascular system presents a high risk because the formation of any blood clots or the release of any particles in the artery will cause a stroke as they are carried toward the brain where they block the arterioles.

The carotid artery bifurcation is another location commonly associated with a higher risk for atherosclerotic lesions. An X-ray can show the presence of calcification but does not provide any information as to the degree of blockage of the artery. Ultrasound is another technique that provides additional information, but it lacks the accuracy needed before one dares to undergo invasive surgery. Cerebral angiography examination (angiogram) provides the most accurate diagnosis but is risky because it is invasive. Any invasive procedure in the carotid artery presents a risk for ischemic stroke.

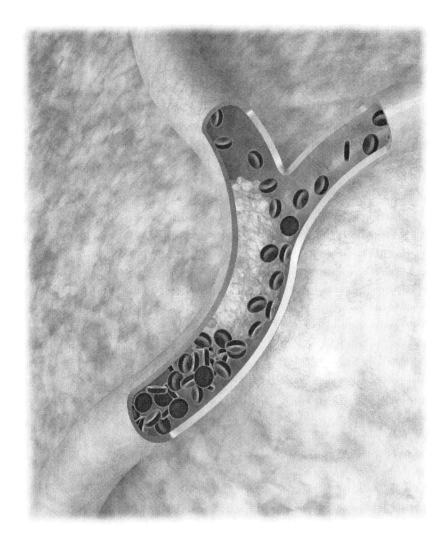

Plaque Deposit Adjacent to an Arterial Bifurcation

The plaque deposit tends to build on the inside of the curve at or prior to the bifurcation. My regimen is very important because a stent cannot be inserted at the bifurcation, and surgery is the only option. My regimen has been shown to remove atherosclerotic lesions and associated calcification throughout the body with virtually no risks and very few side effects.

Chapter 1

What Is Hypertension?

Nearly everyone knows that hypertension is high blood pressure, and most people know that it is an undesirable condition. Pressure within the arteries is measured with two readings, the higher of which is the systolic and occurs during contraction of the heart muscle. The lower pressure, or diastolic reading, occurs between contractions. Arterial pressure is usually taken just above either elbow on the inward side of the arm. Hypertension has many adverse risk factors, including hemorrhagic stroke, kidney, eye, and heart muscle damage, and may contribute to the buildup of atherosclerotic plaque.

Although pressure in the pulmonary artery between the heart and the lungs can be of concern, it is rarely measured because of the invasive procedures required. Heart damage, such as problematic valves, a hole in the septum between the two ventricles, blood clots in the lungs, or disease of the lungs, usually prompts the physician to examine the pulmonary artery pressure. A high measurement is termed *pulmonary hypertension* and can be most accurately measured with a catheter. An abnormally loud sound when the pulmonary semilunar valve closes is a symptom of pulmonary hypertension. The pulmonary venous pressure is measured for consideration and establishment of a diagnosis when symptoms include shortness of breath while sleeping or lying flat. Hypertension in either the pulmonary artery or pulmonary vein can be exhibited in peripheral edema (swelling of the ankles and feet), but this is not an absolute diagnosis because peripheral edema can have many origins.

My regime has greatly reduced edema in my ankles by clearing the ducts of the lymphatic system in the same way as it clears arteries. This allows water to drain from the tissues.

What Is an Irregular Heartbeat, Palpitation, or Arrhythmia?

Normally we cannot feel our hearts beating, but when the rhythm is irregular and becomes noticeable, the condition is called *palpitations*. A more serious condition occurs when an abnormal nerve impulse in the heart produces a pulse rate that is too fast, too slow, or highly irregular. This condition, known as *arrhythmia*, can initiate a medical emergency and life-threatening cardiac arrest.

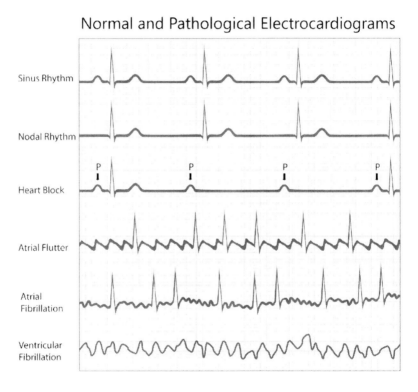

Normal and Pathological Electrocardiograms

The normal pulse rate for a person at rest as shown on an electrocardiogram is in the range of 60–70 beats per minute. The heart monitoring instruments in the intensive care unit of a hospital may typically be set to trigger an alarm at a pulse rate less than 50 or higher than 100. A resting pulse rate higher than 100 is called *tachycardia;* a rate less than 60 is called *bradycardia.* Bradycardia is generally not symptomatic until the rate drops below 50, although professional athletes often have a resting heart rate below 50.

Proper nerve impulses in the heart are highly dependent upon essential nutritional elements, such as essential amino acids, fatty acids, vitamins, minerals, and the level of one or more of the 67 hormones in the body. For example, adrenaline increases the pulse rate, dilates the airways, and contracts blood vessels as it prepares the body for a flight-or-fight response to a disturbing situation. A low or high level of potassium in the blood is life-threatening. The hormones and minerals in the body are very powerful agents that can control the heart rate, blood pressure, muscles, and other organs. They can shut down some organs while diverting the blood supply to other areas of the body. Chapter 5 will provide detailed information concerning essential nutrients and supplements that will help to regulate the hormones and greatly reduce or eliminate heart irregularities such as tachycardia, bradycardia, palpitations, and arrhythmias.

People often become complacent with heart rhythm irregularities because they feel no serious side effects. This complacency is very dangerous because many irregularities can cause blood clots to form within the heart that can then discharge into the arteries and result in a fatal stroke or other serious side effects. Ventricular fibrillation commonly causes fatal strokes.

Heart arrhythmias can be life-threatening.

I will not attempt to list or explain any of the standard practices physicians use to treat heart rhythm irregularities. However, one of the treatments is to cauterize (burn in order to destroy) the nerves in various areas of the heart during a catheterization procedure. Three out of four people I know who have had heart cauterization were thin to the point of malnutrition and ate a low-fat, low-cholesterol diet. Only one had a normal body weight.

A physician also has numerous pharmaceutical drugs available that he can prescribe in an attempt to restore normal heart rhythm. Implanting a pacemaker in combination with a defibrillator is also a very popular treatment. These approaches have a degree of success but present risks and side effects as well. Many pharmaceutical drugs used to treat other conditions have the nasty side effect of creating heart rhythm irregularities.

I will explain in Chapter 5 how to use nutrition and supplements to restore the proper body chemistry needed to improve heart rhythm. This method has proved to be very effective and has many positive results and virtually no undesirable side effects. The primary treatment for correcting heart rhythm irregularities should be through diet and supplementation, but physicians rarely consider this approach. It is simply not according to standard medical practices. The diet and supplement approach gets very little attention because the profit margin is very small, and the United States Food and Drug Administration forbids supplement manufacturers from making any health claims. Remember, this is a science book, not a book written to promote the purchase of products such as essential amino acids, essential fatty acids, vitamins, minerals, other supplements, or drugs. I recommend nutritional supplements that I have found to be beneficial in treating my physical conditions. Much of the information I present has not been confirmed by official medical studies, so follow your physician's advice if you have any questions.

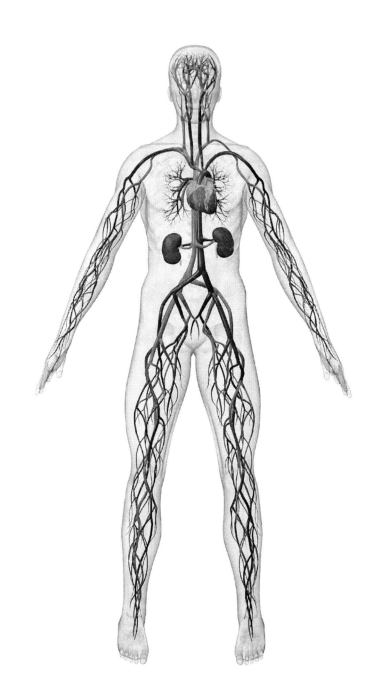

Cardiovascular System

Reversing Heart Disease and Preventing Diabetes

Chapter 2

Dietary Scientific Facts and Human Physiology

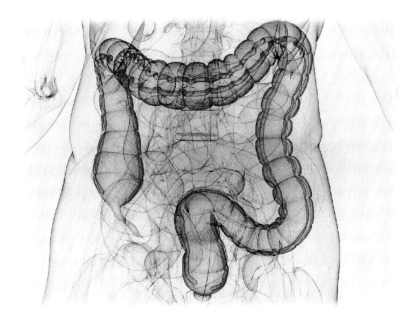

M y first approach to reversing my heart disease was to investigate the scientific truth behind human anatomy and physiology prior to deciding on matters of diet, supplements, and pharmaceuticals. You may think all professional dietitians, physicians, medical clinics, universities, and government departments of health are well versed in how the body works. They are not! We see many false and unscientific statements in books, reports, and studies that are contrary to the anatomy and physiology of the human body. I have already exposed a few of these errors, and in the following chapters, I will continue to expose a multitude of dietary and health claims that violate the known and proven science of human anatomy and physiology. I am not talking about the millions of trivial nuances falsely presented in the mass media. I will focus on major mistakes often presented that can be directly opposite to the actual workings of the human body.

Outrageously false claims have been made that the proper diet for an individual is related to blood type, metabolic typing, metabolic rate, climate or short-term weather differences called *bioclimatology*, seasonal or long-term weather differences called *biometeorology*, continent, elevation, ancestry, affluence, race, sex, environmental accommodation, or religion. All of these theories are false. Human anatomy and physiology are the same for everyone. People react differently because of damage done to the body from an unhealthy diet. The small differences are of no consequence. People are basically the same.

The high-carbohydrate diet will eventually give everyone diabetes, cancer, and heart disease if death doesn't result from an accident or infectious disease first. The diet I present will give everyone a robust, healthy body and prevent and reverse disease because it is based on sound human physiological facts.

Before we discuss the many dietary factors affecting heart disease, we must first understand how the body reacts to and digests the food we eat. Prepare your mind to receive scientific truths that will strongly conflict with the brainwashing that overwhelms us in advertisements, statements by the major media, food manufacturing companies, nutritional supplement salesmen, and religious groups.

The *USFDA Nutrition Facts* are actually worse than what I have already described. Humans certainly require a minimum level of protein for optimal health, but the guidelines do not list any minimum for this essential macronutrient and completely neglect essential fatty acids. You will develop many diseases and die without essential omega-3 and omega-6 fatty acids in the diet, but the *USFDA Nutrition Facts* that are required by law to appear on each manufactured food product in the United States have no listing for essential fatty acids.

Digestion of Protein in Meats

The digestion of meat and natural fats does not require intestinal bacteria and does not promote unhealthy fermentation by bacteria as occurs in the digestion of some carbohydrates. The stomach releases an enzyme called *pepsin* that starts the digestion process by breaking down the protein molecules in meat, eggs, cheese, fowl, fish, and seafood into small groups of amino acid molecules called *peptides*. The enzyme supplement protease can be purchased and taken orally to assist in the efficient digestion of protein. I strongly recommend that a complex enzyme supplement as listed in the supplement section of this book be taken with each meal because some people can be enzyme deficient.

Stomach acid is very good for us.

The stomach also secretes hydrochloric acid (HCL), which helps to break down protein. A multitude of false information has been published on the topic of HCL and the digestion of meats.

Stomach acid is very good for us, but problems surface as we grow older, when the production of HCL in the stomach declines. For this reason, I have suggested that older individuals or anyone suffering from acid reflux should supplement the diet with Betaine HCL. That's right—acid reflux is not caused by excessive stomach acid. It is caused by acid being secreted at the wrong time. Eating my diet will stop acid reflux within a few days if not immediately.

The body is able to digest large quantities of meat without any ill effects. The Big Texan Steak Ranch® restaurant in Amarillo, Texas, offers a meal for $72 that includes a 72-ounce (4.5 pounds or 2.03 kg) steak proudly nicknamed *The Texas King*. The entire dinner is offered free to anyone who can eat all of the steak within one hour. The feat was first accomplished many years ago, and 8,000 people have since succeeded. The record for the shortest time is 8 minutes 52 seconds set by Joey Chestnut, a competitive eating champion. The huge quantity of meat does not make a person sick, and the body handles it reasonably well.

The pancreatic enzymes carboxypeptidace, chymotrypsin, and trypsin are secreted into the small intestine, where they continue to complete the digestion of protein into the individual amino acids. These enzymes can break protein down into peptides and continue to break the peptides down into the different amino acids so that they can be absorbed in the small intestine.

The small intestine produces aminopeptidase, an enzyme that breaks the peptide bond in order to release the terminal amino acid from the amino acid at the end of the peptide. Dipeptidase is another enzyme secreted to separate two amino acids that are joined by a peptide bond so that each can be absorbed individually. The individual amino acids can then pass through the intestinal wall and enter the bloodstream. The human anatomy and physiology are most certainly designed for the consumption of a large amount of meat in one sitting.

The beautiful actress, Angelina Jolie, had a bad experience with her vegetarian diet and returned to eating big juicy steaks. She said,

> "I joke that a big juicy steak is my beauty secret," Jolie said. "But seriously, I love red meat. I was a vegan for a long time, and it nearly killed me. I found I was not getting enough nutrition."

The human digestive tract is definitely designed to digest large quantities of meat easily and quickly. The vegetarians' claim that meat putrefies in the intestines is scientifically untrue. Actually, vegetarian foods such as dietary fiber, starches, and complex carbohydrates can turn the colon into a fermentation tank, where pathogenic bacteria and other creatures create a toxic waste dump that causes leaky gut syndrome, inflammatory bowel diseases, and many other autoimmune diseases. The scientific analysis of this unhealthy process is presented in detail in *Absolute Truth Exposed – Volume 1*.

Remember, amino acids are the building blocks of the body that heal and maintain a strong, healthy physique—from the vitreous gel in the center of the eye, to the immune system's NK (natural killer) cells, to the super-strong Achilles tendon in the calf of the leg. Every part of the human body is made from amino acids that are best obtained from eating meat, eggs, cheese, fowl, and seafood.

Undigested proteins rarely enter the colon and do not appear to cause any ill effects by not doing so. Amino acids in the stool are not a problem either. Amino acids obtained from meat will never make you sick or give you a disease. Amino acids rule!!

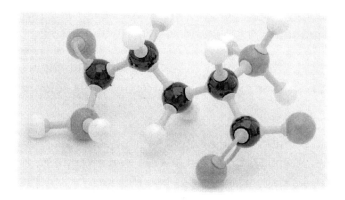

Glutamine Amino Acid Molecule
Take Supplemental Glutamine for Awesome Colon Health

Amino Acids Are the Building Blocks of Life

Amino acids combine in an unlimited number of configurations to make all the proteins of which our bodies are composed. The body uses amino acids to make the following components:

- Flexible, tough skin
- Muscles, Tendons, and ligaments
- The clear gel that fills the eyes
- The clear lenses and retinas of the eyes
- Blood vessels
- Nerves
- Hair, fingernails, and toenails
- Collagen matrix structures in bones
- Natural killer (NK) immune cells
- All other immune cells
- Low-friction surfaces in the joints
- Brain
- Lipoproteins in the blood

The only complete food sources for all of the amino acids used by the body are meat, eggs, cheese, fowl, fish, and seafood. Large amounts of fresh, unprocessed meats should be eaten with every meal. Meat keeps the body healthy. Meat heals the body and prevents disease. Meat causes no diseases. Statements and studies that claim eating meat creates health problems are all false. The 20 major amino acids, plus hundreds of minor amino acids found in meat, keep us alive, vibrant, and healthy. A deficiency in a single amino acid will cause problems for us, and even a single deficiency should be corrected. An essential body tissue that lacks the proper amino acids cannot function as intended and becomes diseased.

If you want a strong immune system, eat meat because all of the immune cells that keep us healthy are made from amino acids. Claims that fruits and vegetables are required to build a strong immune system are scientifically false. In addition to making up all of the protein structures in the body, amino acids have many other numerous functions—far too many to discuss here.

All amino acid molecules in the bodies of humans and animals have a left-hand configuration. For example, amino acids such as taurine may also be designated as L-taurine or simply taurine. Chemists cannot produce left-hand amino acids in the laboratory or factory because half of them have the right-hand configuration. For this reason, all amino acid supplements must be obtained by chemically breaking animal or vegetable protein molecules into the separate amino acids. The body cannot use right-hand amino acids to make protein molecules. This scientific fact makes it impossible for left-hand animal amino acids and protein molecules to have evolved. Chemists can't create animal proteins in the laboratory from an assortment of amino acids, yet our bodies perform this amazing miracle daily.

I will discuss and strongly recommend supplementing the diet with taurine amino acid for heart health. The heart muscle contains a high percentage of taurine, and supplementing the diet with a pharmaceutical grade taurine maintains and rebuilds the heart muscle. The benefits are amazing and truly perform dietary heart therapy.

The dietary deficiency of protein and amino acids is the best kept secret in nutrition and health. I will show you that amino acids are the building blocks for a healthy body and mind. Amino acid supplements can cure diseases and perform nutritional miracles. Physicians or nutritional counselors who underestimate the importance of protein in the diet are harming the patient.

Before each amino acid is discussed, you will read how it is classified within the various categories, such as essential versus non essential, glycogenic versus ketogenic, etc.

Essential - Indicates that the amino acid cannot be made in the body from other amino acids and must be obtained from food. Failure to obtain the full complement of amino acids from food results in an amino acid deficiency accompanied by a resulting health problem or disease.

Amino Acid - Amino acids as found in life forms are molecules that have a left-hand configuration. Because all amino acids are left-hand molecules, the "L" is simply not shown, although some references will show an "L" preceding the name as in L-taurine.

Proteogenic - The term *proteogenic amino acids* is to be understood as meaning all amino acids that are constituents of proteins or polypeptides, specifically the following: aspartic acid, asparagine, threonine, serine, glutamic acid, glutamine, glycine, alanine, cysteine, valine, methionine, isoleucine, leucine, tyrosine, phenylalanine, histidine, lysine, tryptophan, proline, and arginine.

Ketogenic - A term meaning *related to or involving amino acids that the body can convert into ketone bodies by a process called ketogenesis.* Leucine and lysine are the two amino acids in the human body that are exclusively ketogenic and cannot be converted to glucose.

Glycogenic - A term meaning *related to or involving amino acids that can be converted by the body into glucose.* Isoleucine, phenylalanine, tryptophan, and tyrosine are the four amino acids in the human body that are both glycogenic and ketogenic.

Polar - A term meaning *the molecule has an electron polarity.* Non-polar is a molecule that has a balanced polarity.

Uncharged - An amino acid in which the molecule has no electron charge.

Hydrophilic - A hydrophilic molecule or portion of a molecule is one that is typically charge-polarized and capable of hydrogen bonding, enabling it to dissolve more readily in water than in oil or other hydrophobic solvents.

Hydrophobic - Hydrophobic (lipophilic species or hydrophobes) amino acids tend to be electrically neutral and nonpolar and thus prefer other neutral and nonpolar solvents or molecular environments. Hydrophobic is often used interchangeably with *oily* or *lipophilic*.

Aromatic - Aromatic compounds are those in which the main molecule or a branch of the molecule has a group of atoms that close in a circular fashion called an *aromatic ring*. This is not related to aroma or fragrance.

Aliphatic - Aliphatic compounds are non-aromatic, organic compounds in which carbon atoms are joined together in straight or branched chains rather than in rings.

Amidic - Amides are commonly formed from the reaction of carboxylic acids with an amine. This is the reaction that forms peptide bonds between amino acids.

Side Chain - A side chain in organic chemistry and biochemistry is a part of a molecule that is attached to a core structure.

Branched Chain - Branched-chain amino acids are those having aliphatic side chains with a carbon atom branch to more than two other carbon atoms.

The primary and essential amino acids we need to remain healthy are listed below along with the categories, main functions, consequences of deficiencies, responses to overdoses, cautions, and comments. Amino acid supplements can have very powerful, therapeutic (disease curing) properties to greatly improve health. Likewise, some amino acids taken in excess have powerful, unhealthy side effects, and supplementation must be avoided even though the amino acid is considered to be essential in the diet.

A close review of these amino acids and their properties is very beneficial for analyzing dietary deficiencies and treating health problems with supplementation as I strongly suggest in the following chapters.

ALANINE

Non-Essential – Proteogenic – Glycogenic
Non-Polar – Hydrophobic – Aliphatic

Main Functions:

- Supplies energy for muscle
- Functions as the primary amino acid in sugar metabolism
- Boosts immune system by producing antibodies
- Forms connective tissue

Alanine Deficiencies Seen In:

- Hypoglycemia
- Muscle breakdown
- Fatigue
- Viral infections
- Elevated insulin and glucagon levels

Alanine Excess Seen In:

- Low insulin and glucagon levels
- Diabetes mellitus
- Kwashiorkor (starvation)

Caution:

High levels of alanine have been correlated with high blood pressure, energy intake, cholesterol levels, and obesity.

The liver can convert alanine into glucose, a process which is undesirable for preventing heart disease because the goal is to keep blood glucose and insulin low.

Do not supplement the diet with alanine.

ARGININE

Conditionally Essential – Proteogenic – Glycogenic
Basic Side Chains

Main Functions:

- Essential for normal immune system activity
- Necessary for wound healing
- Assists with regeneration of damaged liver
- Necessary for production and release of growth hormone
- Increases release of insulin and glucagon
- Most potent amino acid in releasing insulin
- Assists in healing through collagen synthesis
- Precursor of GABA, an important inhibitory neurotransmitter
- Precursor of nitric acid
- Aids in wound healing
- Decreases size of tumors
- Necessary for spermatogenesis

Arginine Deficiencies Seen In:

- AIDS
- Immune deficiency syndromes, including Chronic Fatigue Syndrome and Gulf War Syndrome
- Candidiasis (systemic yeast or fungal infection)

Caution:

Because arginine gives a powerful boost to the immune system, those suffering from a great variety of ailments may be tempted to experiment with it. Before doing so, make sure you do not have an acute or chronic virus such as Epstein-Barr virus (EBV), Cytomegalovirus (CMV), Human Herpes Virus (HHV-5), or Herpes Simplex I or II.

Arginine will speed up the rate of viral growth that can prove to be dangerous. The amino acid lysine has the opposite effect on viruses because it slows down their growth. I recommend lysine for chronic virus infections.

Arginine has been touted as a heart healthy supplement because it is a precursor of nitric acid that relaxes the blood vessels and improves circulation. Arginine is abundant in meats for optimum health but should never be taken as a supplement because of the negative side effects.

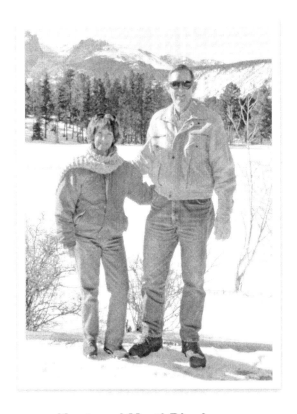

Kent and Marti Rieske
Sprague Lake, Rocky Mountain National Park
January 10, 2010

ASPARTIC ACID

Non-Essential – Proteogenic – Glycogenic
Acid Side Chain

Main Functions:

- Interconvertible with asparagine
- Increases stamina
- Functions with glutamate (glutamic acid) as one of the two main excitatory amino acids
- Protects the liver by removing ammonia
- Aids in DNA and RNA metabolism
- Aids in immune system function by enhancing immunoglobulin production and antibody formation

Aspartic Acid Deficiency Seen In:

- Calcium and magnesium deficiencies

Aspartic Acid Excess Seen In:

- Amyotrophic Lateral Sclerosis (ALS or Lou Gehrig's disease)
- Epilepsy, particularly right after a seizure
- Stroke

Caution:

Aspartic acid is a major excitatory neurotransmitter. Do not supplement the diet with aspartic acid.

Low aspartic acid levels should lead the clinician to test for calcium and/or magnesium deficiencies.

ASPARAGINE

Non-Essential – Proteogenic – Uncharged
Hydrophilic – Amidic

Main Functions:

- Made from aspartic acid plus ATP (adenosine triphosphate)
- Functions as one of the two main excitatory neurotransmitters along with glutamate
- Functions as a neurotransmitter
- Occurs in high concentrations in the hippocampus and hypothalamus along with aspartic acid
- Assists short-term memory in the hippocampus
- Involved in the hypothalamus for the biology of emotion
- Serves as a neurological gate between the brain and the rest of the nervous system
- Aids in removing ammonia from the body
- Increases endurance and decreases fatigue
- Detoxifies harmful chemicals
- Involved in DNA synthesis
- May stimulate the thymus gland

Asparagine Caution:

Asparagine is a major excitatory neurotransmitter. Do not supplement the diet with asparagine.

CYSTEINE & CYSTINE

Non-Essential – Glycogenic – Ketogenic
Uncharged – Hydrophilic – Sulfur-Containing

Main Functions:

- Protective antioxidant against radiation, pollution, and ultraviolet light
- Protective against increased free radical production
- Acts as a natural detoxifier
- Essential in growth, maintenance, and repair of skin
- Provides a key ingredient in hair
- Acts as one of the three main sulfur-containing amino acids, along with taurine and methionine
- Constituent of glutathione, an important tripeptide composed of cystine, glutamic acid, and glycine
- Precursor of the amino acid taurine
- Precursor of chondroitin sulfate, the main component of cartilage

Cysteine/Cystine Deficiency Seen In:

- Chemical sensitivity
- Food allergy

GABA

(Gamma Amino Butyric Acid)
Non-Essential – Non-Proteogenic

Main Functions:

- Acts as one of the two main inhibitory neurotransmitters, the other being glycine
- Precursor of GABA
- Provides a calming, sedative effect but less effective when taken orally
- Raises IQ and treats seizures in mega doses

GABA Deficiency Seen In:

- Seizure disorders

GABA Excess Seen In:

- Anxiety
- Acute mania
- Liver hepatic encephalopathy
- Cirrhosis

Note:

GABA does not easily pass through the blood-brain barrier.

Benzodiazepines such as Valium and Librium activate GABA neurons.

GABA is activity found in glands controlled by the sympathetic nervous system, e.g., the pancreas and thymus.

GLUTAMIC ACID

Non-Essential – Proteogenic – Glycogenic
Acid Side Chain

Main Functions:

- Precursor of glutamine and GABA
- Acts as one of three excitatory neurotransmitters, the others being aspartic acid and asparagine
- Causes brain tissue cell damage in excess
- Provides mechanisms by which strokes kill brain cells through the release of large amounts of glutamic acid
- Helps eliminate alcohol and sugar cravings
- Increases energy
- Accelerates wound healing and ulcer healing
- Detoxifies ammonia in the brain by forming glutamine
- Crosses the blood-brain barrier unlike glutamic acid
- Plays major role in DNA synthesis

Glutamic Acid Deficiency Seen In:

- Vegetarians

Caution:

The high incidence of leaky gut syndrome and inflammatory bowel disease found vegetarians is probably the result of deficiencies of glutamic acid and glutamine.

Glutamic acid is a major excitatory neurotransmitter. Do not supplement the diet with glutamic acid.

GLUTAMINE

Non-Essential – Proteogenic – Glycogenic
Uncharged – Hydrophilic – Amidic

Main Functions:

- Precursor of the neurotransmitter GABA
- Inhibitory neurotransmitter that produces serenity and relaxation
- Essential glycogenic amino acid for maintaining normal and steady blood sugar levels
- Improves muscle strength and endurance
- Essential to gastrointestinal function
- Provides energy to the small intestines as the primary source of energy
- Provides the highest blood concentration of all the amino acids
- Precursor of the neurotransmitter glutamate (glutamic acid)
- Involved in DNA synthesis

Glutamine Deficiency Seen In:

- Bowel diseases
- Chronic Fatigue Syndrome
- Alcoholism
- Anxiety and panic disorders
- Vegetarians

Glutamine Excess Seen In:

- Use of some anticonvulsant medications

Caution:

> The high incidence of leaky gut syndrome and inflammatory bowel disease found vegetarians is probably the result of deficiencies of glutamic acid and glutamine.

Note:

> Glutamine can be supplemented in the diet without fear of an excess conversion to glutamate, which is an unhealthy neuro-exciter. Glutamine supplementation is highly recommended for building strong muscles and other body tissues.

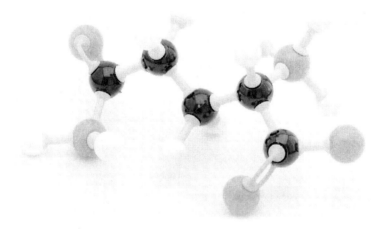

Glutamine Amino Acid Molecule
Promotes Awesome Heart and Colon Health
Take One Heaping Teaspoon Daily with Tomato Juice

GLYCINE

Non-Essential – Proteogenic – Glycogenic
Non-Polar – Hydrophobic – Aliphatic

Main Functions:

- Part of the structure of hemoglobin
- Acts as one of the two main inhibitory neurotransmitters, the other being GABA
- Part of cytochromes, which are enzymes involved in energy production
- Inhibits sugar cravings
- Acts as one of the three critical glycogenic amino acids, along with serine and alanine
- Involved in the production of glucagon, which assists in glycogen metabolism

Glycine Deficiency Seen In:

- Chronic Fatigue Syndrome
- Hypoglycemia
- Anemia
- Viral Infections
- Candidiasis

Glycine Excess Seen In:

- Kwashiorkor (starvation)

HISTIDINE

Essential – Proteogenic – Glycogenic
Basic Side Chains

Main Functions:

- Found in high concentrations in hemoglobin
- Useful in treating anemia due to relationship to hemoglobin
- Has been used to treat rheumatoid arthritis
- Precursor of histamine
- Associated with allergic response and has been used to treat allergies
- Assists in maintaining proper blood pH

Histidine Deficiency Seen In:

- Rheumatoid arthritis
- Anemia
- Dysbiosis (imbalance of intestinal bacterial flora)
- Vegetarians

Histidine Excess In:

- Pregnancy

Special Functions and Predictive Value:

- A high histidine level is associated with a low zinc level.
- A low histidine level is associated with a high zinc level.
- An abnormal histidine level is an indicator that zinc level should be tested.

ISOLEUCINE

Essential – Proteogenic – Glycogenic – Ketogenic
Non-Polar – Hydrophobic – Aliphatic

Main Functions:

- Acts as one of the three major branched-chain amino acids (BCAA), the others being leucine and valine
- Provides muscle strength, endurance, and stamina
- Acts as an energy source for muscle tissue
- Required in the formation of hemoglobin
- Decreased significantly by insulin

Isoleucine Deficiency Seen In:

- Obesity
- Hyperinsulinemia
- Panic disorder
- Chronic Fatigue Syndrome
- Acute hunger
- Kwashiorkor (starvation)
- Vegetarians

Isoleucine Excess Seen In:

- Diabetes mellitus with ketotic hypoglycemia

Note:

Dietary sugar or glucose causes the release of insulin, which in turn causes a drop in BCAA levels. Therefore, do not ingest foods high in glucose before exercise.

LEUCINE

Essential – Proteogenic – Ketogenic
Non-Polar – Hydrophobic – Aliphatic

Main Functions:

- Acts as one of the three branched-chain amino acids (BCAA), the others being isoleucine and valine
- Provides the same properties as isoleucine since it pertains specifically to the branched-chain amino acid functions
- Potent stimulator of insulin
- Helps with bone healing
- Helps promote skin healing
- Modulates release of enkephalins, which are natural pain reducers

Leucine Deficiency Seen In:

- Hyperinsulinemia
- Depression
- Chronic Fatigue Syndrome
- Acute hunger
- Kwashiorkor (starvation)
- Vitamin B-12 deficiency in pernicious anemia
- Vegetarians

Leucine Excess Seen In:

- Ketosis

LYSINE

Essential – Proteogenic – Glycogenic
Ketogenic – Basic Side Chains

Main Functions:

- Inhibits viral growth
- Forms collagen in ligaments, tendons, and joints
- Assists in the absorption of calcium
- Essential for children
- Critical for bone formation
- Involved in hormone production
- Lowers serum triglyceride levels

Lysine Deficiency Seen In:

- Herpes
- Epstein-Barr virus
- Chronic Fatigue Syndrome
- AIDS
- Anemia
- Hair loss
- Weight loss
- Irritability
- Vegetarians

Lysine Excess Seen In:

- Excess of ammonia in the blood

Comment:

Lysine is another amino acid that I highly recommend you add to your supplement program as listed in the following chapters. Lysine discourages and reduces the effects of chronic viral infections. Since early childhood, I have suffered from the common Herpes Simplex Type II virus that causes oral cold sores. A cold or sunburn would stimulate the virus and cause an outbreak. Lysine has virtually stopped these outbreaks, and when one rarely occurs, it is very minor and disappears quickly.

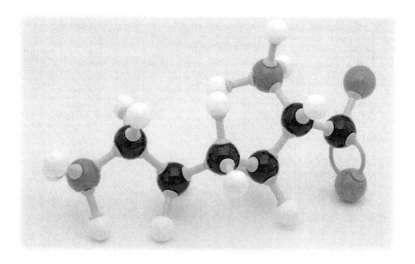

Lysine Amino Acid Molecule
Fights Viruses
Take One or Two 500 mg Capsules Daily

METHIONINE

Essential – Proteogenic – Glycogenic
Non-Polar – Hydrophobic – Sulfur-Containing

Main Functions:

- Assists in breakdown of fats
- Precursor of the amino acids cysteine (and cystine) and taurine
- Reduces blood cholesterol levels
- Acts as an antioxidant
- Assists in the removal of toxic wastes from the liver
- Acts as one of the sulfur-containing amino acids, the others being cysteine and the minor amino acid taurine
- Prevents disorders of hair, skin, and nails due to sulfur and antioxidant activity
- Precursor of carnitine, melatonin (the natural sleep aid) and choline (part of the neurotransmitter acetylcholine)
- Involved in the breakdown of epinephrine, histamine, and nicotinic acid
- Required for synthesis of RNA and DNA
- Natural chelating agent for heavy metals such as lead and mercury

Methionine Deficiency Seen In:

- Chemical exposure
- Multiple chemical sensitivity (MCS)
- Vegetarians

Methionine Excess Seen In:

- Severe liver disease

Caution:

Do not supplement the diet with methionine. The metabolism of methionine produces homocysteine, which is a sulfur-containing amino acid. It exists at a critical biochemical juncture between methionine metabolism and the biosynthesis of cysteine and taurine.

Homocysteine is used to build and repair tissues, but an excess of homocysteine has been shown to be a major factor in the hardening and obstruction of the arteries, leading to full-blown heart disease.

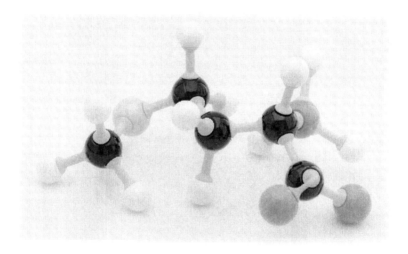

Methionine Amino Acid Molecule
Essential in the Diet but Very Harmful in Excess
Never Take Supplemental Methionine

PHENYLALANINE

Essential – Proteogenic – Glycogenic – Ketogenic
Non-Polar – Hydrophobic – Aromatic

Main Functions:

- Precursor of tyrosine, which is the precursor of the neurotransmitter, dopamine, and the excitatory neurotransmitters, norepinephrine and epinephrine
- Precursor of the thyroxine hormone
- Enhances mood, clarity of thought, concentration, and memory
- Suppresses appetite
- Promotes collagen formation
- D and DL forms used to treat pain, particularly from arthritis
- Powerful antidepressant
- Used in the treatment of Parkinson's disease

Phenylalanine Deficiency Seen In:

- Depression
- Obesity
- Cancer
- AIDS
- Parkinson's disease

Caution:

Phenylalanine should be avoided in:

- High blood pressure due to its hypertensive properties.
- Urination difficulties caused by benign prostate hyperplasia (BPH or enlarged prostate).
- Pregnancy. The excitatory neurotransmitters could harm the baby.

- Pigmented melanoma. Melanoma is the deadliest form of skin cancer.
- PKU (phenylketonuria), a disorder related to improper phenylalanine metabolism.
- Panic disorder and/or anxiety attacks.

Note:

Tyrosine is more powerful and safer in raising the level of norepinephrine for treating depression.

Diet sodas containing aspartame are a major source of phenylalanine in the diet. These should never be consumed because aspartame breaks down into an excess of phenylalanine during digestion. High-calorie drinks or regular sodas containing sugar or high-fructose sweeteners should not be consumed either.

Do not eat any foods sweetened with aspartame. The body converts aspartame to phenylalanine, the precursor of tyrosine which, in turn, is the precursor of dopamine and the excitatory neurotransmitters epinephrine (adrenalin) and norepinephrine (noradrenalin). These neurotrans-mitters are powerful vasoconstrictors that constrict the blood vessels and raise blood pressure dramatically. Aspartame hypes the hormonal system, which results in hunger, anxiety, and insomnia. Do not take phenylalanine and tyrosine supplements except as part of a low-carb whey protein powder. Phenylalanine and tyrosine are both helpful in treating depression, but both should be avoided by those with hypertension.

This is not simply a prejudice against aspartame. Most of the negative claims about aspartame are false. Most critical sources claim that aspartame turns to formaldehyde in the blood. This is basically false. The body can convert 10% of the aspartame into methanol in the small intestines, and this could possibly be converted to formaldehyde. But this does not occur because formaldehyde is not found in the blood of a person who consumes drinks and foods sweetened with aspartame. However, it is a scientific fact that aspartame is broken down into phenylalanine during digestion. Diet drinks containing aspartame give this warning for those with phenylketonuria (PKU). This is a rare genetic disorder in which a baby is born without the ability to properly break down the phenylalanine amino acid molecule.

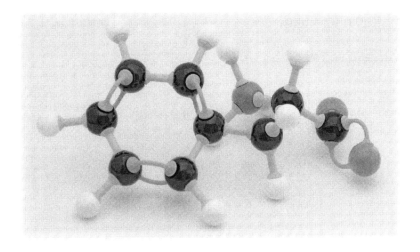

Phenylalanine Amino Acid Molecule
Major Molecule in Aspartame Low-Calorie Sweeteners
Precursor of Neuroexciter Hormones
Promotes Panic Disorder and/or Anxiety Attacks
Dangerous for People with PKU

PROLINE

Non-Essential – Proteogenic – Glycogenic
Non-Polar – Hydrophobic – Aliphatic

Main Functions:

- Critical component of cartilage and hence the health of joints, tendons, and ligaments
- Involved in keeping heart muscle strong
- Can be made from glutamate, a primary precursor
- Can be made from ornithine, a secondary precursor
- Works in conjunction with vitamin C to keep skin and joints healthy

Proline Excess Seen In:

- Chronic liver disease
- Sepsis (infection of the blood)
- Acute alcohol intake

SERINE

Non-Essential – Proteogenic – Glycogenic
Uncharged – Hydrophilic – Hydroxylic

Main Functions:

- Acts as one of the three most important glycogenic amino acids, the others being alanine and glycine
- Critical in maintaining blood sugar levels
- Boosts immune system by assisting in production of antibodies and immunoglobulins
- Component of the myelin sheath (the fatty acid complex that surrounds the axons of nerves)
- Performs several important functions within the central nervous system in the form of phosphotidylserine
- Required for growth and maintenance of muscle
- Interconvertible with glycine

Serine Deficiency Seen In:

- Total body gamma and neutron irradiation
- Hypoglycemia
- Candidiasis

Serine Excess Seen In:

- Vitamin B-6 deficiency

Note:

Phosphoserine, a minor amino acid and a modification of serine, is a good predictor of vitamin B-6 deficiency, particularly the pryidoxal-5-phosphate (P5P) form of vitamin B-6.

If plasma phosphoserine levels are abnormally high, it is a clear indication of P5P deficiency. P5P is critical in amino acid processes.

For example, tyrosine cannot be converted into the neurotransmitter norepinephrine if there is not enough P5P. Likewise, tryptophan cannot be converted into the neurotransmitter serotonin if there is not enough P5P.

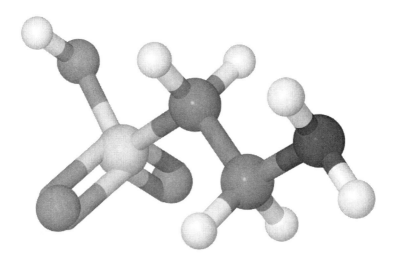

Taurine Amino Acid Molecule
Builds Strong Immune System Cells
Most Important Heart Supplement
Builds Strong, Healthy Heart Muscles
Take Two or Three 850 mg Capsules Daily

TAURINE

Conditionally-Essential – Non-Proteogenic
Sulfur-Containing

Main Functions:

- Stabilizes cell membranes in the nervous system, which raises the seizure threshold
- Treats epileptic seizures and is long lasting
- Acts as an inhibitory neurotransmitter and is as potent as glycine and GABA
- Slows down the aging process as an antioxidant that neutralizes free radicals
- Reduces risk for gallstones by combining with bile acids to make them water soluble
- Treats congestive heart failure (CHF)
- Strengthens neutrophils (white blood cells) in their ability to kill bacteria
- Treats brain injury
- Decreases cholesterol levels along with lysine, carnitine, and tryptophan

Taurine Deficiency Seen In:

- Parkinson's disease
- Anxiety
- Candida
- AIDS
- Cardiac insufficiency
- Hypertension
- Depression
- Kidney failure

Taurine Excess Seen In:

- Vitamin B6 deficiency

83

- Rheumatoid arthritis
- Zinc deficiency
- Liver disease

Note:

High concentrations are found in the heart and eyes.

Taurine is involved in stabilization of heart rhythm, and the loss of intracellular taurine in the heart leads to arrhythmias.

Predictive Value:

The taurine level, whether high or low, indicates if further lab work is needed. For example, if the taurine level is low and the clinical picture is suggestive of candidiasis, one should test for the candida fungus through comprehensive stool analysis and/or anti-candida antibodies.

If the taurine level is high, zinc and vitamin B6 levels should be tested. P5P, an important form of vitamin B6, is necessary for many amino acid reactions to take place.

Supplementing the Diet with Taurine:

Taurine is the best supplement available for maintaining and building a strong heart muscle, and taking taurine as a nutritional supplement is highly recommended. This is especially true for anyone who has suffered heart muscle damage as a result of a heart attack or for older people who have very little human growth hormone, which will prevent the body from repairing itself in a robust manner. Therefore, all older people should supplement the diet with taurine. This powerful amino acid cannot be too highly praised.

THREONINE

Essential – Proteogenic – Glycogenic
Uncharged – Hydrophilic – Hydroxylic

Main Functions:

- Required for formation of collagen
- Prevents fatty deposits in the liver
- Aids in production of antibodies
- Convertible to glycine (a neurotransmitter) in the central nervous system
- Acts as detoxifier
- Promotes a healthy gastrointestinal tract
- Provides symptomatic relief in ALS (Amyotrophic Lateral Sclerosis [Lou Gehrig's disease])
- Increases thymus weight in laboratory experiments with animals
- Treats depression

Threonine Deficiency Seen In:

- Depression
- AIDS
- Muscle spasticity
- ALS (Amyotrophic Lateral Sclerosis)
- Vegetarians
- Epilepsy

Threonine Excess Seen In:

- Alcohol ingestion
- Those treated with sedative anticonvulsant medication (animal studies)
- Vitamin B6 deficiency
- Pregnancy
- Liver cirrhosis

TRYPTOPHAN

Essential – Proteogenic – Glycogenic – Ketogenic
Non-Polar – Hydrophobic – Aromatic

Main Functions:

- Precursor of the key neurotransmitter serotonin, which exerts a calming effect
- Effective sleep aid due to conversion to serotonin
- Reduces anxiety
- Effective in some forms of depression
- Treats migraine headaches
- Stimulates growth hormone
- Lowers cholesterol along with lysine, carnitine, and taurine
- Converts into niacin (vitamin B3)
- Lowers risk for arterial spasms
- Only plasma amino acid bound to protein
- Passes through the blood-brain barrier as do tyrosine, phenylalanine, leucine, isoleucine, and valine, identified as Large Neutral Amino Acids (LNAA)
- Combines with pyridoxal-5-phosphate (P5P), a form of vitamin B6, for conversion into serotonin

Tryptophan Deficiency Seen In:

- Depression
- Insomnia
- Chronic Fatigue Syndrome
- ALS (Amyotrophic Lateral Sclerosis)
- Vegetarians

Tryptophan Excess Seen In:

- Increased intake of salicylates (aspirin)
- Increased blood levels of free fatty acids

- Sleep deprivation
- Niacin intake

Caution:

Simultaneous treatment with tryptophan and Prozac or other SSRI antidepressants such as Paxil and Zoloft can produce Serotonin Syndrome, an irreversible brain disorder. Avoid this treatment combination.

P5P deficiency will lower serotonin levels even if tryptophan levels are normal.

Note:

Standard AMA, APA (American Psychiatric Association), FDA, and pharmaceutical industry positions have been that tryptophan is not an effective treatment of serotonin-depletion depressions when compared to Prozac and other SSRIs.

Clinical experience has shown that some people respond well to Prozac while others respond well to tryptophan in the treatment of serotonin-depletion depressions.

When the FDA banned tryptophan several years ago, thousands of people who only had a positive response to tryptophan (and not to Prozac) decompensated psychologically and never recovered.

L-tryptophan is again available as an over-the-counter supplement.

TYROSINE

Conditionally Essential
Proteogenic – Glycogenic – Ketogenic
Uncharged – Hydrophilic – Aromatic

Main Functions:

- Precursor of neurotransmitters dopamine, norepinephrine, epinephrine (adrenaline), and melanin
- Antidepressant for norepinephrine-deficient depressions
- Preferred over phenylalanine, which is also a precursor of all of the above neurotransmitters
- Precursor of thyroxine and growth hormone
- Improves energy, mental clarity, and concentration
- Combines with pyridoxal-5-phosphate (P5P), a form of vitamin B6, to be converted into norepinephrine

Tyrosine Deficiency Seen In:

- Depression
- Chronic Fatigue Syndrome
- Gulf War Syndrome
- Hypothyroidism
- Parkinson's disease
- Drug addiction and dependency

Tyrosine Excess Seen In:

- Hyperthyroidism
- Chronic liver disease and cirrhosis

Note:

P5P deficiency will lower norepinephrine levels even if Tyrosine levels are normal.

VALINE

Essential – Proteogenic – Glycogenic
Non-Polar – Hydrophobic – Aliphatic

Main Functions:

- Acts as one of the three major branched-chain amino acids (BCAA), the others being leucine and isoleucine
- Involved with muscle strength, endurance, and muscle stamina
- Causes release of insulin, which in turn causes a drop in BCAA levels as a result of high dietary sugar or glucose intake
- Competes with tyrosine and tryptophan in crossing the blood-brain barrier
- Actively absorbed and used directly by muscles as an energy source
- Not processed by the liver before entering the bloodstream
- Needed for acute physical stress, including surgery, sepsis, fever, trauma, or starvation

Valine Deficiency Seen In:

- Kwashiorkor (starvation)
- Hunger
- Obesity
- Neurological deficit
- Elevated insulin levels
- Vegetarians

Valine Excess Seen In:

- Ketotic hypoglycemia
- Visual and tactile hallucinations

Note:

The higher the valine level, the lower the brain levels of tyrosine and tryptophan. One of the implications of this competition is that tyrosine and tryptophan supplements need to be taken at least one hour before or after meals or supplements that are high in branched-chain amino acids.

Deficiency causes all of the other amino acids (and protein) to be less well absorbed by the GI tract.

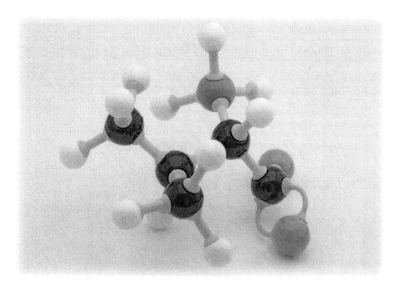

Valine Amino Acid Molecule
Supplement for Trauma, Surgery, and Heart Muscle Energy
Increases Insulin, a Negative Side Effect

BRANCHED-CHAIN AMINO ACIDS

Comments:

Branched-chain amino acids (BCAA) are the three unique amino acids - leucine, isoleucine, and valine.

BCAAs are essential, which means that they must be consumed in the diet since the human body cannot make them from other compounds. Our bodies use these three amino acids to build lean muscle proteins, promote muscle synthesis, and provide fuel for the muscle cells. They increase endurance and support anabolic hormone production. All of these functions are extremely beneficial for building a robust, strong, and healthy body, including the heart muscle.

BCAAs are highly touted by bodybuilders for lean muscles, strength, energy, and endurance. BCAAs are perfect for older people who suffer from low energy, low endurance, and weak muscles. The *USDA Food Guide Pyramid* suggests eating carbohydrates for energy, but carbohydrates make people fat, shrink muscles, and give them diseases such as diabetes, cancer, and heart disease.

BCAAs are metabolized in the muscles rather than the liver so the benefit is direct.

BCAA deficiencies in chronic fatigue syndrome, gulf war syndrome, and fibromyalgia are associated with muscle weakness, fatigue, and post-exertion exhaustion.

BCAAs are needed for acute physical stress, including surgery, sepsis, fever, trauma, or starvation that requires higher amounts of valine, leucine, and isoleucine than any other amino acid.

Digestion of Lipids (Fats)

The average person refuses to eat a chunk of white fat on his dinner plate or a smear of oily fat that has solidified. He immediately separates the piece of fat from the rest of the food and pushes it aside for later disposal. His apprehension is worse when the fat is solidified because it is associated with saturated fats. He fears the fat will cause instant harm to his health because he has been convinced that the fat will immediately begin to plug his heart arteries. This paranoia shows us the extent of the mass brainwashing that has occurred throughout the English-speaking world. It is hilarious to me because this is the food that he must eat in order to reverse or prevent heart disease. Fat phobia, the fear of eating fat, is a major psychological disorder in our society.

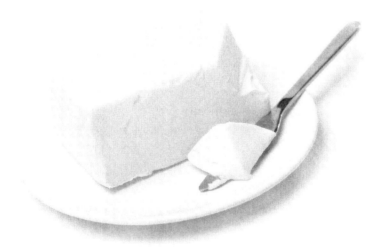

Butter Is Your New Health Food

Visible fats in foods are generally triglycerides, which are most abundant in animal and vegetable fats. A triglyceride molecule consists of three fatty acid molecules connected together with a glycerol molecule. Phospholipids, another type of fat, are the major components of body cell membranes that are connected to form lipid layers. The majority phospholipids are diglyceride or diacylglycerol (DAG) molecules. The diglyceride molecule consists of two fatty acids connected to a glycerol molecule.

Fat phobia, the fear of eating fat, is a major psychological disorder of our society.

The glands of the tongue secrete an enzyme called *lingual lipase* that begins the digestion of fats by splitting some of the triglycerides and phospholipids into individual fatty acids. Lipase secreted by the small intestine continues to break the lipids into molecules that are small enough to pass through the intestinal wall into the bloodstream. Chyme (partially digested stomach contents) discharges into the duodenum, where it mixes with bile acids that are discharged from the gallbladder. These acids break globules of triglycerides into small droplets in a process called *emulsification*. This is similar to the action of soap when it breaks up oils and fats.

The pancreas also secretes an enzyme called *pancreatic lipase* that assists in breaking the triglycerides into individual fatty acid molecules. This completes the digestion process, and the individual fatty acid molecules can pass through the lining of the small intestine into the bloodstream. The body digests lipids without the need for bacteria or other microorganisms.

Individuals with bowel disease are able to digest short-chain saturated fats more easily than other fats. When the disease is severe, those with the inability to digest fats are given medium-chain triglycerides (MCT oil) in the hospital as an energy source. These MCTs are very helpful when carbohydrates cause severe intestinal distress as is common in people with inflammatory bowel diseases. To understand the complete pathology of inflammatory bowel disease and diet therapy to improve your digestion, please read *Absolute Truth Exposed – Volume 1*.

The healthy individual can easily digest a large quantity of lipids. The only symptom is a full feeling that totally shuts down the appetite and prevents overeating. On the other hand, primitive people who had not been brainwashed to avoid fat always preferred the fattiest pieces of meat and often consumed large quantities of pure animal fat. The fatty brains of animals were often treated as delicacies. The Indians and white explorers preferred the tongues and ribs of North American bison because of the high fat content.

Undigested lipids that enter the colon do not cause any serious health issues. In fact, lipids in the colon tend to suppress pathogens because they get trapped in the fat and are removed from the bowel in the stool.

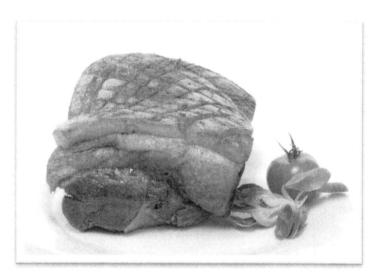

High-Fat Roasts Helped Me to Reverse Heart Disease

Digestion of Nucleic Acids RNA and DNA

Deoxyribonucleic acid (DNA) is an extremely long molecule in all living organisms, including vegetables, animals, and simple microorganisms. DNA holds the genetic information necessary to duplicate, operate, and control the organism. DNA is a double-stranded molecule of nucleotides that looks like a very long string and contains a set of blueprints or instructions that are necessary for the complete development and growth of the organism. Our DNA defines who we are down to the smiles on our faces and the wrinkles on our foreheads. One DNA molecule from our body is able to provide the instructions for making an identical clone. Identical twins are created when the first cell divides to form two separate bodies.

DNA is capable of copying itself and can synthesize ribonucleic acid (RNA). RNA is a single-stranded molecule that can remain as a single strand in many biological roles or fold onto itself in other roles. RNA is a much shorter chain of nucleotides than DNA.

Pancreatic secretions contain two nucleases for the digestion of nucleic acids RNA and DNA. The first nuclease, deoxyriboncuclease, is for the breakdown and digestion of DNA. The second, ribonnuclease, is for the digestion of RNA.

The digestion of DNA and RNA helps to prevent animal DNA and RNA from entering the bloodstream, where the immune system senses that an invader is setting up an attack. The pancreatic nucleases keep us from being contaminated with foreign DNA and RNA, genetic blueprints of vegetables, animals, and microorganisms. We don't want tadpoles swimming in our bloodstreams after finishing a delicious dinner of frogs' legs.

Chapter 2

Nutritional Labeling of Manufactured Foods

The three nutritional macronutrients are fats, proteins, and carbohydrates. Fats have nine calories (actually kilocalories) per gram, proteins have four calories, and carbohydrates have four calories. Honey is almost 100% carbohydrates, butter is almost 100% fats, but pure protein is rare. Fatty steaks, eggs, and cheese are on the order of 25% protein and 75% fat. A low-fat diet is always a high-carbohydrate diet. There are no other choices because fats and carbohydrates are essentially interchangeable in the diet. Protein, the only other macronutrient, has a smaller degree of variation between 0% and 25%. Lettuce and other low-carbohydrate vegetables have almost no calories and can be ignored when counting food calories in each category.

The USFDA requires the Nutrition Facts label to be placed on packages of all manufactured foods in accordance with the *Food Labeling Guide*. The minimum requirements known as *Daily Values* are based on the *USDA Food Guide Pyramid* and show the amount of fats, proteins, carbohydrates, fiber, cholesterol, primary minerals, and primary vitamins in the food product. The daily value for carbohydrates based on a 2000-calorie diet is 300 grams. This is a strange daily requirement because the scientific essential requirement for carbohydrates in the human diet is zero.

The *USFDA Nutrition Facts* are actually worse than what I have described. Humans certainly require a minimum level of protein for optimal health, but the guidelines do not list any minimum for this essential macronutrient. The *Food Labeling Guide* also neglects essential fatty acids. You will develop many diseases and die without the essential omega-3 and omega-6 fatty acids in the diet, but the Nutrition Facts required by law to appear on each manufactured food product in the United States have no listing for essential fatty acids.

Carbohydrates should be avoided like the plague.

The Nutrition Facts do have one good feature in that carbohydrates are identified. Instead of selecting foods that will provide the daily value of 300 grams of carbohydrates per day, you are able to select those foods that have almost no carbohydrates. The avoidance of carbohydrates is the standard that I used to reverse my heart disease. The following chapters will tell you why carbohydrates are to be avoided like the plague.

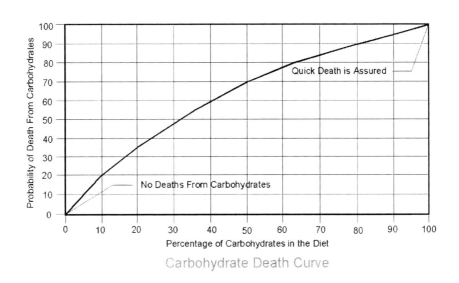

Carbohydrate Death Curve

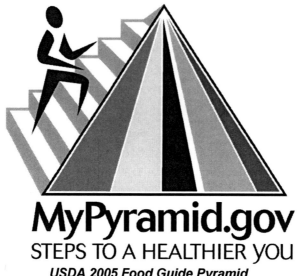

MyPyramid.gov
STEPS TO A HEALTHIER YOU
USDA 2005 Food Guide Pyramid
Source: United States Department of Agriculture
Carbohydrates: 50–60% Depending on the Individual

The 2005 *USDA Food Guide Pyramid* above added more confusion with many different pyramids to choose from. The high-carbohydrate pyramid plans have caused the obesity, cancer, diabetes, and heart disease epidemics to become worse.

Carbohydrates are not essential in the human diet. The *Food Guide Pyramid* is scientifically wrong.

The pathogenic effects of carbohydrates are slow but sure. The label, *20-Year Rule,* was given to describe the length of time between the start of the high-carbohydrate diet and the onset of disease. The separate diseases, severity, and time needed to develop these diseases are directly related to the percentage of carbohydrates in the diet. In the advanced stage, several different diseases are present before death occurs.

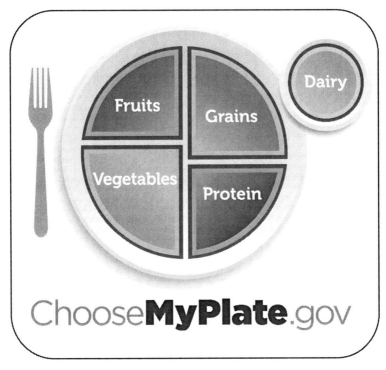

USDA

2010 My Plate
Source: United States Department of Agriculture
Carbohydrates: 50–60% Depending on the Foods Eaten

The icon represents the revised U.S. government's dietary guidelines that have been changed from a pyramid to a food plate. Calorie guidelines and limits are buried deep within the program and have been replaced with verbal descriptions of the desirable foods and lists of those to be avoided. The emphasis is on a balanced diet of vegetables, fruits, grains, protein, and dairy even though the balanced diet concept is devoid of scientific verification. You are instructed to enjoy your food, eat less, and avoid oversized portions; but no quantities are given. Exercise is recommended, but exercise is not represented on the icon.

The *USDA 2010 My Plate* advises against eating saturated animal fat from meat, poultry, cheese, and milk. The diet program says,

"Meat and poultry choices should be lean or low-fat." It recommends monounsaturated and polyunsaturated vegetable oils. The diet focuses three-quarters of the plate on vegetables, fruits, and grains—all high-carbohydrate and high-sugar foods. The saturated fat has been cut from 10% to 7% of calories. The side dish labeled as dairy represents no-fat or low-fat milk, yogurt, or cheese. Milk is another high-sugar food—lactose.

The *USDA 2010 My Plate* diet recommendations are high-carbohydrate and low-fat foods.

As you can see from the icon, the new government dietary recommendations are 25% fruit in which all of the calories are fructose and glucose sugars. Foods that are naturally high in sugars are considered to be very healthy and highly recommended by the program, but refined sugars are strongly discouraged. Honey is neither recommended nor condemned, and it appears to be missing from all of the lists even though honey is 95% identical to common table sugar—a food strongly shunned by the government program.

Type 2 diabetes mellitus is 100% preventable, but I can clearly project that our present obesity and diabetes epidemics will continue to soar as people attempt to follow the new guidelines that can contain more calories from sugars than previously. The obesity and diabetes epidemics around the world tend to be concentrated in English-speaking countries where governments are actively involved in giving dietary advice to the citizens. People in many cultures live at elevations and climates where no vegetables, fruits, or grains can grow, yet they are in better health than people in the U.S., U.K., and Australia.

Dietary Scientific Facts and Human Physiology

Digestion of Carbohydrates

All carbohydrates are broken down into sugars, after which the sugar molecules enter the bloodstream one at a time. The *USDA Food Guide Pyramid* and *2010 USDA My Plate* with the caloric consistency of 50–60% carbohydrates are actually 50–60% sugar in one form or another. Scientifically, it comes as no surprise that obesity, diabetes, heart disease, and cancer are epidemic in all countries where the government promotes the *USDA Food Guide Pyramid*.

Carbohydrate molecules consist of individual sugar molecules, simple chains of sugar molecules, complex chains of sugars, or cross-linked complex chains of carbohydrates called *starches*. However, all are classified as carbohydrates. Cellulose is also a complex molecule of sugars, but the human body does not produce the enzyme necessary to digest cellulose as do the bodies of goats and some other animals. Remember, all carbohydrates become sugars after digestion. The following are examples of common foods that consist primarily of carbohydrates:

- Potatoes consist primarily of starches in the form of complex molecules of glucose which form long chains that are also cross-linked to each other by covalent glycosidic bonds. Potatoes become glucose when digested.

- Grains such as wheat, rice, cassava, and maize (corn) consist primarily of complex carbohydrate chains of glucose and starches that become individual glucose molecules upon digestion.

- Fruits consist primarily of individual fructose and glucose molecules that are quickly absorbed from the small intestine directly into the bloodstream. Fructose travels directly to the liver where it is converted into triglycerides. The liver allows glucose to travel throughout the body to be metabolized in the cells as a fuel. The liver converts excess glucose into triglycerides.

- White table sugar consists of molecules that contain one fructose molecule bonded to one glucose molecule. This bond is easily broken into the two individual sugars.

- Honey is essentially the same as white table sugar with the addition of several other types of sugar molecules and is digested in the same way. The claim that honey is healthy food while with table sugar is unhealthy is false. Both are unhealthy foods.

- Milk contains a high level of lactose (a disaccharide sugar) which consists of one molecule of galactose bonded to one molecule of glucose. The bond is quickly broken by the lactase enzyme produced by the villi (small protrusions of the small intestines) for absorption into the bloodstream. The liver processes the galactose and glucose into triglycerides. Lactose intolerance, a deficiency of the lactase enzyme, is common and leads to inflammatory bowel diseases.

- Legumes, nuts, seeds, and other foods also contain varying levels of different types of carbohydrates that digest into various sugars, primarily glucose.

The digestion of carbohydrates begins immediately in the mouth when the salivary glands secrete alpha-amylase, an enzyme that begins the digestion of starches to produce glucose. This immediate digestion of food gives it the sweet taste, which can easily lead to a sugar addiction. A sugar high begins before the food or candy is swallowed. Sublingual (under the tongue) glucose tables are often given to diabetics during a hypoglycemic episode in order to get glucose into the bloodstream as quickly as possible. The stomach can also absorb some of the glucose before it reaches the small intestine.

Starches are further digested by the amylase pancreatic enzyme in the small intestine to produce alpha-dextrin that continues to be digested by glucoamylase into maltose and maltotriose, both of which are sugars. Other carbohydrates are attacked by sucrase, isomaltose, and lactase enzymes in the brush border section of the small intestine until the smallest basic sugar molecule called a *monosaccharide* can pass through the intestinal lining into the bloodstream. Common sugars such as glucose, galactose, fructose, ribose, and xylose are examples of monosaccharides. When two monosaccharides are attached to each other, they are called *disaccharides,* which can also pass through the intestinal lining to the bloodstream.

Unhealthy High-Carbohydrate Foods		
Grains	Cereals	Bagels
Legumes	Fruits	Breads
Pastas	Potatoes	Yams
Sugars	Ice Creams	Candies

The digestion of carbohydrates usually occurs in the upper section of the small intestine as it moves through the brush border of the epithelium, but more resistant molecules are digested in the lower ileal portion of the intestine. Carbohydrates such as highly resistant starches move undigested into the colon where they are attacked by bacteria, candida yeast, fungi, protozoa, and other pathogens that cause inflammatory bowel diseases as I discussed in great detail in *Absolute Truth Exposed – Volume 1.* The fermentation of carbohydrates in the colon produces toxic gases, acids, and other chemicals that attack the lining of the colon and cause inflammation, disease, and the leakage of the toxins into the bloodstream.

Chapter 2

Excessive Carbohydrates Can Make You Sick

Fruit pie-eating contests are good examples of what happens when a person eats a large quantity of carbohydrates in one sitting. The contestants soon begin to get sick as the stomach involuntarily rejects the load of sugar. The expulsion of the entire contents is uncontrolled even when the cameras are running as occurred in the television series *The Bachelor Pad* in August 2010.

> "*The Bachelor Pad* ladies found this out firsthand, in a setup reminiscent of *Stand by Me*'s famous barf-o-rama scene, only with sports bras and bikinis instead of county-fair attire."

Stand by Me was a Chinese television series that had a gross puking scene during a classic fruit pie-eating contest.

Because fruit pies make contestants sick, pie-eating contests made famous in the United Kingdom usually consist of meat and potato pies. Some fruit pie-eating contests limit the contestant to only one piece, and the winner is determined by the shortest time taken to eat the piece of pie, not the quantity eaten during a fixed time limit. Fruit pie-eating contests based on the amount of pie eaten in a given time have been done with common supermarket pies made from fruit and sugar. These contests can put the participants in the hospital or worse, in the grave.

Carbohydrates Are Highly Addictive

Carbohydrates are highly addictive, unlike protein and lipids. People diagnosed with eating disorders are actually addicted to carbohydrates. They should restrict all carbohydrates the same way that drug addicts and alcoholics must restrict drugs and alcohol. Attempting to cure an addict is doomed to failure if he is allowed to consume even a small amount of the substance to which he is addicted.

Carbohydrate addicts soon learn they can return to eating again by purging the contents of the stomach and waiting a few minutes for the craving/appetite to return. This cycle leads them to become addicted to gorging on carbohydrates and deliberately purging the contents so they can do it all again. Carbohydrates are like a sweet, poisonous drug. Children often eat Halloween candy until they make themselves sick. The result is either to throw up or suffer from diarrhea later as the colon tries to flush the undigested sugars along with the pathogens.

Carbohydrates enter the bloodstream as sugars.

Carbohydrates digest into sugars and create the same metabolic response in the body as candy. Eating a baked potato will actually raise blood sugar levels faster than eating straight white table sugar. Potatoes are candy. Organic, all natural, pure honey is digested exactly the same as white table sugar. Honey is nature's candy. Bagels and whole wheat bread are 70% carbohydrates that digest into sugars, and they affect the body in the same way as many candy bars. Fruits and fruit juices are 100% candy. This is why people who eat the high-carbohydrate diet that includes whole wheat bread, bagels, pasta, cereal, fruit, and potatoes will develop diabetes as frequently as people who eat a similar quantity of candy.

I must make a correction here. I have seriously maligned candy. Some candy is 100% sugar as is fruit. However, *Dove*® dark chocolate *Silky Smooth Promises*® made by Mars are only 43.4% sugar after digestion. I will recommend this treat as a *cheat* later in this book, but the quantity must be restricted. People who have an inflammatory bowel disease that has been in remission for several months according to the diet regimen detailed in *Absolute Truth Exposed – Volume 1* can test this candy in small amounts as a special treat. They cannot do the same with French bread as it most likely will cause a severe flare of their disease.

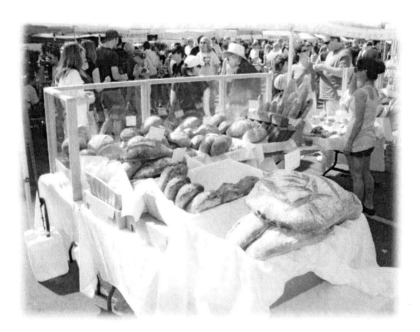

Bread Is Delicious but Contains 76% Sugars
I Reversed My Heart Disease by Avoiding Bread

Acid/Alkaline Diet Theory for the Stomach and Blood

A considerable amount of false information has been published about the effects of food on the acid/alkaline balance of the stomach and blood. The claim is often made that some foods cause the body to enter an unhealthy inflammatory, acidic state, while other foods make the body more alkaline, which the proponents claim is healthier. The recommended alkaline foods are from vegetarian sources and leave an ash residue when completely digested. We know from chemistry that ash is alkaline. People who avoid meat typically condemn high-acid foods because the stomach secretes hydrochloric acid in the natural process of digesting meat, and meat leaves no alkaline ash residue. This entire fictitious topic was contrived and continues to be promoted by vegetarians to discourage people from eating meat.

The acid/alkaline diet theory is not scientific.

The body controls the chemical acid/alkaline balance (pH), within a very narrow range. Contrary to the dozens of books, articles, and scientific reports, the pH remains within the extremely narrow range of 7.35–7.45 as can be seen in a standard blood test report. It doesn't matter how much meat you eat. The acid produced naturally in the stomach is immediately neutralized prior to entering the small intestines. The stomach produces bicarbonate (alkaline or base) when the stomach pH gets too low, and the duodenum produces bicarbonate in large amounts as necessary to completely neutralize the stomach acid in the chyme so that damage to the lower intestines will not occur. The body does this naturally in a healthy way. Eating meat will not give you acid reflux disease, but eating the high-carbohydrate diet outlined on the *2010 USDA My Plate* certainly will because carbohydrates digest into sugars that activate insulin production. The parietal cells in the stomach are stimulated by insulin to increase the secretion of gastric acid—chemically, hydrochloric acid. People with acid reflux disease find immediate relief by switching to a low-carbohydrate diet because insulin is kept low.

My diet therapy eliminates acid reflux disease, but I go one step further by recommending that you take Betaine HCL (hydrochloric acid) with every meal. Many people have verified that it is effective, so I urge you to try it before making a judgment.

Our bodies can quickly and easily adjust the pH of the blood to keep it within controlled limits by automatically increasing or decreasing our breathing since the amount of carbon dioxide (CO_2) in the blood greatly affects the pH. If the body lacks oxygen, the pH of the blood will become lower or more acidic, and the pH will move higher or more alkaline when we hyperventilate. The automatic homeostatic system provides physiological internal control of certain body parameters, including the acid-based homeostasis, to properly control the balance between acids and bases (alkaline or pH). The acid/alkaline diet theory has no basis in science and cannot be confirmed by practical measurements.

Table salt has been found to increase acidity and deplete bone mass as verified in tests conducted at the International Space Station. The same holds true for people on Earth, especially those who are bedridden. This is another of the many reasons why you should avoid salt.

Dietary Scientific Facts and Human Physiology

Physiology of Humans Versus Goats and Cows

We can easily decipher the correct diet for humans based on a close examination of the physiology of the digestive tract. The *2005 USDA My Pyramid* and the new *2010 USDA My Plate* recommend that people eat a diet with lots of fruits, vegetables, and whole grains, while they recommend that we eat only a small amount of meat, if any, and avoid fats, particularly saturated animal fats. People who avoid eating meat and fat have a diet very similar to ruminant herbivores, such as goats, cattle, giraffes, elk, deer, bison, and sheep. The human physiology is similar to that of carnivorous lions and tigers, not herbivorous cows and goats.

Human physiology is similar to that of carnivorous lions and tigers, not herbivorous cows and goats.

Let's compare the adult ruminant herbivore's digestive tract to that of the human. We only have one stomach, classified as *monogastric* (mono=one). Ruminant herbivores have four compartments, classified as *polygastric* (poly=many), that function as four separate stomachs. Vegetarian foods that the animal eats enter the first and largest compartment called the *rumen* that functions as a big fermentation chamber. The rumen contains bacteria and protozoa to break down the fiber in the food. Goats also produce the cellulace enzyme that allows them to digest cellulose as found in paper. You may have seen the insurance advertisement on television that shows a goat munching on paper. Goats like paper because it is food for them, and they will quickly snatch a piece of paper out of your hand or pocket at the farm or petting zoo, chew it up, and swallow it.

These animals also regurgitate the food in the rumen to further break down the fiber by chewing and swallowing it again. This is called *chewing the cud*. The fermentation process produces gas that makes the animal belch and can cause bloating and death if it eats too much rich fodder like alfalfa grass. The fermentation also produces heat to keep the animal warm as occurs in Arctic caribou and moose that live well in temperatures as low as 50 degrees below zero.

After fermentation and chewing the cud, the food particles become small enough to pass into the second compartment called the *reticulum,* where indigestible trash and other objects accidentally swallowed by the animal are separated into the honeycomb structure in the wall of the reticulum. This section of the animal's digestive system is sometimes referred to as the *hardware stomach*.

The fermented food then passes on to the third compartment called the *omasum,* which removes the excess water and absorbs some of the nutrients, such as volatile fatty acids (e.g., acetate, butyrate, lactate, and propionate) and proteins that were made by the bacteria and protozoa in a process called *microbial protein synthesis*. This is the process by which an animal such as a goat or cow can produce milk with a high-fat, high-protein content even though its food contained very little fats or proteins.

The fourth compartment in the animal's stomach is called the *abomasum* and is referred to as the true stomach, which functions in a similar manner to the human stomach. It is here that hydrochloric acid is produced to break down the protein into various amino acids. The digested food then passes into the small intestines in a manner similar to that in humans.

Dairy farmers and cattle ranchers make a high-quality fodder for ruminant animals called *silage* from grass hay, corn stalks, or sorghum by using a fermentation process very similar to that in an animal's stomach. Special bacteria and water are added to the chopped hay that is then placed in the silo or in a plastic covered storage pile where the fermentation takes place. The final product has a higher level of volatile fatty acids and proteins that are produced by the bacteria. This is a very nutritious food for ruminant animals.

The human digestive tract is more like that of a lion, tiger, wolf, cat, or dog, and the stomach does not function as a fermentation vat. It produces hydrochloric acid for the digestion of meat. Sugars are tolerated but produce unpleasant symptoms such as belching or flatulence. Health authorities recommend dietary fiber as the foundation of the ultimate diet program. This recommendation is wrong. Humans cannot digest fiber, but it is digested by pathogenic microbes in the colon and results in inflammatory bowel diseases and damage to the delicate tissue. This is discussed in great detail in *Absolute Truth Exposed - Volume 1*. The **Perfect Diet – Perfect Nutrition** for humans is 100% meat with the associated animal fats, but a very small percentage of the population in English-speaking countries has ever eaten a single such meal and certainly not a diet of 100% meat and animal fat as a lifestyle.

Perfect Diet – Perfect Nutrition

Fermentation will begin immediately in the stomach after eating fruits like grapes or grain products because some bacteria or yeasts are present in the body or in the food. The fermentation produces carbon dioxide gas and ethanol (drinking alcohol). The gas produces burping, and the ethanol creates an alcoholic addiction to the fructose and glucose. The fermentation continues into the small intestines and colon, resulting in water retention, bloating, flatulence, and a frequent loose stool. The human digestive tract does not function properly when fermentation is taking place. Fermentation of sugars, starches, and other carbohydrates occurs in the colon because of malabsorption in the small intestine. The fermentation can become volatile because bacteria, yeasts, molds, and fungi are easily cultured by undigested sugars, carbohydrates, and dietary fiber. The colonic floras also produce hydrogen gas, carbon dioxide gas, alcohol, acetaldehyde, lactic acid, acetic acid, and a host of other toxic chemicals. The results of fermentation are leaky gut syndrome, inflammatory bowel diseases, and autoimmune diseases as discussed in detail in *Absolute Truth Exposed – Volume 1.*

The low-fat, low-protein, high-carbohydrate diet promoted by the *USDA 2010 My Plate* allows hydrochloric acid in the stomach to be released at the wrong time. People often misdiagnose acid reflux into the esophagus as the excess production of stomach acid. This is not true, and taking antacids is not the proper treatment.

Fruits and whole grains cause acid reflux disease.

Digestive health will immediately improve with the diet I present in this book. Negative symptoms, such as bloating, flatulence, burping, stomach acid reflux, and pain, will immediately return when carbohydrates and fiber are reintroduced into the diet in a direct relationship to the percentage consumed. The discomfort may begin within minutes.

Vegetarians falsely claim that meat putrefies in the intestines. Putrefaction is the decomposition of protein and other organic matter by microorganisms that produce foul smelling gases. People on a high-protein diet do not have these symptoms, but they are common in those on a high-carbohydrate vegetarian diet in which the digested sugars are promoting fermentation by microorganisms in the intestinal tract. Fruits, vegetables, sugars, and fiber are the foods that cause obesity, heart disease, diabetes, inflammatory bowel diseases, and a catalog full of autoimmune ailments. Carbohydrates make people fat and sick. Meat heals the body.

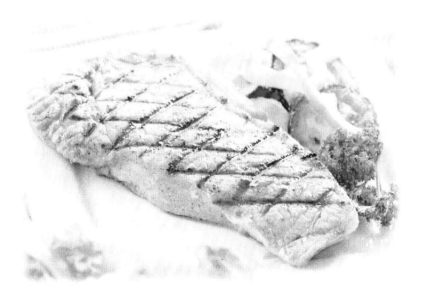

Grilled Steak Heals the Body and Prevents Disease

Food Digestion by Feedlot Steers Versus Humans

The following compares the digestion process of feedlot steers that are fed whole grains and vegetable grasses to people who eat whole grains and vegetable salads.

Feedlot Steer

Whole grains and grasses →→ fermentation with bacteria →→ amino acids and fatty acids →→ bloodstream

Result: Amino acids and fatty acids enter the animal's bloodstream.

Human

Whole grains and vegetables →→ digestion with enzymes →→ glucose and other sugars →→ bloodstream

Result: Sugars enters the bloodstream.

This is the most important scientific fact concerning nutrition and human physiology. All carbohydrates become sugars after digestion and enter the bloodstream as sugars. You must understand this scientific fact in order to correctly understand the proper connection between diet and health. If you are unsure, continue reading. After you have finished this book, return to the first page and read it all again. The science is irrefutable but often denied.

Obviously, humans do not receive the same micronutrients into the bloodstream as do herbivorous animals even though both eat the same foods. Animals receive nutritious proteins and fats in the bloodstream upon digestion, but humans receive mostly sugar in the bloodstream. Whole grains and vegetables make feedlot steers strong and healthy, but whole grains and vegetables make people obese and give them diseases. People obtain only a small amount of essential amino acids and essential fatty acids from the same meal.

Fruits, whole grains, and vegetables all become sugars after digestion and enter the bloodstream.

The digestive systems of herbivorous animals function the same way as the process for making hard cheeses. Fermentation with bacterial cultures converts the lactose in milk into cheese. The result is a product that contains only proteins and fats. The percentage of carbohydrates (lactose) in the final cheese product is zero. Do humans have a vegetarian digestive system? No! Human physiology shows our digestive system is more suited toward a diet containing high levels of meat and animal fats.

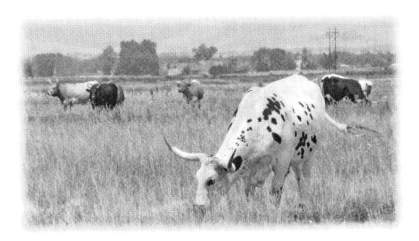

Texas Longhorn Cattle Grazing
Boulder County, Colorado, July 27, 2010

Swine have monogastric, nonruminant digestive systems as do humans. The digestive system of swine is not like that of a cow or goat. Swine are omnivores like humans, and they will eat meat given the chance. They have been known to eat other animals and even become cannibalistic. As one expert said,

> "Farmers can't let anything go to waste, so they often throw dead livestock that can't be processed to the hogs. It saves on feed."

A girl who was raised on a farm said,

> "My stepdad is a hog farmer. He says that pigs are cannibals and will eat each other. Another pig farmer in the area must have fallen into the pig pen because he was "missing" and later they discovered only his bones and his clothing in the pig pen. The pigs ate him up."

Whole grains and vegetables fed to swine result in the animal become very fat—obviously. Farmers in the past attempted to make swine fat by feeding them fat but it didn't work. The swine became skinny. Carbohydrates make swine fat the same way carbohydrates make people fat.

Someone wrote to me to complain that swine should not be kept in pens because they get manure on their feet, and the manure could make them sick. She thought that swine should be raised in a *free range* manner. Oh, poor little piggy! A nearby farm must be owned by someone with the same concern. He fenced a large area of prime grass pasture and released a herd of swine to allow them the free range openness of the pasture. This is something I had never seen. The pigs completely decimated the pasture in less than a month. They ripped up the grass sod in large areas, preferring the corners. Now the rain has come, and the piggy-plowed sod has become a mud hole. They have reverted back to the hog pen all by themselves.

Pigs gone wild do the same thing. The hogs tear up the ground to make a mud hole, defecate in the mud, and then roll in it. Domestic swine released into the wild become mean, dangerous animals. They will come into suburban yards and literally destroy the lawns, flower beds, and vegetable plots. They will attack people and pets. Sorry! Pigs must be kept in pens with manure on their feet.

Actually, swine grown in commercial hog factories live in a pristine environment. The feces fall through grates in the floor and are recycled as fertilizer or can be processed into bio-gas as an energy source. The hogs remain perfectly clean and healthy, although rolling in the mud hole did not make them sick either.

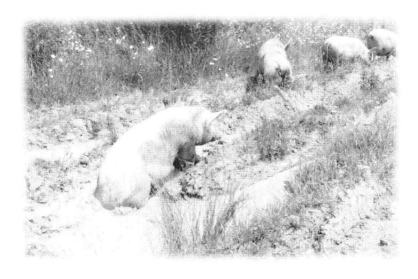

Free Range Pigs Enjoying a Mud Hole

Arctic Explorers Prove 100% Meat Diet Is Healthy

We often hear doctors or professors with PhD degrees in nutritional science admit that fruits and vegetables are mostly devoid of essential amino acids and fatty acids. This is indeed true, but they insist that everyone should eat a balanced diet with an abundance of fruits in order to obtain the essential vitamins and minerals. This is statement is scientifically false. A 100% meat diet with all of the natural animal fats is the perfect food for humans and carnivorous animals because it contains all of essential amino acids, fatty acids, vitamins, and minerals. Meat is the perfect food. Nothing else need be eaten to maintain perfect health. The vitamins and minerals in meat, fish, seafood, and fowl are deliberately underrated or literally erased from nutrition count books and references. Some references claim that meat does not contain vitamin C, but it certainly does. In fact, fresh meat has enough vitamin C to cure scurvy (a disease caused by vitamin C deficiency) as was proved over and over again in the Arctic, where people ate a 100% meat diet with all of the natural animal fats. The Arctic expedition led by Captain Sir John Franklin, an officer in the British Royal Navy, proved overwhelmingly that eating fresh meat will prevent scurvy.

In 1845, the Franklin Expedition sailed from England across the Atlantic Ocean with 128 men in two ships. They sailed around the southern tip of Greenland and along the coast of northern Canada to the Arctic Ocean in an attempt to find the Northwest Passage from the Atlantic to the Pacific Ocean. Franklin hoped enough of the polar ice cap would have melted near the mainland in summer to allow passage. They were fully loaded with supplies, including the prized lime juice that was supposed to provide vitamin C for the prevention of scurvy. As he had planned, Franklin's two ships became frozen in the ice as winner approached. Eskimos who had none of these advanced provisions waved at the sailors as they passed by the ships that were locked in the winter ice. The Eskimos, who ate a 100% meat diet with the natural animal fats, never developed scurvy, but all of the sailors died from the dreaded disease or from other diseases caused by nutritional deficiencies as a result of eating the food stored on the ships. The sailors could not survive even though they had firearms for hunting, but the Eskimos lived reasonably well with their handcrafted spears and bows and arrows.

Eskimos hunting with bows and arrows lived well. Englishmen hunting with guns could not survive.

In the 1920s, Dr. Weston A. Price found the Maasai people in central Africa living in extraordinarily good health on their traditional diet of the meat, milk, and blood from cattle they herded. The Maasai shunned grains and grass seeds because they considered grains and seeds to be food for the animals rather than people. The Maasai were extremely tall, up to 7 feet (2134 mm) and rarely less than 6 feet (1829 mm), and had perfect teeth and bones. The Maasai men would stroll through lion country carrying their long spears without concern. Recently, the government of Kenya restrained the Maasai warriors from killing lions because they are now considered to be endangered. Unfortunately, influence from *educated* foreigners has changed the Maasai diet to their detriment. The Maasai have seen a decrease in health since they included grains and beans in their diet and began eating less meat.

The Plains Indians of North America lived in excellent health for centuries, if not millennia, on a diet consisting primarily of buffalo (bison) meat and fat. They prepared a mixture for long-term storage by cutting the lean portions of meat into strips that they hung on racks to dry in the sun. The fat was half internal hard fat and half external soft back fat. The big slabs of fat were cut into pieces and heated in stone bowls over a fire to boil off the water trapped in the fat. The Indians observed the connection between diet and health very closely, and they learned that moisture left in the fat would cause the mixture to become rancid. The dried meat was ground between rocks and added to the fat at a 50% ratio before being placed in the storage containers made from the animal intestines. They called the mixture *pemmican* and relied on it as their sole food source during the harsh winter months. The pemmican lasted for years and through the summer heat without deterioration. This diet grew tough, strong, and healthy children. The content was 80% fat on a calorie basis, which contradicts the erroneous statements in numerous books that the Indians ate lean meat. These writers came to this hasty conclusion because buffalo flesh is leaner than modern feedlot beef.

The Hudson Bay Company (founded in 1670 as Adventurers of England Trading) and North West Company (incorporated in 1783) were fur trappers and traders who purchased pemmican from the Indians by the ton to supply the fur trappers throughout North America. These companies were large enough at that time to trade shares on the London Stock Exchange. The Indians received rifles, ammunition, and knifes in exchange for the pemmican, and they rode horses that the Spaniards introduced into North America in the 16th century. Because the horses made killing buffalo easy, the trade volume in pemmican greatly increased. The Indians and the whites were both responsible for the demise of the buffalo, contrary to modern claims that the white man annihilated the buffalo for sport. The buffalo were becoming scarce when the Mormon pioneers and others crossed the plains in 1847.

The United States government moved the Indians to reservations to protect the pioneers and provided the Indians with grains for their food instead of meat. The awesome health the Plains Indians enjoyed for centuries was decimated overnight when they were placed on reservations where their diet was forcefully changed to organic whole grains. The Indians are now free to leave the reservations, but they have retained the high-carbohydrate, whole grain-based diet that has caused them to suffer dreadfully. The incidence of diabetes, heart disease, and cancer among the once healthy North American Indians is epidemic.

North American Plains Indians lived in perfect health for unknown millennia on a diet of 80% fat.

Vilhjalmur Stefansson and Rudolph Martin (Karsten) Anderson explored northern Canada beyond the Arctic Circle in two expeditions during 1906–1912. On the first expedition, they found Eskimos living in superior health on the Mackenzie River Delta, consuming a diet that was almost 100% salmon caught from the river. Stefansson could not find a single dental caries in any of the living individuals or in any of more than 2000 skulls of the deceased he examined. They had excellent health, and by his own examination or by questioning the people, he could not detect anyone who had ever had cancer. They never reported anything that resembled heart disease and certainly never exhibited anything that could be diagnosed as diabetes. The primary cause of death, as it had been in people worldwide for millennia, was from infections. The people also suffered from the hazardous climate in which they lived.

On his second expedition, Stefansson and an Eskimo companion ventured onto the frozen Arctic Ocean during midwinter, where they found Eskimos who have never seen a white man. They were living in excellent health on a diet consisting entirely of seal meat and blubber with a calorie content that was approximately 80% fat. The Eskimos' husky dogs consumed the very same diet. The seals were caught with a tethered spear through a hole in the ice they used for breathing. Occasionally, the men were lucky enough to encounter a polar bear, which they considered to be a great prize because of the meat and valuable skin. They would quickly gather the dogs, spears, and bows and arrows to go charging after the bear. Their spear tips and knives were made from pure native copper found on the nearby island.

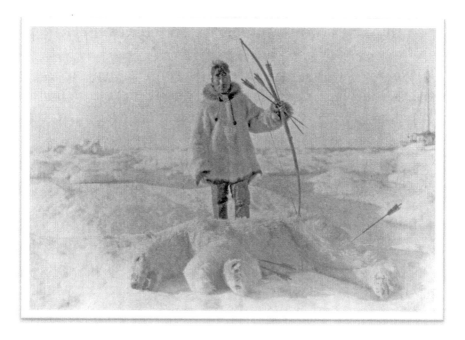

Eskimo Kills a Polar Bear
Place and Date Unknown

The Eskimo women often prepared a soup made from blood and water. They melted snow, boiled the water in small stone bowls, and added the seal blood slowly so it would not curdle. The meat and fat were also boiled and often eaten raw. The small fire consumed seal blubber and provided light as well as some heat for the igloo, which reached a comfortable temperature when many people were inside.

Eskimos lived in perfect health for unknown millennia on a diet that was 80% fat.

The people knew that plants with berries grew on some of the islands in the summer but never bothered to pick any berries because they didn't consider them to be food. In the spring prior to the ice melt, the Eskimos ventured south onto the mainland of northern Canada to search for wood that was used to make frames and runners for their dog sleds and to hunt caribou for the desirable meat and hides. These people never ate fruits, vegetables, or whole grains, and they were not obese as depicted in cartoons. They would not have considered vegetation to be food for humans. It was caribou food.

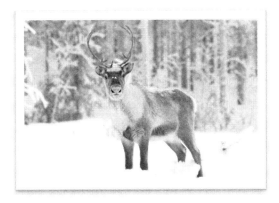

Reindeer in Scandinavia or Caribou in North America

Vegetarians Expose Poor Health on Message Boards

I enjoy reading other books, reference materials, studies, and websites in order to see the nutrition and health information being disseminated to the public. I joined a vegetarian message board where the people were allowed to ask questions about nutrition and health and receive answers from the professional nutritionists and doctors who monitored the board. The other members of the board were also permitted to make comments. I made several comments that were scientifically accurate, but they were instantly deleted by those who monitored the board. They only allowed comments with which they agreed and did not allow scientific references. Examples like this have led to severe nutritional brainwashing in our society.

Alice was a member and vegetarian on a message board. Her husband who was 48 years old became her work-in-progress, or should I say, "negligent-homicide-in-progress." She bragged constantly about her sister-in-law (husband's sister) who was a *professional nutritionist*. The two of them had taken it upon themselves to use the poor unsuspecting husband and brother-in-law as a research animal for their vegetarian lifestyle. She described him as a large, muscular man with a job that required a lot of physical labor, and the two women believed that he needed a substantial amount of carbohydrates in his diet in order to provide the energy needed to perform his work. He was overweight, his cholesterol readings were atrocious, his total cholesterol and LDL cholesterol were high, and his HDL cholesterol was very low. His triglycerides were out of sight, and he had high blood pressure. In addition, they described him as hypoglycemic. In actuality, he was most likely already diabetic. She bragged that he was on a vegetarian diet of 85% carbohydrates. These two self-proclaimed diet experts, one with a college degree, were attempting to solve his health problems through diet therapy, but his diet was not much better than that of the fictitious people whose plane was forced to land on a South Pacific island. He did obtain some amino acids from grains and beans, but the fatty acids in his diet were mainly from unhealthy omega-6 vegetable oils. The two women were perplexed because his health continued to deteriorate.

Alice and her husband's sister are killing him with a diet of 85% carbohydrates and bragging about it.

This was approximately four years ago, and perhaps he has since died. They were attempting to make him better, but because they believed the false information taught to those who are studying to become professional nutritionists, they were actually killing him.

Another vegetarian on the message board posted his frustration at the bad numbers he received in his blood test report. He thought his nearly vegan diet should have given him the awesome cholesterol readings that the professional nutritionists on the message board had promised. Neither he nor his physician understood that his high-carbohydrate, low-fat diet was the cause of his high triglycerides and dreadfully low HDL cholesterol. So, what did the message board experts tell him? They pulled the standard excuse from the hat, "It must be genetic because your distant relative died from a heart attack." They never blamed it on the high-carbohydrate diet because it didn't fit the false predetermined paradigm they had accepted. This vegan lost body fat and muscle, but the fat in his blood is still high. Not one of the individual readings on his blood test was good. They were all either neutral or bad.

He posted the following on the message board:

"I'm surprised and upset by the results of my blood work. I'm a vegetarian, and am nearly vegan. I eat vegan most of the time, occasionally allowing a pizza with real cheese and sometimes having a veggie burger that includes an egg white. However, the pizza has only been one or two per month. I used to drink a lot of sugary soda pops, but I quit that starting about June of '10. I've also lost about 30 pounds since January.

However, unfortunately, I still have high cholesterol. Here are my numbers from my recent blood work:

Cholesterol:	200	< - neutral
Triglyceride:	177	< - high = bad
HDL:	37	< - very low = bad
Non-HDL Cholesterol:	163	< - neutral
VLDL Calc:	35	< - neutral
LDL Calc:	128	< - neutral
LDL/HDL Ratio:	3.5	< - high = bad
Cholesterol/HDL Ratio:	5.4	< - high = bad

The doctor said if I don't improve by December, I should go on cholesterol-lowering drugs. I don't want to do that if I don't have to. I asked how it was possible for me to have bad numbers like this even though I'm a vegetarian and he said I may be genetically predisposed to heart disease, and that if I weren't vegetarian, these numbers may be off the

> charts. My maternal grandfather died of heart disease."

The vegetarian in the above example must not have read the Nutrition Facts on the package of veggie burgers he has been eating. Check them yourself. I noticed some frozen veggie burgers on sale at the store with the proud proclamation on the front, *100% Vegan*. I turned the package over and checked the Nutrition Facts, which listed the contents as they appear in the following table. I proceeded to the candy section of the store, where the Nutrition Facts on the chocolate, peanut, and caramel candy bars show the following:

Nutritional Macronutrients	100% Veggie Burger	Chocolate Candy Bar
Calories	172	172
Fats	8 gm	8 gm
Carbohydrates	21 gm	23 gm
Protein	4 gm	2 gm

The 100% veggie burger is almost identical in composition to the chocolate candy bar. Both are 100% vegan and both have a very high level of carbohydrates. The 100% veggie burger was pumped up with a little soy protein, but the nutritional result is almost identical. He could have eaten the chocolate candy bar for lunch with a sprinkle of soy protein powder and his body would have never known the difference. He could have called it a health bar because this is exactly how they are made. His triglycerides are high because the liver converts fructose in both foods directly into blood triglycerides.

The following young adult female was perplexed to find that her vegetarian diet, daily jogging, and ice skating did not result in a good blood cholesterol report, so she pulled out the standard excuse, "It's genetics, not my diet." She failed to realize that her high level of exercise did not help either.

> *"I am 23 years old and female. I recently got back my first cholesterol test. I had it done because I know high cholesterol runs in my family. I have 250 mg/dL total cholesterol and 208 mg/dL triglycerides. I believe that these numbers are very high. I am shocked considering I run every day and ice skate almost every night. I am a vegetarian and do not eat any fried foods... Is there anything I can do? I do not want to take meds...*
>
> *Thanks"*

Vegetarians are perplexed when their low-fat diet causes high cholesterol and triglycerides.

This vegetarian's report shows the degree of brainwashing that has spread throughout the vegetarian community. She thinks fried foods are to be avoided, but the scientific facts show that the liver converts fructose in fruit directly into triglycerides. Her high triglycerides are consistent with her vegetarian diet, but she doesn't understand why.

Breakfast Menu in the Hospital Cardiac Unit

The cardiac unit in the local hospital serves heart patients a breakfast consisting of two large whole wheat pancakes, syrup, vegetable oil margarine, cooked oatmeal, and a small piece of sausage. A food count analysis would put the range of carbohydrates at about 70–80% of the calories. You will see as you read this book why everything in the meal, including the sausage, is on my list of **Forbidden Foods** that must be avoided in order to reverse heart disease. I believe the breakfast served in the cardiac unit of the local hospital is giving patients heart disease.

An out-of-state visitor was in the cardiac unit to see her friend who was a patient. The visitor, who is also a nurse, bragged that her new dietary guidelines allow free fruit, which means she can eat as much fruit as she wishes. The guidelines were issued by a company that charged her an expensive membership fee, and she hoped that the recommended diet and nutrition program would reverse her many ailments and reduce her weight. She admitted that she loved fruit. Well, no wonder! The calories in fruit are half fructose sugar and half glucose sugar. Fructose has the highest sweetness rating of all of the common sugars. Yes, sugar addicts love fruit.

The common recommendation to eat lots of fruit and the extensive addition of high-fructose corn syrup in manufactured foods has skyrocketed parallel to the increase in diabetes. These examples illustrate the nonsense that has polluted the professional nutrition programs recommended by hospitals, nurses, physicians, and companies that charge fees for nutritional and weight control diet programs.

Is Fructose in Fruit a Savior or an Executioner?

Fructose has become the latest fad in the fight against diabetes because the body produces insulin at a lower rate than during the metabolism of glucose. Fructose is absorbed directly into the bloodstream in the small intestine without the need for an enzymatic reaction or digestion and is delivered by the hepatic portal vein directly to the liver where it is metabolized by synthesis into glycogen and further into fatty acids and triglycerides. In plain English, consuming fructose from fruit results in an increase in triglycerides—a major risk factor for heart disease. This occurs without insulin, thus reducing the glucose and insulin surge that occurs when high-glycemic foods are eaten. (The glycemic index is a measure of the amount and time required for the body to produce blood glucose from the digestion of carbohydrates and starches.) Fructose is highly recommended in nearly every diet and special food designed and sold for the diabetic, but fructose has two deadly properties.

- It causes insulin resistance in the cells of the body—the major cause of diabetes.

- The liver instantly converts it into blood fats.

Fructose is the diabetic's worst enemy.

Fructose has become the new health food fad even though researchers have known for decades that mice are fed high levels of fructose in order to deliberately make them diabetic for research purposes. Actually, fructose obtained from eating fruit is metabolized into triglycerides in the blood faster than you can swallow. Fruit is nature's candy.

Reversing Heart Disease and Preventing Diabetes

Chapter 3

Scientific Causes of Cardiovascular Diseases

Healthy
artery

Build-up
begins

Plaque
forms

Plaque
ruptures;
blood clot
forms

Chapter 3

This book will give the scientific etiologies of heart disease, not the propaganda offered by government health organizations to fit their agendas. My first book, *Absolute Truth Exposed – Volume 1*, contains a chapter that explains why brainwashing the human psyche is awesomely easy. In addition to being slaves who are brainwashed by other people, the general public brainwashes themselves by studying all the false propaganda they can find instead of testing both sides of the issue. We must be constantly on guard in order to discover the absolute truth.

I will show why the studies cited by major media, university researchers, numerous health and medical associations, and government agencies do not report many of the scientific causes for coronary artery disease. The studies are conducted in a manner that supports the sacred low-fat agenda rather than looking at all dietary options. These organizations have been unable to prevent or reverse coronary artery disease because the low-fat, high-carbohydrate diet they advocate is the actual cause of heart disease.

As you read other books about reversing heart disease, look for references to scientific studies, accurate descriptions of human physiology, my scientific method for reversing heart disease, actual laboratory test results, and cardiologists' findings that verify the degree of reduction in arterial plaque. I have provided all of this data for your review. A 5% or 10% reduction in the size of arterial plaque is not a reversal of heart disease when the patient has lost 10% of his body weight. I would expect some reduction in arterial plaque with weight loss, but this is not reversing heart disease. The plaque will return as the weight returns. True reversal of heart disease is a major reduction of plaque even though the patient has not lost any weight.

Erase Your Brain

You may find it virtually impossible to comprehend what you are about to read because of the vast amount of false data that has been presented to the general public for the last century. An individual will enter a state of confusion when the scientific facts conflict with his long-held beliefs. He begins to feel insecure, disoriented, and fearful when his brain tries to embrace two opposing positions. Is the low-fat diet wrong? If he accepted the low-fat diet dogma but now rejects it, he must admit that he was tricked into believing lies. The human mind rebels against any suggestion that it might be wrong, and the mind strongly rebels against making a change that disrupts its foundational understanding of a healthy diet. The brain locks up because of this conflict, and people simply proceed in error for the rest of their lives rather than accept a drastic change. They want to believe the scientific truth but are terrified of being tricked again.

Are you in the learning stage, or has your brain locked up from false understanding?

You must take the same approach that William Banting did in the 1850s. He was suffering from obesity, degenerative diseases of his joints, and many other ailments. He almost certainly had undiagnosed diabetes and heart disease. Hoping to restore his health, he saw a physician, presented his symptoms and complaints, and followed the doctor's advice. When his conditions did not reverse, he went to the next physician and continued until he finally consulted a doctor who placed him on a relatively low-carbohydrate diet. When Banting's health dramatically improved in a very short time, he wanted to tell the world about it. He wrote a booklet titled, *Letter on Corpulence,* and sold copies for a very small price. He was shocked when physicians and lay people largely ignored him, and his testimony was summarily dismissed. His booklet is now available as a free download from Internet websites and has been recently republished since no copyright exists.

Heart Disease Is Caused by Atheromatous Plaque

Most medical references and medical societies describe the etiology of atheromatous plaque in coronary artery disease (CAD) by listing risk factors, such as high cholesterol, smoking, obesity, diabetes, and high blood pressure. Since half of the heart attack victims don't have any of these risk factors, something else is the primary cause of CAD. These factors may be symptoms of heart disease or a separate disease that has the same etiology as heart disease. I believe that most of these so-called risk factors have one common source—the high-carbohydrate diet.

Which came first, heart disease or diabetes? The first time many patients receive their heart disease and diabetes diagnoses is in the hospital emergency room. I will tell you the scientific etiology for coronary artery disease, but it's not the result of eating red meat, eggs, cheese, saturated animal fats, butter, or coconut oil. Let's look at scientifically based heart disease risk factors often missing from health and medical literature.

Scientific Heart Disease Risk Factors:

- High insulin
- High glucose
- Bacterial infections
- Viral infections
- High Triglycerides

- High LDL$_b$ Cholesterol
- Low HDL Cholesterol
- Diabetes Mellitus
- Omega-6 Fatty Acid

Insulin Causes Coronary Artery Disease and Cardiovascular Disease

Insulin is the number one contributing factor to coronary artery disease because it promotes the formation of plaque in the arteries of the heart. It also produces plaque formation in other arteries of the body and leads to peripheral artery disease, stroke, and kidney disease. You may think this is puzzling because it is an essential natural hormone. We cannot live without insulin, but high levels will give you cardiovascular disease. This should come as no surprise since many of the essential nutrients such as potassium will kill us if they are too high or too low.

We cannot live without insulin, but high levels will give you cardiovascular disease.

Insulin is a hormone made by the beta cells in the islets of Langerhans in the pancreas. Insulin is needed to move glucose from the blood into the cells of the body, where the glucose is consumed as fuel in the mitochondria (the power plant of the cell) to produce energy and heat. Glucose is unable to cross the outer membrane of the cell without the aid of insulin.

Insulin is a powerful anabolic hormone that builds muscles, tendons, ligaments, and bones. The word *anabolic* means *to build up*, and insulin certainly does this in a powerful way. Insulin is needed to convert excess glucose to triglyceride fatty acid, and insulin moves triglycerides from the bloodstream into body fat cells for storage. Many people don't understand that the body can convert fructose in orange juice into body fat on the tummy and hips. Yes, the liver can and does convert orange juice into saturated and monounsaturated fats.

135

The body is very sensitive to blood glucose levels that are too high or too low, and this is why physicians monitor the glucose level whenever blood chemistry measurements are taken. Physicians recommend that diabetics purchase a glucose meter to monitor their glucose levels. You can do the same.

Glucose is the most common sugar obtained from the digestion of carbohydrates and starches. The liver can also make it by metabolizing fats and proteins. However, the body reacts very differently to these two sources of glucose. Carbohydrates and starches are broken down into individual glucose molecules during digestion, and the glucose must be moved in large quantities into the bloodstream whether it is needed or not. The liver will make glucose from amino acids and lipids only when the level of glucose in the blood is low or in the early morning when we awake from a long night of fasting. These two differences are very important. The glucose produced by the liver in the morning gives us the energy we need to start our day prior to eating breakfast. Many people lack an appetite in the morning and simply skip breakfast because their glucose levels are high. Type 1 diabetics who do not produce insulin may require an insulin injection in the morning to reduce the level of glucose in the blood even though they have not eaten food all night.

Insulin makes us feel energetic when glucose and insulin levels are both high. People incorrectly believe the high-carbohydrate diet is wonderful because they feel energetic. They think the glucose and insulin rushes are healthy because they have high metabolisms. There is no end to the books that advise people to eat a high-carbohydrate diet in order to increase their metabolisms and drop their weight. The high-metabolism diet works for those who are already thin because they have zero insulin resistance, but the obese find the same diet only serves to make them fatter. This is why weight loss diets based on increasing the metabolism are always a failure for the obese.

Eating carbohydrates produces glucose and insulin that may make you feel energetic, but that doesn't necessarily mean you have a high metabolism. People who are obese simply do not have high metabolisms. If they did, they would be skinny. Many of the diets recommended by professional nutritionists deliberately attempt to increase the metabolism with the false impression that you will lose weight, but when you don't lose weight, they pass it off to the weight-loss scapegoat—exercise. They blame you by saying, "You didn't exercise enough." More will be said about exercise in Chapter 7, *Learn When Exercise Can Kill You*.

Insulin is a deadly hormone we can't live without.

Insulin causes cardiovascular disease because it forces LDL cholesterol, triglycerides, calcium, heavy metals, glucose, and free radicals to bind to the arteries throughout the body. Free radicals are undesirable chemical compounds with free electrons or vacant electron sites that bind easily to body cells in an unhealthy manner. This binding produces a mixture of these compounds in plaque, which does not coat the inside of the artery as many believe. The insulin literally pushes LDL cholesterol and these other molecules through microscopic openings in the thin internal lining of the artery. The plaque is between the lining, called the *tunica intima,* and the muscular layer, called the *tunica media* or *smooth muscle cells*. The outer third layer of the artery is called the *tunica externa*, also known as the *tunica adventitia*. This outer layer is primarily made of collagen, a fibrous tissue similar to that found in bones, ligaments, and tendons.

Because the plaque is trapped between these layers of the arterial wall where it is not easily dislodged, reversing heart disease is very difficult. It requires special methods that can draw the components of the plaque away from the deposit one small molecule at a time until the deposit is gone. This is the scientific process I used to reverse my heart disease, and I will give you the complete regimen that I used to do it.

I have stated that insulin causes coronary artery disease and peripheral artery disease, but let's see what the major professional association says about the cause of CAD.

The American Heart Association® lists the following as major risk factors for heart disease:

- Increasing age
- Sex – male
- Heredity, including race
- Tobacco smoke
- High blood cholesterol
- High blood pressure
- Physically inactive
- Obesity and overweight
- Diabetes mellitus

We typically interpret these risk factors as the causes of coronary artery disease, but they are risk factors, not causal factors. This list does not include hyperinsulinemia (elevated blood insulin levels), which I believe is the primary contributor to coronary artery disease. In fact, none of the etiologies of coronary artery disease identified in this book is listed by the American Heart Association®. Can you reverse coronary artery disease like I did by following the dietary, health, and medical advice of the American Heart Association®? I seriously doubt it. I could not find any data, studies, or personal testimonies to prove that following the American Heart Association® guidelines and reducing their risk factors have reversed coronary artery disease.

It is interesting that the American Heart Association® says that males are at a greater risk for CAD than females, but the statistics have changed in the U.S. since men now die from cancer at a higher rate than heart disease. Men tend to be more concerned about heart disease and nonchalant about cancer, and women are terrified of getting cancer but less concerned about heart disease. The number one cause of death in women has shifted to heart disease with cancer moving to second. The public's misconceptions are a result of health officials' inaccurate statements as illustrated here.

Individuals are often jolted to the core when they get coronary artery disease and have a heart attack without any of these risk factors. It is shocking to see that the American Heart Association® does not list insulin or elevated insulin as a risk factor, but I have it listed as the number one cause of coronary artery disease by scientific analysis.

Carbohydrates are more deadly than smoking.

The world's oldest living person was Jeanne Louise Calment, who died August 4, 1997, at the age of 122. She was born in Arles, France, on February 21, 1875, and lived her entire life in France. She said that she smoked from age 21 until age 117, but she claimed she smoked no more than two cigarettes a day. She quit only because her eyesight was failing and she didn't want to bother others by asking them to light her cigarettes. Smoking was once ranked as the primary cause of heart disease until the public reduced their smoking. Now we find that the heart disease rate did not decrease. Officials misled the public by overstressing the connection between smoking and heart disease. I do not recommend that people smoke because it raises the cancer risk and is a small contributor to heart disease due to the increased free radicals in the blood. Smoking is certainly a risk factor for lung cancer, but smoking has decreased in the United States and cancer has increased. Could it be that cancer and heart disease have not decreased along with the smoking rate because people are more strictly complying with the *2004 USDA Food Guide Pyramid*, *2005 USDA My Pyramid*, or *2010 USDA My Plate*? Yes, it is the increase in the consumption of carbohydrates according to these guidelines.

The American Heart Association® says, "But by losing even as few as 10 pounds, you can lower your heart disease risk." This statement is very misleading because I personally know several very skinny people who exercise regularly, run in competitive races, and yet developed severe heart disease. I also know people who are 100 pounds overweight, 85 years of age, get no exercise, and appear to have no signs of heart disease. I reversed my heart disease and reduced my heart artery plaque in two places by 50% in 25 months while actually gaining 10 pounds. Yes, I reversed heart disease and gained weight at the same time. How did I do this? I reversed my heart disease because it is carbohydrate intake that is correlated with CAD, not body weight or changes in body weight. Yes, carbohydrate intake correlates with weight gain and CAD. That is the relationship.

Carbohydrate intake is correlated with biomarkers for coronary heart disease in a population of overweight premenopausal women

The Journal of Nutritional Biochemistry
2005 Apr;16(4):245-50

Department of Nutritional Sciences, University of Connecticut, Storrs, CT 06269, USA

"Abstract

The associations between macronutrient intake and plasma parameters associated with increased risk for coronary heart disease (CHD) were evaluated in 80 overweight premenopausal women. We hypothesized that higher carbohydrate intake would be associated with a more detrimental plasma lipid profile. Dietary data were collected using a validated food frequency questionnaire (FFQ). Plasma total cholesterol (TC), triglycerides (TGs), high-density lipoprotein cholesterol (HDL-C) and low-density lipoprotein cholesterol (LDL-C) were determined from two fasting blood samples. In addition, selected apolipoproteins (apo) and LDL peak size were measured. Values for TC, TG and HDL were not in the range of risk classification; however, the mean values of LDL-C, 2.7 +/- 0.7 mmol/L, were higher than the current recommendations. Carbohydrate intake was positively associated with TG and apo C-III (P < .01) concentrations, and negatively associated with LDL diameter (P < .01). Participants were divided into low (<53% of energy) or high (> or = 53% energy) carbohydrate intake groups. Individuals in the <53% carbohydrate group consumed more cholesterol and total fat, but also had higher intake of polyunsaturated and monounsaturated fatty acids (SFAs). In contrast, subjects in the > or =53% group consumed higher concentrations of glucose and fructose than those in the low-carbohydrate (LC) group. In addition, subjects consuming <53% carbohydrate had lower concentrations of LDL-C and apo B (P < .01) and a larger LDL diameter (P < .05) than the > or =53% group. These results suggest that the lower LDL-C in the LC group may be related to both the amount of carbohydrate and the type of fatty acids consumed by these subjects."

Insulin packs glycated LDL cholesterol, glycated proteins, glycated hemoglobin, and oxidized polyunsaturated omega-6 vegetable fatty acids into arteries of the heart, neck, and legs, causing blockages and death. Deposits in the neck arteries cause strokes. Insulin causes heart disease, and a high level of blood insulin produces many unhealthy body reactions which eventually lead to diseases of all types. The first obvious symptom of high insulin is the increase in body fat when the excess carbohydrates are converted to glucose, which promotes insulin production and body fat deposits.

Over many years, the onslaught of carbohydrates results in glucose intolerance and insulin resistance. Carbohydrates drive insulin production which leads to cardiovascular heart disease. Heart attack patients may not be told about the close relationship between their newly diagnosed heart condition and diabetes. Blood insulin reaches high levels, remains high, and progresses from hypoglycemia to Type 2 diabetes. Glucose rises uncontrollably because the beta cells in the pancreas are unable to maintain insulin production, and insulin-dependent Type 2 diabetes occurs as the pancreas becomes fatigued from many years of excessive insulin production. This makes diabetes appear to be age related, but it is actually the cumulative effect of the over consumption of carbohydrates. The resulting high levels of glucose and insulin also lead to diseases of the eyes, kidneys, blood vessels, and nerves.

Insulin also pushes omega-6 vegetable fatty acid molecules into the artery walls to begin the process of atherosclerosis. The omega-6 vegetable fatty acid molecule is pushed between the "gap-junction" of the endothelial cells where it gets stuck. The omega-6 vegetable fatty acid molecules become oxidized and are attacked by free-radicals. The immune system attacks the decaying omega-6 vegetable fatty acid molecules and sets off inflammation. The body then deposits cholesterol at the site in an attempt to repair the injury.

Insulin stimulates the unhealthy growth of arterial smooth muscle cells and causes arteriosclerosis and hypertension. It stimulates the unhealthy growth of fibrous tissue and forms plaque in the arteries. It also stimulates the unhealthy growth of fibrinogen that thickens the blood and forms clots. The entire process occurs rather suddenly as insulin resistance peaks and insulin levels skyrocket. I call this sudden appearance of heart disease the *Rieske Instant Atherosclerosis Cycle (IAC)*.

Insulin resistance is rarely mentioned as a heart disease risk even though diabetics have four times the risk for heart disease. Sixty-five percent of diabetics die from heart disease, but doctors rarely measure insulin resistance or the blood insulin level during a health checkup. Insulin is a major risk factor for many diseases, but it is mostly ignored. Carbohydrate consumption is the culprit behind most age-related diseases.

Insulin causes heart disease, but it is rarely checked in blood tests.

Eating a low-carbohydrate diet brings unhealthy insulin-related body processes to a screeching halt. All humans react the same way. People are not different from one another as the myth implies, and the metabolic typing diet is a myth. The high-carbohydrate diet is not healthy for anyone even though some people may remain thin. The variable is the amount of damage that carbohydrates and insulin have already done to the body, but this damage is often incorrectly diagnosed as genetic.

The scientific proof that insulin triggers many age-related diseases is beyond question, yet professional medical practitioners rarely measure their patients' insulin levels. Many diabetics have never had their insulin levels measured. Professional heart disease organizations rarely mention insulin as a heart disease risk or promote a low-insulin diet as a method of preventing heart disease. The carbohydrate - glucose - insulin cycle is getting away with mass murder while these professional organizations are saying, "Don't eat red meat or saturated fat." A few brave individuals like Dr. Robert C. Atkins have promoted the science of health while enduring a constant assault from professional organizations such as the American Heart Association® and American Medical Association®. Professional medicine almost universally ignores mountains of scientific evidence against dietary carbohydrates in favor of unproven myths against dietary saturated fats.

The average cardiologist will tell you that heart disease is caused by cholesterol and fat in the diet. This is because the medical establishment and the American Medical Association® think carbohydrates are innocent and necessary dietary requirements. However, the scientific and nutritional requirement for carbohydrates in the diet is zero—absolutely none. Most professional nutritionists and the *USDA Food Guide Pyramid* falsely claim that carbohydrates are required in the diet. Studies have consistently shown that the lower the dietary intake of carbohydrates, the better the long-term health. Heart disease is caused by the excessive consumption of carbohydrates in combination with a deficiency of protein and fat from animal sources.

The dirty little secret in nutritional health is the high rate of heart disease among vegetarians, who are continually falling away from their diet because they realize it is harming their health. The vegetarians of southern India eat a low-calorie diet very high in carbohydrates and low in protein and fat. They have the shortest life span of any society on Earth, and their bodies have an extremely low muscle mass. They are weak and frail, and the children clearly exhibit a failure to thrive. Their heart disease rate is double that of the meat eaters in northern India.

The dirty little secret in nutritional health is the high rate of heart disease among vegetarians.

Vegetarians have been brainwashed to think that their diet is healthy, but in online forums that deal with osteoporosis, Crohn's disease, ulcerative colitis, and other inflammatory bowel diseases, approximately 80% of the sufferers are vegetarians or people who have highly restricted their intake of meat in the past. This is shocking since only 6% of the people in the United States are vegetarians. The protein-deficient, vegetarian diet will cause degenerative disc disease, inflammatory bowel diseases, autoimmune diseases, and raise the risk for cancer and hemorrhagic stroke. Amino acids found in meat are the building blocks of life, and the body becomes thin and frail with an almost ghostly gray cast to the skin when amino acids are deficient. The diet I present in this book builds strong, robust, healthy bodies in everyone from infants to the elderly.

Chapter 3

**Anthropological Research Reveals Human
Dietary Requirements for Optimal Health**
H. Leon Abrams, Jr., MA, EDS
Associate Professor Emeritus of Anthropology, ECJC,
University System of Georgia, Swainsboro, Georgia.
Journal of Applied Nutrition, 1982, 16:1:38-45

"No cultures or people in the world have ever been 100% vegetarians; however, a number, such as the Masai of Africa, Plains Indians, the Eskimo and the Lapps, in their traditional culture, subsist almost entirely on meat and have been very healthy. When they adapted to our modern diet which is high in refined carbohydrates, their health deteriorated rapidly; they developed a high incidence of degenerative diseases characteristic of our modern civilization, especially heart disease.

Michael DeBakey, world renowned heart surgeon from Houston, who has devoted extensive research into the cholesterol coronary disease theory, states that out of every ten people in the United States who have atherosclerotic heart disease, only three or four of these ten have high cholesterol levels; this is approximately the identical rate of elevated cholesterol found in the general population. His comment: "If you say cholesterol is the cause, how do you explain the other 60 percent to 70 percent with heart disease who don't have a high cholesterol?" In 1964 DeBakey made an analysis of cholesterol levels from usual hospital laboratory testing of 1,700 patients with atherosclerotic disease and found there was no positive or definitive relationship or correlation between serum cholesterol levels and the extent or nature of atherosclerotic disease.

A comparative study of men in Crete and the village of Crevalcore, Italy, indicates that there is probably no relationship between serum cholesterol and coronary heart disease when the level is 245 mg of cholesterol per 100ml.

146

The men in Crete show serum cholesterol levels of 200mg/dl and have an incidence of less than one coronary heart disease per 100 men in five years. In contrast, the men in Crevalcore with similar serum cholesterol levels suffer an incidence of approximately six cases of coronary heart disease in five years.

Many questions are being asked about the generally accepted and greatly advertised theory that consumption of saturated fatty acids (beef, lamb, mutton, butter, and pork) are major factors contributing to hypercholesterolemia and heart disease, while the consumption of polyunsaturated fatty acids (vegetable oils) will prevent coronary heart disease. Rivers states that the trend toward eating so much margarine and other vegetable oil products may be "exactly the wrong thing," and explains that because polyunsaturates are very unstable, extra polyunsaturated fatty acids are added by substituting soft margarines and stabilized vegetable oils for animal fats and butter. The difficulty is, he continued, that the two changes lead to a dramatic increase in the eating of trans-fatty acids that results in hypercholesterolemic effects that far outweigh the reported benefits of polyunsaturated fats.

It seems that the human body requires some essential polyunsaturated fatty acids such as linoleic and arachidonic acid, but the established requirement seems to be only approximately 1% of calories. Studies strongly indicate that large consumption of margarine, and other polyunsaturated vegetable fats, may be conducive to cancer. Animal experiments found that rats fed a chemical carcinogen in addition to 20% vegetable polyunsaturated fat and a much higher incidence of tumors than when fed a carcinogenic with animal fat. In a similar experiment, rats treated with a carcinogen and given 5% corn oil had a 3.5 times higher incidence of colon tumors that did rats who were maintained on 5% lard.

Studies have also linked a high intake of polyunsaturates, which is probably over 10% of the average American's diet, with vitamin deficiencies, liver damage, premature aging, nutritional muscular dystrophy, cancer, and severe blood disease in infants. Polyunsaturated fatty acids are believed to be highly reactive chemical compounds that render them possibly harmful; they can be oxidized by ordinary cooking in one's body when they react with nitrous oxide in smog, from X-rays and sunlight and some trace metals such as iron. Passwater states that of fourteen tests conducted, all showed a high correlation between eating high amounts of polyunsaturates in the form of corn oil, peanut oil, margarines, soybean oil, et al., and notes that presently Americans eat two to three times more vegetable oils than were consumed sixty years ago. He stresses that only from two to four percent of one's diet should consist of vegetable fats.

Most hunting and gathering societies eat a large amount of meat. The classical example is the Eskimo who lived almost entirely on land and sea mammals, fish and birds. Anthropologist Vilhjalmur Steffansson, who spent many years living with the Eskimo around the turn of the century, found that they were in excellent health and remained so as long as they maintained their traditional diet. It was discovered that as long as they ate fresh meat, they obtained an ample supply of vitamin C which was previously thought to come only from plant sources. However, cooking at high temperatures destroys vitamin C in both meat and plant foods.

Although it was accepted that the Eskimo thrived in a high state of good health on an almost complete meat diet, authorities stated that the diet would probably be harmful for Europeans. To prove the thesis that a 100% meat diet is sufficient for sound health, Vilhjalmur Steffansson and Karsten Anderson submitted themselves to an experiment conducted by The Russell Sage Institute of Pathology at Bellevue Hospital, an affiliate of the Medical College of Cornell University. For a period of one year, they ate only fresh meat in the ratio of two pounds of fresh lean meat to one-half pound of fat per day. Steffansson, who had been on the Eskimo diet for years, remained in good health, while Anderson was found to be in much better physical condition than when he began the experiment. Steffansson continued to live on the Eskimo diet for many decades, in very good health, until his death at the age of 83.

Otto Schaeffer, a specialist in internal medicine and director of the Northern Medical Research Unit at Charles Campbell Hospital, Arctic Canada, found that as long as the Eskimo lived on his native diet in the traditional manner, he remained in sound health and was practically free from degenerative diseases, especially those that afflict Americans. He reports that with the adoption of the white man's diet, which consists largely of refined carbohydrates (sugar, white flour), processed polyunsaturated fats, and other processed foods, the Eskimo is widely afflicted with all the degenerative diseases common to our modern society."

William and his wife are good examples of those who religiously followed the low-fat diet as outlined by the American Heart Association® and the *USDA Food Guide Pyramid*. William would have loved eggs for breakfast and a big, fatty, medium-rare beef steak for dinner, but his wife would not allow it. He was henpecked, and she was domineering. She insisted that they eat the low-fat diet. Breakfast consisted of whole grain cereals with fruit, low-fat milk, and low-fat yogurt. Lunch could have been whole grain bread, whole grain pasta with tomato sauce, and salad with olive oil. Dinner was a soy veggie burger and lots of fruit. She said her diet was "the best in the world." She claimed the smell of meat cooking made her sick, and she could not swallow the smallest piece of fat without gagging. She was proud of the title, *Health Nut*, but her low-fat diet made them and their son fat as they became part of the obesity epidemic that plagues all English-speaking countries. William's doctor gave him the cholesterol-lowering drug because his LDL was "a little high." He had a heart attack followed by quadruple artery bypass surgery after taking a cholesterol-lowering statin drug for five years. The program his doctor prescribed did not stop the progression of heart disease. Actually, his heart disease escalated because the low-fat, high-carbohydrate diet his doctor recommended is the real cause of coronary artery disease. The cholesterol-lowering drug did not prevent his heart disease.

William had two strokes after the bypass surgery, suffered horribly, and died several months later. He was diagnosed with diabetes while in the hospital recovering from his heart attack, and this diagnosis totally surprised his family. His doctor had never tested him for blood glucose irregularities and never measured his insulin level. If his doctor had understood the disastrous effects of his diet, William would be alive today. Sixty-five percent of diabetics die from heart disease because insulin causes heart disease, not cholesterol or saturated fats.

William's wife hasn't fared too well on her low-fat diet either. She has also been diagnosed with diabetes that has progressed to the point where oral drugs are not sufficient. She will soon be taking insulin shots. She has also had two cancer surgeries, had her gallbladder and appendix removed, and suffers from inflammatory bowel disease and degenerative spine disease.

Carbohydrates Cause Diabetes, Heart Disease, and Cancer

I describe diabetes, heart disease, and cancer as *Carbohydrate Addicts' Syndrome*. Carbohydrates cause heart disease by raising the blood level of triglycerides, raising LDL cholesterol, and lowering the level of HDL cholesterol. All of these measurements increase CAD risk factors. These are the results you will get on the low-fat, high-carbohydrate diet as proposed by the *USDA Food Guide Pyramid* and *2010 USDA My Plate*.

> "High triglyceride levels, in conjunction with high LDL and low HDL, significantly increase the risk for developing cardiovascular disease. Controlled carbohydrate nutrition effectively lowers triglycerides while raising HDL cholesterol. Lowering the LDL to HDL ratio in conjunction with lowering triglycerides will significantly reduce the risk of coronary heart disease." Dr. Robert C. Atkins.

The following study shows that carbohydrates should not replace saturated fats as occurs on the low-fat diet. Contrary to the advice of the *2010 USDA My Plate*, replacing saturated animal fats in the diet with whole grains, legumes, fruits, and starchy vegetables actually increases coronary heart disease risk factors, Syndrome X, diabetes, and cancer.

> **High-Carbohydrate Diets, Triglyceride-Rich Lipoproteins, and Coronary Heart Disease Risk**
> Abbasi F, McLaughlin T, Lamendola C, Kim HS, Tanaka A, Wang T, Nakajima K, Reaven GM.
> American Journal of Cardiology 2000 Jan 1;85(1):45-8
> http://www.ncbi.nlm.nih.gov/pubmed/11078235?dopt=Abstract
>
> Stanford University School of Medicine, California, USA
>
> "In this study we compared the effects of variations in dietary fat and carbohydrate (CHO) content on concentrations of

triglyceride-rich lipoproteins in 8, healthy, nondiabetic volunteers. The diets contained, as a percentage of total calories, either 60% CHO, 25% fat, and 15% protein, or 40% CHO, 45% fat, and 15% protein. They were consumed in random order for 2 weeks, with a 2-week washout period in between. Measurements were obtained at the end of each dietary period of plasma triglyceride, cholesterol, low-density lipoprotein (LDL) cholesterol, high-density lipoprotein (HDL) cholesterol, remnant lipoprotein (RLP) cholesterol, and RLP triglyceride concentrations, both after an overnight fast and throughout an 8-hour period (8 A.M. to 4 P.M.) in response to breakfast and lunch. The 60% CHO diet resulted in higher (mean +/- SEM) fasting plasma triglycerides (206 +/- 50 vs 113 +/- 19 mg/dl, p = 0.03), RLP cholesterol (15 +/- 6 vs 6 +/- 1 mg/dl, p = 0.005), RLP triglyceride (56 +/- 25 vs 16 +/- 3 mg/dl, p = 0.003), and lower HDL cholesterol (39 +/- 3 vs 44 +/- 3 mg/dl, p = 0.003) concentrations, without any change in LDL cholesterol concentration. Furthermore, the changes in plasma triglyceride, RLP cholesterol, and RLP triglyceride persisted throughout the day in response to breakfast and lunch. These results indicate that the effects of lowfat diets on lipoprotein metabolism are not limited to higher fasting plasma triglyceride and lower HDL cholesterol concentrations, but also include a persistent elevation in RLPs. Given the atherogenic potential of these changes in lipoprotein metabolism, it seems appropriate to question the wisdom of recommending that all Americans should replace dietary saturated fat with CHO."

My conclusion: This study proves that saturated fat in the diet should not be replaced with carbohydrates. Coronary heart disease risk factors are increased with an increase consumption of carbohydrates and a reduction in saturated fat in the diet."

Scientific Causes of Cardiovascular Diseases

The following study shows that a carbohydrate-restricted, high-fat diet achieves more favorable changes in cardiovascular disease risk factors than the low-fat diet.

The science is clear.
Heart disease risk increases when
saturated fats are replaced with carbohydrates.

In other words, cardiovascular disease risk factors move in the wrong direction when dietary fat is avoided. The low-carbohydrate, high-fat diet group had greater reductions in diastolic blood pressure, triglyceride levels, and very-low-density lipoprotein (VLDL) cholesterol levels, along with lesser reductions in low-density lipoprotein (LDL) cholesterol levels. The beneficial high-density lipoprotein (HDL) cholesterol levels increased a whopping 23% in the high-fat diet group after two years.

Weight and Metabolic Outcomes After 2 Years on a Low-Carbohydrate Versus Low-Fat Diet
Annals of Internal Medicine, August 3, 2010
http://www.annals.org/content/153/3/147.abstract?aimhp

A Randomized Trial

"Background: Previous studies comparing low-carbohydrate and low-fat diets have not included a comprehensive behavioral treatment, resulting in suboptimal weight loss.

Objective: To evaluate the effects of 2-year treatment with a low-carbohydrate or low-fat diet, each of which was combined with a comprehensive lifestyle modification program.

Design: Randomized parallel-group trial. (ClinicalTrials.gov registration number: NCT00143936)

153

Setting: 3 academic medical centers.

Patients: 307 participants with a mean age of 45.5 years (SD, 9.7 years) and mean body mass index of 36.1 kg/m^2 (SD, 3.5 kg/m^2).

Intervention: A low-carbohydrate diet, which consisted of limited carbohydrate intake (20 g/d for 3 months) in the form of low–glycemic index vegetables with unrestricted consumption of fat and protein. After 3 months, participants in the low-carbohydrate diet group increased their carbohydrate intake (5 g/d per wk) until a stable and desired weight was achieved. A low-fat diet consisted of limited energy intake (1200 to 1800 kcal/d; ≤30% calories from fat). Both diets were combined with comprehensive behavioral treatment.

Measurements: Weight at 2 years was the primary outcome. Secondary measures included weight at 3, 6, and 12 months and serum lipid concentrations, blood pressure, urinary ketones, symptoms, bone mineral density, and body composition throughout the study.

Results: Weight loss was approximately 11 kg (11%) at 1 year and 7 kg (7%) at 2 years. There were no differences in weight, body composition, or bone mineral density between the groups at any time point. During the first 6 months, the low-carbohydrate diet group had greater reductions in diastolic blood pressure, triglyceride levels, and very-low-density lipoprotein cholesterol levels, lesser reductions in low-density lipoprotein cholesterol levels, and more adverse symptoms than did the low-fat diet group. The low-carbohydrate diet group had greater increases in high-density lipoprotein cholesterol levels at all time points, approximating a 23% increase at 2 years.

Limitation: Intensive behavioral treatment was provided, patients with dyslipidemia and diabetes were excluded, and attrition at 2 years was high.

Conclusion: Successful weight loss can be achieved with either a low-fat or low-carbohydrate diet when coupled with behavioral treatment. A low-carbohydrate diet is associated with favorable changes in cardiovascular disease risk factors at 2 years."

Primary Funding Source: National Institutes of Health."

Cancer cells are gluttons for glucose. A high insulin level raises the risk for cancer as revealed in the higher cancer rate in those who are diabetic, obese, or have insulin resistance. Cancer cells don't become insulin resistant, so insulin acts as a supercharger, stuffing the cancer cells with glucose. The result of force feeding glucose to the cancer cells is an increased growth rate.

During digestion, carbohydrates are broken down into the basic glucose molecules that enter the bloodstream and cause the body to automatically increase the insulin level. Cancer cells utilize the glucose at a rate higher than normal cells to propagate, grow, and increase in temperature. Thermal imaging is a technique used to find these higher temperature cancer cells among the normal cells that are lower in temperature.

Carbohydrates also increase the risk for candida yeast and fungal infections, particularly in the colon, where these infections flare out of control. Inflammatory bowel diseases and a higher risk for colon cancer occur when the immune system is ineffective in controlling the infestation overload.

Tests have shown that carbohydrate foods have high quantities of acrylamide (a chemical classified as a human carcinogen) at levels hundreds of times higher than the maximum carcinogen exposure limit listed by the U.S. Environmental Protection Agency. Stockholm University researchers, in collaboration with experts at Sweden's National Food Administration, panicked when research revealed that carbohydrate foods contain acrylamide. The U.S. Food and Drug Administration simply ignored the study and expected that food manufacturers would somehow dismiss the claim. This is another cancer cover-up. A study of primitive cultures shows that those who ate a higher level of carbohydrates increased the cancer rate, and cancer has recently become the number one cause of death in the United States.

Contrary to the false propaganda that states otherwise, animal fats actually prevent cancer. Saturated fats and a high-fat diet of fresh or fresh frozen meats have no effect on cancer risks as is falsely claimed. Natural saturated fatty acids from animals provide healthy cell membranes and protect against cancer. Cell membranes are made from diacylglycerol phospholipids (two fatty molecules connected by a glycerol molecule) in two layers with embedded protein molecules. Saturated fats produce strong cell membranes that resist intrusion by heavy metals and free radicals into the center of the cell where the DNA can be damaged and result in the cell becoming cancerous. Yes, saturated animal fats prevent cancer.

Yes, saturated animal fats prevent cancer.

Studies that suggest saturated animal fats are a cancer risk are always distorted because they include saturated hydrogenated vegetable oils (trans fatty acids) or processed meats. Researchers combine trans fatty acids with animal fats in the studies in order to condemn animal fats. Studies have become so fraudulent that they can't be trusted. The harsh criticisms of red meat and saturated fats are not supported by scientific research or anthropological surveys.

The Diet That Fights Cancer
NewsMaxHealth
Thursday, October 21, 2010 10:20 AM
http://www.newsmaxhealth.com/dr_blaylock/diet_fights_canc er/2010/10/21/357532.html

"A ketogenic diet — one that is high in fat and low in carbs — can slow the growth of cancer. One case reported in the journal Nutrition & Metabolism involved a 65-year-old woman who had one of the most malignant primary brain tumors known to medicine (glioblastoma multiforme). The survival rate for this terrible tumor has not changed since I was a resident in neurosurgery 30 years ago.

The tumor wasn't completely removed, which invariably leads to a recurrence within months. The patient placed herself on a standard, low-calorie, high-fat, 4-to-1 ketogenic diet before standard radiation/chemotherapy was begun.

Within two-and-a-half months, her MRI scan and a more accurate PET scan demonstrated no evidence of any tumor or brain edema. Remember, she had an incomplete removal of the tumor, meaning that the combined diet and traditional treatment completely eliminated it.

When she decided to no longer follow her strict caloric restriction (her daily intake was 600 calories), the tumor recurred.

While this was the first report of the elimination of a highly malignant brain tumor in an adult due to ketogenic diet, several reports described similar success in children with malignant brain tumors.

Evidence suggests that ketogenic diets also have a dramatic effect on the growth of other cancers. By limiting proteins and carbohydrates, the cancer cells are actually starved of glucose, the main fuel they use to grow.

Patients with high blood glucose levels experience rapid growth and invasion of their tumors. High glucose levels also increase angiogenesis — the growth of new blood vessels from existing vessels — which is essential for tumor growth and invasion.

Ironically, many cancer clinics tell their patients to eat lots of sweets to prevent weight loss during therapy. Instead, cancer patients should be eating a low-calorie, high-fat ketogenic diet."

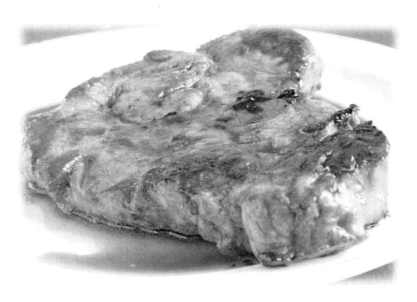

Grilled High-Fat Pork Shoulder Steak

President Bill Clinton Has Become the False Poster Boy of Heart Disease

People who have already had heart artery bypass surgery are at an increased risk on the low-fat diet because it promotes the deadly combination of high glucose and high insulin, yet the American Heart Association® recommends that these patients be placed on a low-fat, high-carbohydrate diet. Many of them are devastated when they find the bypass arteries can become plugged in as little as one or two years. President Bill Clinton is a good example.

Bill Clinton was elected Governor of Arkansas in 1979 at age 33 and went on to become the third youngest president of the United States in 1993 at age 46. From the time he was 33 years old, he enjoyed fully-paid government health care at prestigious medical centers, private professional nutritionists, and free food. Prince Charles of the United Kingdom was never pampered as much as President Clinton. It comes as no surprise that President Clinton developed heart disease at a very early age after being surrounded by government health and nutrition experts most of his adult life.

President Clinton and others have made the excuse that their heart disease was caused by the fast food they ate. They draw a double arch with one finger as they state, "This caused President Clinton's heart disease." Such a lame excuse is ridiculous. He hasn't eaten in a fast food restaurant since he was a teenager. As the president, he was constantly followed by the nagging press corps, unable to sneeze without dozens of camera flashes blinding everyone and his spokesmen shouting, "You'd better not print that!" The rare pictures that show him entering or leaving a fast food restaurant were taken when he ordered only coffee, not regularly gorging himself on "greasy burgers" that are blamed for his heart disease. Any picture of President Clinton at a fast food restaurant has become a valuable collector's item, and I have been unable to find any picture of him eating a fatty burger or steak.

President Bill Clinton obviously had some very bad cholesterol test results during his first term because he became a health nut. Good reports would not have been kept secret from the press and public. His medical examination must have been stamped *TOP SECRET*. He was obviously overweight, and the appearance of his face easily proved he was pushing high glucose and insulin. He could not hide that from the public or the press. He just looked all puffed up, but maybe that was his body's reaction to being the "leader of the world" and not from the diet. Well, it must have been both.

Jogging did not prevent President Clinton from developing heart disease.

For eight years, we saw President Clinton jogging with the Secret Service agents who were forced to plod along behind him. We are told that exercise prevents heart disease. "Run, run, run!" was the cry, but his face and body screamed warnings about his high blood insulin levels as a result of his high-carbohydrate diet. His blood pressure must have been high as well. But he forced himself to plod along, sweating, smiling, and waving at the dozens of cameras as if he were the first health genius to live in the White House. His world-class medical care professionals most likely didn't bother to measure his blood insulin level because they don't see insulin as the health hazard.

He proved beyond any doubt that exercise does not prevent heart disease, and it didn't make him thin either. He was fat and remained fat throughout the eight years that he jogging around Washington, DC. The nightly news on the major media never failed to show a quick clip of him jogging, surrounded by specially selected Secret Service agents who could also keep up the pace and run faster if needed for security reasons. Washington is humid year round and everyone was drenched in sweat. This was his doctor's advice for keeping him healthy, but it failed.

Disaster struck President Bill Clinton like a stealth Air Force jet fighter. He developed coronary artery plaque in several arteries at the same time, and the best doctors in the world didn't have the slightest clue. He didn't have just one small plaque that ruptured unexpectedly. His heart was plugged from one side to the other! On September 6, 2004, three years after leaving office on January 20, 2001, he was rushed to Columbia University Presbyterian Hospital, where doctors performed a quadruple artery bypass in order to save his life. Bypasses are veins taken from the legs and grafted into the arterial system to provide blood to the heart artery on the downside of the restriction. They are used as arteries, but they can be problematic because veins are naturally weaker than arteries.

What happened to the theory that exercise prevents heart disease? Now they say it was the fatty fast-food burger he ate at one time in the past. The fact is, the White House had a professional dietitian and a carefully chosen kitchen staff who prepared food fit for a king—King of the *USDA Food Guide Pyramid.* Remember, President Clinton was the boss of the U.S. Department of Agriculture, U.S. Food and Drug Administration, and the U.S. National Institutes of Health. His annual signature on the United States' budget provided billions of dollars for the operation of these government agencies involved in "keeping

Americans healthy" and funding university grants for health research. These hundreds of thousands of government employees and university researchers could not prevent President Clinton from plugging his heart. In fact, they caused it.

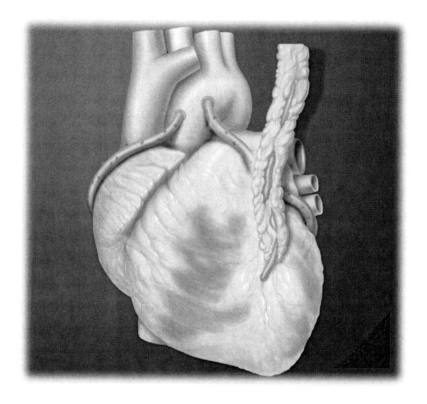

Heart with Three Bypass Artery Grafts

He was now in a panic. During his two presidential terms, he followed the low-fat, high-carbohydrate diet promoted by the government health departments that he supervised. They recommended that meat be limited to one small three-ounce piece per day no larger than the palm of the hand with all the visible fat removed. Well, that didn't work. He plugged all four of his main heart arteries while eating that way.

Scientific Causes of Cardiovascular Diseases

We can be sure that the White House professional nutritionist had forbidden him to eat a big, fat, delicious rib-eye steak with all of the fat left on. His guardians believed beef fat meant instant death, while they stuffed him with 60–80% carbohydrates according to the *USDA Food Guide Pyramid.* Yes, President Bill Clinton was the master of the U.S. Department of Agriculture and dictator of the pyramid. He could have ordered the *USDA Food Guide Pyramid* to be corrected, but he wrongly thought it was the gospel.

The medical and health experts were wrong again. President Clinton's doctors gave him the regimen that causes heart disease, but they still think heart disease is caused by eating saturated animal fats. How did that piece of saturated animal fat sneak past the Secret Service and get into the White House?

President Clinton had the best health care in the world and it was free. So why did he suddenly develop quadruple heart artery blockages that required bypass surgery? The answer is simple. His doctors didn't know that insulin causes heart disease. They blamed it on saturated fat. President Clinton is just one of millions of people worldwide who suffer from heart disease because of the incorrect recommendations of the American Medical Association®, American Heart Association®, U.S. National Institutes of Health, U.S. Food and Drug Administration, and the U.S. Department of Agriculture. He was brainwashed, and it nearly cost him his life as it does millions of people every year.

After his close brush with death, President Bill Clinton became more determined than ever to avoid the hidden piece of saturated animal fat that must have given him heart disease. His doctors insisted he be more careful in adhering to the American Heart Association's® low-fat diet. President Clinton knew that wasn't enough. He abandoned the United States Department of

Health dietary guidelines after his sad discovery that the low-fat diet did not prevent coronary artery disease and contacted a popular diet health guru. His new doctor promised a vegetarian diet would prevent the future buildup of arterial plaque, and it would cure his heart disease. Thirteen months after his quadruple bypass surgery, he told news reporters at CNN that he was improving his diet. The reporter wrote on August 7, 2005:

> "Clinton has made changes since his health scare. He said he has cut down on french fries, eats more fruits and vegetables and incorporates exercise into his mornings. He said he wants to teach that lesson to American children."

Why is he avoiding French fries? The calories in potatoes are carbohydrates just like the calories in fruits are carbohydrates. Oh, yes, French fries are cooked in fats. He is determined to reduce dietary fats and increase carbohydrates even more. He and his team of medical and nutrition experts were really on fire to give him perfect health. He will not be allowed to even look at a piece of fat or red meat let alone chew it. He and his daughter, Chelsea, became vegetarians, and he became very fond of the Asian Indian vegetarian cuisine. His new diet was devoid of all meat and animal fats. His brainwashing continued.

President Bill Clinton has abandoned the *USDA Food Guide Pyramid* he once promoted.

People worldwide have been brainwashed to believe that vegetarians don't get heart disease. This is a lie. Actually, vegans are more likely to get heart disease than non-vegetarians according to a recent study in India. Notice that the researchers in the following study were surprised at the results, indicating they too had been brainwashed.

Vegetarian Indians more likely to suffer heart disease
The Med Guru, September 26, 2010
http://www.themedguru.com/20100926/newsfeature/vegetari
an-indians-more-likely-suffer-heart-disease-study-
86140640.html

"On the occasion of World Heart Day (September 26) there's a bad news for vegetarians Indians. As per a new research report presented by a Pune-based bariatric Dr. Shashank Shah, vegetarian Indians are more prone to suffer from heart ailments.

To come to this startling conclusion Dr Shah along with his colleague Dr Todkar, studied the data collected from about 300 patients from Hiranandani Hospital, Powai, over the period of one year.

They were startled to find out that 70 percent of these patients had suffered from a cardiac disease or are at greater risk of cardiac attack in near future.

Nearly all of them were found to be suffering from vitamin B12 deficiency.

'When vitamin B12 levels fall, homocysteine levels increase. The latter is known to cause atherosclerosis (hardening and narrowing of the arteries), as well as an increased risk of heart attacks, strokes and blood clot formation,' noted Dr Shah in his study report."

People throughout the world have been brainwashed to believe that vegetarianism is a healthy way of eating. Actually, vegetarianism is a religion in India, where they worship cattle and other animals. Their religion teaches that dead ancestors are reincarnated as one of the animals. A quick review of vegetarian authors reveals many of them to be of Indian ancestry. A closer investigation confirms their backgrounds and education to be

Indian. If they want to sacrifice their bodies to save a cow, fine, but they should not encourage other people to eat a diet that has been shown to cause the shortest life span on Earth.

President Bill Clinton, at only 63 years of age, was rushed into the hospital cardiac care unit on February 11, 2010, with another heart attack. The bypass arteries were plugging with plaque, and doctors inserted two stents to open the restrictions and save his life once again.

I guess the vegan Indian food didn't prevent the continuing buildup of arterial plaque. What is a multi-millionaire to do? Certainly money was no object, and besides, President Clinton has had all of his medical procedures and health consultations provided totally free of charge. He is covered 100% by the generous U.S. Department of the Treasury—no co-pay and no minimums. It's 100% gratis!

How did his new Indian vegetarian diet work for him? Well, it also plugged two of the bypass arteries. He was rushed into surgery to have two new plaque deposits reopened with stents. It looks like President Bill Clinton hit the Rieske Instant Atherosclerosis Cycle (IAC) not once but twice.

President Clinton's White House lifestyle most likely caused his heart disease or made it worse. Certainly, the initial cause could have been a bacterial or viral infection but nobody knows. The multiple artery blockages in both episodes are the typical results of his high-carbohydrate diet that is the actual cause of heart disease.

He must have thought that little piece of meat plugged his arteries as many vegetarians claim. Neither he nor his health advisors understands that cutting out the meat and natural animal fats results in a huge boost in carbohydrate intake that results in higher levels of glucose and insulin, the very cause of his heart disease. The science relating to heart disease is not difficult to understand for those who are not brainwashed.

President Clinton did not abandon his vegetarian diet or the diet guru who was counseling him. Instead, he summoned a second vegetarian diet guru to assist the first. Having a team of doctors is no problem when the United States Government is picking up the tab. This time the two doctors put him on a very low-calorie, low-fat, vegetarian diet—starvation.

At Chelsea's wedding, the press went crazy when they saw President Clinton. Some papers suggested that he had cancer because he was pathetically thin and his skin was gray. He reassured them he did not have cancer and said that his weight loss was achieved by his new diet. Yes, vegetarians and cancer victims have a lot in common—they look alike.

He has made yet another change in his diet, but is it in the right direction? Finally, he realized that the USDA Food Guide Pyramid had given him heart disease, but what was this new diet? It can best be described as starvation. Not only is it vegetarian, but the vegetable fats and vegetable carbohydrates have been slashed as well.

He presented the details of his new diet in his interviews with the major media. Vegetarians around the world were thrilled, and the video was splashed all across the Internet. Starvation is the new mantra for the prevention of heart disease. If you're skinny, you won't get heart disease, right? No! Wrong!

The doctors who are directing President Clinton's new diet parade him around as if his heart disease has been reversed. This is not the case. His new diet has proved nothing. His data are being kept secret. The few weeks of starvation have proved nothing. Does he have some artery or bypass plaque that can be used as a baseline measurement for appraising his new diet? We don't know. His doctors know, but we certainly can't trust them to present the truth. His previous heart problems were kept secret until it was impossible to hide them from the public. His failures to provide details about his health are continuing. He doesn't provide copies of any of his blood tests, but I provide several of my blood test reports in this book to prove that my diet therapy for reversing heart disease has given me awesome results.

Has President Bill Clinton proved that his new diet reverses heart disease and will prevent plaque from coming back into his coronary arteries? Absolutely not! He has not proved anything. Even so, President Clinton has become the Vegetarian Poster Boy for Reversing Heart Disease.

President Bill Clinton has become the Vegetarian Poster Boy for Reversing Heart Disease.

Actually, the starvation diet that he has embraced may keep the plaque deposits from coming back as long as he can endure the agony of being hungry 24 hours a day. His glucose is kept fairly low simply because he restricts carbohydrates. Starvation also controls the insulin, which is the primary cause of coronary artery disease. He may be diabetic, and his low glucose intake will help there as well. The big problem with President Clinton's starvation diet is that others who have heart disease are unable to starve themselves this way. This program would never be effective for the general public.

In a television interview on September 24, 2010, he was almost in tears as he described his fear of having stents placed in the weaker veins used as artery bypasses. He was told that the expansion of the stents upon installation could have caused the weaker veins to rupture.

What Is President Clinton's New Vegetarian Diet?

President Clinton and his two doctors described his new diet program as restricting the following:

- Anything with a mother
- Anything with a face
- Dairy products
- Refined grains
- Chicken
- Meat
- Nuts
- Fish

Note: President Clinton did say he ate "a little fish" but not often. This violates his doctors' recommendations because a fish has a mother and a face. Now he has another excuse if the starvation diet doesn't prevent further heart problems. He can blame it on the fishes.

President Clinton's new diet consists of the following:

- Plant based foods only
- Legumes (beans)
- Whole grains
- Vegetables
- Flax seed
- Fruit
- Protein powder
- Almond milk

Note:

"Plant-based foods only" indicates that this is a vegetarian diet, but he and his doctors avoid using this most descriptive word in the interview.

We must assume the protein powder is soy protein in accordance with the above restrictions because egg protein and whey protein powders are from animal sources.

Perhaps almond milk is one of the many commercial products with that same name. It is probably not 100% almond milk and may contain various sugars and gum thickeners. He mixes the almond milk, protein powder, and fruit to make a shake.

President Clinton and his doctors identified the following supplemental vitamins and pharmaceuticals that he is taking:

- Multivitamin tablet
- Vitamin B_{12}
- Vitamin D_3
- Calcium
- Statin drugs

I must assume that he has more restrictions that have been kept secret. Allowing unlimited carbohydrates in the form of whole grains, fruits, and starchy vegetables can make you fat in a month, not skinny. He certainly has severe calorie restrictions in all of these other foods (that don't have a mother or a face). What about honey? No mention of that either! Do vegans make bees work for honey? Probably not!

Vegetarian diets are usually accompanied by yoga exercises and Transcendental Meditation (TM), but I don't believe President Clinton has mentioned these in formal interviews. They are of no scientific value either physically or mentally. They are performed as Hindu religious rituals and should not be interpreted as health related.

Yoga exercises and Transcendental Meditation have certainly not improved the health of Hindus in southern India who are known to be extremely skinny, frail, and sickly. Their society has the shortest lifespan of any on Earth, and no one from this region has ever won a gold medal in a World Olympic competition.

Don't Attempt President Clinton's New Vegan Diet

Run when you hear or read something that tells you not to eat anything that "has a mother or a face." You are about to join a religion in which animals are worshipped and the individual is asked to sacrifice his body to the creatures. History shows that all major vegetarian groups were motivated by their religions.

This is a science book that details my research and personal experience. I studied the science first without restricting any food. I then applied the scientific results to outline a regimen of diet therapy, nutritional supplements, and pharmaceuticals that have reversed my heart disease. The result has been exactly as predicted by the scientific facts. It works because it's true. President Clinton's starvation diet has yet to be proved.

A starvation diet may prevent the accumulation of arterial plaque but at what cost?

So, is President Bill Clinton's health finally on the mend? Not so fast! A scientific analysis of his new diet shows the potential for many health problems other than heart disease. He now faces the same threats that other vegetarians have faced. I will address the health problems that those on a calorie-deficient, protein-deficient, vegetarian diet can expect.

- Cancer is a risk for all organs of the body, particularly the colon, liver, lungs, prostate, and brain.

- Ischemic stroke caused by a moving clot is now at an elevated risk.

- Aneurysm and hemorrhagic stroke caused by weakening and bursting of the blood vessels in the brain are a risk.

171

- Aneurysm or ruptured aorta may occur as a result of thinning of the wall of the aorta.

- Thinning of all protein structures in the body is common.

- Heart valve leakage or regurgitation as a result of thinning of the delicate cusps of the valves from lack of protein can occur.

- Inflammatory bowel diseases, such as leaky bowel syndrome, systemic candida yeasts, colon fungal infection, and pathogenic bacterial infection of the colon are promoted.

- Degenerative disc disease is a real threat, as a high percentage of members of the Seventh-day Adventist Church on a similar vegetarian diet have experienced. The body starts to eat the spinal discs in its search for protein. I don't know why the body prefers cervical discs for lunch, but I do know a woman whose husband was forced into disability retirement at age 45. A friend and bodybuilder became vegan only to have his spinal discs begin to disappear.

- Hip or bone fractures become a higher risk as the body consumes the protein bone collagen matrix structure that gives the bone tensile strength.

- There is a higher risk for irregular heart rhythm and atrial and ventricular fibrillation. These heart ailments cause blood to pool and clot and lead to the ischemic stroke described above.

- Sudden cardiac arrest is a risk. The heart simply stops beating from lack of proper nutrition that will lead to a severely catabolic state. Sudden cardiac arrest is a common cause of death in people on a starvation diet.

I received an email from an ex-vegetarian who described how her spine degenerated as a result of the vegetarian diet she ate in her younger years. She also ate very little meat during the 10 years that followed and experimented with the raw vegan diet as well. She is a perfect example of someone who suffers from a protein deficiency. The following is her description of her current condition:

> *"Hi,*
>
> *I went a few years when I was younger without meat. Then, when I went back to it, I only ate it occasionally. I've played with different ways of eating in the past 10 years, even doing raw for weeks at a time.*
>
> *I have had pain for months down my left leg. It radiates from my left buttock down through the side of (but toward the back of) my left leg, running down through the calf.*
>
> *My x-ray report shows the following:*
>
> *Lateral lumbar view, loss of disc height at L5 S1, osteohyte formation anterior vertebral body L5 and accompanied by IVD thinning and L3 anterior vertebral body. Lateral cervical view; reversal of cervical curve. Disc space thinning at the levels of C5-C6 and C6-C7. Osteophyte formation at C5-C6 and C6-C7."*

The vegan starvation diet results in a catabolic state in which the body robs protein from all the muscles including heart muscles. Arms and legs are usually very thin, and problems develop with joints, ligaments, tendons, bones, and cervical discs. President Clinton's body has begun to devour itself because of his starvation diet and drastic weight loss. He has lost more than body fat. He has also lost muscle, tendons, and ligaments throughout his body as well as protein collagen from his bones. Elderly women are at a higher risk for hip fractures because they tend to shun meat, not because they lack calcium in the diet. The body eats away the collagen matrix in the bones that gives them tensile strength. The vegan starvation diet can result in a plunge in bone density and a hip fracture. President Clinton's new catabolic diet is directly opposite to the anabolic diet used by professional bodybuilders to build strong, healthy bodies.

Professional bodybuilders build strong muscles and strong bones by eating meat.

Our present medical system has many physicians who will only treat a patient for a condition that falls within his specialty. This may have unintended consequences by placing the patient at risk for other health problems. Preventing another plaque deposit at the expense of developing a stroke or cancer is certainly not desirable. The goals of my diet regimen are maximum physiological nutrition, a superior immune system, and the prevention of all diseases. President Bill Clinton has not reversed heart disease in any way. I have reversed my heart disease as confirmed by one of the best cardiologists in the nation.

My doctor measured the two small plaque deposits in my coronary artery on two separate occasions and found them to be reduced 50% in only 25 months. This proves that my scientifically developed regimen as detailed in this book has reversed my heart disease while I ate two eggs for breakfast every day, two double-stack burgers with cheese (minus the bun) for a midmorning snack, a big pork chop with all the fat for lunch, and a 20-ounce slab of prime rib (including the fat) for dinner—add to this steamed veggies with lots of real butter. Starvation is not required to reverse heart disease. My diet of 70% fat on a calorie basis of which 30% is saturated fat has reversed my heart disease. I am confident that saturated fat does not cause heart disease. Don't believe the brainwashing delivered to the public by prestigious medical schools, medical clinics, and National Institutes of Health of the U.S. Department of Health and Human Services. I reversed my heart disease while gorging myself on saturated animal fats.

Reversing heart disease must be confirmed by a 50% reduction of plaque within 25 months.

I developed the regimen in this book by scientific research and used it to reverse my heart disease. It is based on a diet that sharply restricts fruit, fruit juices, all other forms of sugar, whole grains, starchy vegetables, carbohydrates, soy protein, milk, cereals, breads, pasta, fiber, and all products labeled "low-fat" or "low-cholesterol." In addition to reversing heart disease, I believe this regimen will prevent Type 2 diabetes 100% of the time; stop the progression of Type 2 diabetes; ease the symptoms of Type 1 diabetes by controlling blood sugar naturally; reduce the incidence of fatty liver disease; reduce the incidence of strokes; reduce cancer risks; build strong bones; heal muscles, tendons, and ligaments; and may reduce the prevalence of Alzheimer's disease. This regimen, along with a few other restrictions, allows autoimmune diseases to enter remission as detailed in *Absolute Truth Exposed – Volume 1*.

You may read books, articles, or studies in which a person loses 15% of his body weight and his arterial plaque deposit shrinks by 15%. Is that reversing heart disease? Absolutely not! His legs lost 15% of their weight as well. Shall we call that "reversing leg disease or shrinking leg disease?" The arterial plaque simply went on a diet also. A 15% reduction in the thickness of the walls of the arteries increases the risk for rupture. Shrinkage of the arterial membrane over the plaque deposit increases the risk that the deposit will rupture and allow a blood clot to form that could lead to a heart attack. Starvation diets greatly increase the risk for brain aneurisms, hemorrhagic strokes, heart attacks, and cancer.

Review the following checklist before you accept claims that people have reversed heart disease:

- Check the scientific basis and supporting scientific facts based on nutrition and human physiology—not conjecture or emotional appeal.

- Check the actual blood test reports for lipids, cholesterol, insulin, and other factors. Check the results for liver and kidney function tests.

- Check the patient's weight loss versus the reduction in the size of arterial plaque deposits. A 15% weight loss and 15% shrinkage of a plaque deposit do not qualify as reversing heart disease. The plaque simply went on a diet.

- Check to see if the patient's arterial plaque deposit was reduced 50% in only 25 months as mine was when I reversed my heart disease.

The general public is unable to reverse heart disease because they follow the recommendations of the prestigious medical schools, medical clinics, and National Institutes of Health. These organizations are fighting science.

Glucose Causes Cardiovascular Disease

Animal research with insulin proved many years ago that the artery will plug with plaque just downstream from the point of insulin injection. Insulin causes glucose to be chemically combined with cell membranes, LDL lipoprotein, blood hemoglobin, protein, and other cells in an unhealthy process called *glycation*, which is similar to the caramelization process used to make candy. Atheromatous plaque is composed primarily of macrophage cells, cholesterol, glycated LDL cholesterol, glycated proteins, glycated hemoglobin A1c, calcium, oxidized polyunsaturated omega-6 triglycerides, and fibrous tissue. Oxidized unsaturated fats are said to be rancid. High levels of blood glucose (hyperglycemia) caused by glucose intolerance in the presence of high levels of blood insulin (hyperinsulinemia) make polysaccharide sugar chains attach to serum proteins, artery proteins, serum hemoglobin, and LDL molecules in the glycation process.

Glycation turns your arteries into caramel candy.

The glycated molecules and rancid omega-6 fatty acids form a fatty deposit of atheromatous plaque between the endothelial lining of the interior surface of blood vessels and the smooth muscle layer. White blood cells known as *immune system macrophages* ingest the glycated and rancid molecules and swell to form foam cells that narrow the artery and restrict blood flow. These conditions are brought about by a diet high in carbohydrates, and the process occurs rather suddenly in people who are hyperglycemic, hypoglycemic, or diabetic. Clear arteries can become plugged and lead to a heart attack in as little as one year—the Rieske Instant Atherosclerosis Cycle (IAC).

In other words, dietary carbohydrates cause cell membranes, LDL lipoprotein, hemoglobin, and protein cells to become coated with sugar and prevent them from performing their proper function. Carbohydrates can and will kill you over time. Glycation damages cells throughout the body and disrupts the proper function of major organs and systems.

- Blood vessel walls become stiff and weak.
- Retina, lens, and collagen cells in the eye are damaged.
- DNA damage accumulates over time.
- Beta cells in the pancreas are damaged.
- Nerve cells are damaged.
- Cholesterol molecules are damaged.
- Fibrinogen growth in the blood leads to clots.
- Tendons and ligaments become damaged.

Glycation has also been shown to be involved in carpal tunnel syndrome. In these cases, the tendons and ligaments in the wrist become cross linked with glycated molecules to adjoining tissue, producing rigidity and pain.

Eating carbohydrates can make you go blind.

Glycation is a scientifically proven condition that can be easily measured in the laboratory. One test for diabetes is to measure the concentration of glycosylated (or glycated) hemoglobin A1c, a measure of blood hemoglobin that has been attached to glucose molecules and is accelerated in the presence of high insulin levels. Since the life span of red blood cells is about 120 days, this test indicates the long-term levels of blood glucose and insulin. Glycated hemoglobin is one of the major causes of the coronary artery disease that kills 65% of diabetics. Following a heart attack, people are frequently surprised when the doctor tells them they are in a middle stage of diabetes.

Hyperglycemia, Lipoprotein Glycation, and Vascular Disease – Angiology

July/August 2005 vol. 56 no. 4 431-438
http://ang.sagepub.com/content/56/4/431.abstract?rss=1

Arvindan Veiraiah, MRCP
Llandough Hospital, Penarth, Wales, UK

"Hyperlipidemia and its treatment are currently recognized as important modulators of cardiovascular mortality in the presence of disordered glucose control. On the other hand, the effects of hyperglycemia and its treatment on hyperlipidemia are not widely appreciated. Hyperglycemia is commonly associated with an increase in intestinal lipoproteins and a reduction in high-density lipoprotein (HDL). This could be a consequence of hyperglycemia-induced glycation of lipoproteins, which reduces the uptake and catabolism of the lipoproteins via the classical low-density lipoprotein (LDL) receptor. A high dietary carbohydrate load increases the glycation of intestinal lipoproteins, prolongs their circulation, and increases their plasma concentration. Hyperglycemia also leads to inhibition of lipoprotein lipase, further aggravating hyperlipidemia. Circulating advanced glycation end-products (AGEs) also bind lipoproteins and delay their clearance, a mechanism that has particularly been implicated in the dyslipidemia of diabetic nephropathy. As uptake via scavenger receptors is not inhibited, glycation increases the proportion of lipoproteins that are taken up via inflammatory cells and decreases the proportion taken up by hepatocytes via classical LDL receptors. This promotes the formation of atheromatous plaques and stimulates inflammation. Hyperglycemia increases the formation of oxidized LDL and glycated LDL, which are important modulators of atherosclerosis and cardiovascular death. The risk of cardiovascular death is increased by even short-term derangement of blood sugar control, owing perhaps to the glycation of lipoproteins and other critical proteins. Glycated

LDL could prove very useful in measuring the effect of hyperglycemia on cardiovascular disease, its risk factors, and its complications. Comparing different glucose-lowering and lipid-lowering drugs in respect to their influence on glycated LDL could increase knowledge of the mechanism by which they alter cardiovascular risk."

The endothelial cells become inflamed because the rancid polyunsaturated omega-6 fatty acids, glycated LDL, glycated hemoglobin, and glycated protein in the atheromatous plaque are prompting an attack by the immune system. Inflammation is a normal body response and does not cause heart disease, but it can cause the endothelial lining to rupture and release some of the plaque into the bloodstream. The body responds by releasing fibrinogen, a blood-clotting factor, to form a clot at the site. This is a normal body healing response. The clot, which forms more readily in the presence of hyperinsulinemia, blocks the blood flow in the artery and results in a sudden heart attack. The blood clot can also break loose to flow downstream in the artery until the natural narrowing of the artery causes a blockage and sudden heart attack. The buildup of atheromatous plaque need not be extensive for this type of heart attack to occur. The point of rupture can be at a location where the plaque buildup is not large enough to cause symptoms, and in these cases, the sudden heart attack can occur without any prior warning. You can get an awesome health checkup by your cardiologist and have a heart attack on the way home. It happens all the time.

Heart disease is rampant because prestigious medical clinics, medical schools, health associations, and government authorities are fighting science.

Glucose Causes Type 2 Diabetes Mellitus

My scientific research proves that excess glucose consumption causes Type 2 diabetes mellitus, yet one of the most prominent medical clinics in the world gives the following advice to diabetic patients.

> "Contrary to popular perception, there's no diabetes diet. You won't be restricted to a lifetime of boring, bland foods. Instead, you'll need plenty of:
>
> - Fruits
> - Vegetables
> - Whole grains
>
> These foods are high in nutrition and low in fat and calories. You'll also need to eat fewer animal products and sweets."

Warning!

Did you notice the prestigious medical clinic says that there's no diabetes diet yet recommends a diet that is 85% sugars and shuns animal products? This is shocking because diabetes is a disease of insufficient sugar metabolism. Do not follow the above advice because it recommends too many carbohydrates, which are the scientific cause of Type 2 diabetes, heart disease, fatty liver disease, and cancer. Why they shun animal products is an absolute mystery to me since most animal products other than milk have no carbohydrates, and diabetes is the inability to properly metabolize carbohydrates.

Type 2 diabetes mellitus is epidemic in the general public because the prestigious medical schools, medical clinics, and National Institutes of Health are fighting science.

Chapter 3

Glucose Causes Alzheimer's Disease

Evidence is mounting that glycation is involved in Alzheimer's disease. The high-carbohydrate diet raises glucose and insulin levels, causing glucose molecules to bond to cerebrospinal fluid (CSF) proteins in the brain. Glycation produces an intermediate to the advanced glycation end products (AGE) that is called an *Amadori product*. The following study shows that this action has solid scientific evidence.

Increased Protein Glycation in Cerebrospinal Fluid of Alzheimer's Disease
Neurobiology of Aging - 2001 May-Jun;22(3):397-402
http://www.ncbi.nlm.nih.gov/pubmed/11378244

"Abstract

Accumulation of advanced glycation end products occurs in the brain with ageing and was proposed to be involved in pathogenesis of Alzheimer's disease. We studied changes in the level of an early glycation product, an Amadori product, in cerebrospinal fluid (CSF) in ageing and in late-onset Alzheimer's disease. The work was carried out on 99 consecutive patients. The concentration of Amadori product in CSF correlated with CSF glucose concentration but was not changed with age (n = 70). In contrast, level of CSF Amadori product was 1.7-fold higher in Alzheimer's disease patients (n = 29) as compared with non-demented age-matched control group (n = 20; $P < 0.0005$), although CSF glucose concentration was similar in both groups (4.1 +/- 1.3 vs. 3.8 +/- 0.6 mmol/liter, resp.). An increased accumulation of Amadori products was found in all major proteins of CSF of Alzheimer's disease including albumin, apolipoprotein E and transthyretin. We propose that the increased early glycation of CSF proteins in the Alzheimer's patients may stimulate the formation and the consequent deposition of

182

advanced glycation end products as well as oxidative stress in the brain."

President Ronald Reagan died from Alzheimer's disease because he continually ate sugary jelly beans. It is an unrecognized scientific fact that carbohydrates cause Alzheimer's disease, but the prestigious medical organizations are too busy attacking meat and saturated fats to figure it out. Friends, visitors, and foreign dignitaries continually brought him jelly beans to feed his famous addiction, and he always kept jars of them in front of him. His son has campaigned vigorously for stem cell research in the false belief that stem cells will be the future cure for Alzheimer's disease. A jar of the jelly beans was placed in the Reagan Library as a reminder of his favorite snack food. His family has failed to realize that his killer is being honored.

Carbohydrates cause Alzheimer's disease.

Glucose, either from the digestion of carbohydrates or eaten directly as sugar, leads to heart disease. Glucose in the dry granular form can be purchased in the supermarket just like common table sugar. Diabetics rely on it in a hypoglycemic emergency because it enters the bloodstream quickly without the need for digestion. Glucose is also obtained when any of the many different types of molecules of carbohydrates and starches are broken down by digestion in the small intestine.

Glucose causes coronary artery disease in two ways. First, it requires insulin in order for the body to utilize it, and second, it wreaks havoc by combining with other molecules and bonding to various cells.

Unhealthy High-Carbohydrate Foods		
Grains	Cereals	Bagels
Legumes	Fruits	Breads
Pastas	Potatoes	Yams
Sugars	Ice Creams	Candies

Whole Grains Are a Major Dietary Source of Glucose

Whole grains are by far the major source of glucose in the diet. Breakfast cereals are examples we can easily analyze because the nutritional information is posted on the sides of the boxes as shown in the following table. One popular brand has 100% whole wheat without any added sugars.

Serving size: 2 biscuits (47g)
Amount Per Serving

	2 biscuits	1 biscuit
Calories	160	80
Calories from Fat	10	5
Calories from Saturated Fat	0	0
Amount Per Serving and/or % Daily Value*		
Total Fat	1g (2%)	1%
Saturated Fat	0g (0%)	0%
Polyunsaturated Fat	0.5g	0.25g
Monounsaturated Fat	0g	0g
Trans Fat	0g	0g
Cholesterol	0mg (0%)	0%
Sodium	0mg (0%)	0%
Potassium	180mg (5%)	3%
Total Carbohydrate	37g (12%)	6%
Dietary Fiber	6g (24%)	12%
Soluble Fiber	<1g	<1g

Scientific Causes of Cardiovascular Diseases

Insoluble Fiber	5g	2.5g
Sugars	0g	0g
Sugar Alcohol		
Other Carbohydrate	31g	15.5g
Protein	5g	2.5g
Amount Per Serving and/or % Daily Value*		
Vitamin A	0%	0%
Percent of vitamin A present as beta-carotene	0%	0%
Vitamin C	0%	0%
Calcium	2%	0%
Iron	6%	4%
Vitamin B6	4%	2%
Thiamin	8%	4%
Zinc	10%	4%
Niacin	15%	8%
Folic Acid	4%	2%
Magnesium	15%	8%
Phosphorus	15%	8%
Copper	8%	4%

*Percent Daily Values are based on a 2,000 calorie diet. Your daily values may be higher or lower based on your calorie needs.

Carbohydrates:	31 g x 4 cal/g =	124 calories or 81%
Fats:	1 g x 9 cal/g =	9 calories or 6%
Protein:	5 g x 4 cal/g =	20 calories or 13%

This breakfast cereal has 81% of the calories as carbohydrates that are converted to glucose and fructose in the blood after digestion, yet the scientific minimum essential amount of carbohydrates in the diet is zero. Glucose causes diabetes, heart disease, and cancer and is the fuel for cancer cells. Glucose stimulates the growth of yeasts and fungi that have been implicated in many diseases, including several inflammatory bowel diseases and more than four dozen autoimmune diseases. The scientific proofs that dietary carbohydrates are hazardous to your health are listed in detail in *Absolute Truth Exposed – Volume 1, Chapter 1, Absolute Scientific Proof Carbohydrates are Pathogenic (Disease Causing).*

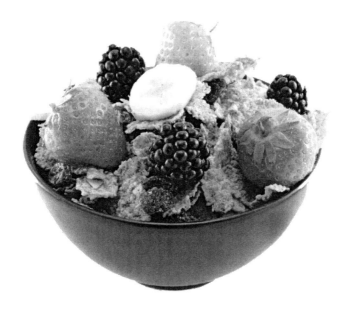

Breakfast Cereal, Fruits, and Low-Fat Milk
Become 85% Sugars After Digestion

Breakfast bran cereals have a high percentage of fiber, and other cereals have extra fiber added. The claim has been made that fiber reduces cholesterol, but that does not necessarily equate to reversing or preventing heart disease. Fiber is not the health panacea that most professional nutritionists, health authorities, and physicians would like you to believe. It does not pass through the digestive tract unchanged as falsely claimed. The body does not have the enzyme necessary to digest the complex carbohydrate molecules in fiber, but bad bacteria in the colon certainly do. For this reason, fiber is a **Forbidden Food**. Fiber causes inflammatory bowel diseases; it does not prevent them as many gastroenterologists claim. See *Absolute Truth Exposed – Volume 1, Chapter 2 – Absolute Scientific Proof Dietary Fiber is Unhealthy.*

Unhealthy High-Fiber Foods			
Bran Cereals	Oats	Rice	Soybeans
Legumes	Split Peas	Lentils	Apples
Broccoli	Potatoes	Grapefruits	Pears

Other breakfast cereals also have every type of sugar and starch (complex glucose) that could possibly be added, including:

Sucrose (table sugar)

- Modified corn starch
- Wheat starch
- Honey
- Brown sugar syrup
- Dehydrated cane juice
- Malt syrup extract
- Rice starch
- High fructose corn syrup

Added sugars can be identified because the name ends with "ose" as in glucose, fructose, sucrose, maltose, isomaltose, maltulose, turanose, kojibiose, erlose, theanderose, and panose. It has been rightfully stated that breakfast cereals contain more sugar than desserts such as cake, pie, and ice cream.

The added sugars in breakfast cereals do not change the percentage of carbohydrates on the nutrition label because whole grains such as wheat, corn, oats, and spelt have the same amount of carbohydrates per gram as the sugars in the above list. Parents of young children get very upset about added sugars in breakfast cereals when the marketing is targeted directly at the kids, but they fail to realize that a bowl of cereal without added sugars and a glass of orange juice give the child the same amount of glucose and fructose sugars as the sugar-laden cereals. A bowl of cereal with low-fat milk and a glass of orange juice become 85% sugar after digestion.

One brand of whole grain oat cereal has a big red heart on the front of the box and the red Heart-Check Mark logo of the American Heart Association® on the side, indicating that the product is considered to be *heart healthy*. Shoppers look at the labels and fill their shopping carts with cereal boxes that display the healthy Heart-Check Mark with the expectation that they will prevent or reverse heart disease because the labels say "zero cholesterol." The nutrition label shows that the second largest ingredient is sugar, third is modified corn starch, forth is honey, and fifth is brown sugar syrup. May I remind you that frosted cakes and fruit filled pies also have zero cholesterol? How about eating dessert for breakfast and calling it *heart healthy*? All of the carbohydrates in breakfast cereals turn to sugars after digestion.

The Glycemic Index Has Become the New Diet Mantra

The latest fad in dietary guidelines is called the *glycemic index*. This is a measure of the amount of glucose that appears in the blood measured over a two-hour period after eating 50 grams of a particular food in which pure glucose equals 100 on the glycemic scale. The claim is made that foods with a lower glycemic index are healthier than foods with a higher index. As discussed earlier, fructose in fruits and fruit juices enters the blood through the walls of the small intestine as fructose. It is never converted to glucose; instead, the liver converts fructose into triglycerides. The glycemic index for fruits and fruit juices is 50 because only half of the sugars are glucose. People who select foods based on the glycemic index are tricked into thinking fruits and 100% fruit juices are exceedingly healthy.

Fruit juices are 100% sugars.

Triglycerides are major contributors to coronary artery disease. The nutrition label on a bottle of 100% pure orange juice correctly shows almost zero fat (4 calories of fat per 112 calories per serving), but more than half of the calories in orange juice are converted directly into blood fats after digestion. The public has been brainwashed again by the claim that orange juice is heart healthy because it's organic, natural, practically fat-free, cholesterol-free, and has a low 50 glycemic index. Common table sugar also has a glycemic index of 50, so why is table sugar brutalized as the health scourge of the century while orange juice is promoted as the perfect food? Brainwashing! The body reacts to table sugar and orange juice in exactly the same way. Okay, let's make them equal by putting vitamin C in table sugar. Actually, they are both unhealthy foods.

> **Wiki Answers**
> http://wiki.answers.com/Q/Is_there_fructose_in_orange_juice
>
> "The sugar content of an orange is only about 30% fructose, along with 50% sucrose and 20% glucose. But since sucrose breaks down to fructose and glucose in 1-1 ratio that would make the effective ratio 55% fructose to 45% glucose."

Fruit juices have the same sugar content as white table sugar (sucrose), so they fall into both categories (glucose and triglycerides) as being a cause of coronary artery disease. Honey must stand alongside of fruit juices and table sugar. They are all sugars.

Honey is essentially the same as white table sugar.

Professional nutritionists cringe at the thought of eating white sugar and insist that children be given orange juice in the school lunch programs, but orange juice has the same amount of glucose and fructose as white sugar. Children are becoming Type 2 diabetics because professional nutritionists, pediatricians, and parents incorrectly think that fruits, fruit juices, dried fruits, whole grain breakfast cereals, bagels, pastas, breads, potatoes, whole grain pancakes, waffles, and baked potato chips are wonderful foods. The more parents concentrate on following the *USDA Food Guide Pyramid*, the higher the rate of childhood diabetes.

The glycemic index for lean meat is zero. It's a wonderful snack food for diabetics because the body converts some of the amino acids to glucose in a natural way in order to maintain normal blood glucose levels without a glucose surge, but diet recommendations for diabetics simply ignore this perfect food. Animal fats, however, actually have a negative glycemic index. Eating natural animal fats will lower the blood glucose levels in both diabetics and healthy individuals.

Unhealthy High-Fructose Foods			
Oranges	Peaches	Grapes	Pineapples
Mangos	Apples	Apricots	Blackberries
Pears	Cherries	Plums	Raspberries
Bananas	Kiwis	Dates	Nectarines

Fructose Causes Heart Disease

Health authorities keep more secrets that I will reveal. I believe I have already convincingly established that the fructose and glucose composition of fruits, fruit juices, and honey is exactly the same as the composition of fructose and glucose in white table sugar. I will now present the scientific connection between these foods and heart disease.

Fructose is obtained mainly from fruits, fruit juices, honey, white table sugar, high-fructose corn syrup, and other syrups. It is also available in a dry granular form very similar to common table sugar. It has become the sweetener of choice for food manufacturing companies and is highly touted by professional nutritionists, medical clinics, and government health authorities because it produces a very small insulin response. This free pass is a very dangerous assumption. The liver metabolizes fructose into blood triglycerides faster than you can swallow. Triglycerides are fats in the blood and have been identified in plaque deposits in the arteries of the heart, legs, kidneys, neck, and brain. High triglycerides are a risk factor for heart disease.

The liver converts fructose from fruit juices into blood fats faster than you can swallow.

The liver's conversion of fructose into triglycerides is a multi-step scientific process that is well understood and proved. This fact illustrates that health authorities ignore scientific truth and instead pursue nutritional dogma that they falsely spew and propagate as a healthy lifestyle. I have searched and found the scientific truth, and I encourage you to seek the truth before you reject this information.

Triglycerides that the liver produces from fructose are usually comprised of one molecule of saturated fatty acid and two molecules of monounsaturated fatty acids. The liver can't produce polyunsaturated fatty acids. Yes, the body quickly turns fructose in orange juice into saturated fatty acids and monounsaturated fatty acids that appear in the blood as triglycerides and on the waistline as body fat. Fruit will make you fat and give you Type 2 diabetes, heart disease, fatty liver disease, and cancer—guaranteed. All of these diseases are in a strong upward trend that corresponds directly to the availability of fruits from around the world 365 days of the year.

Fructose Causes Fatty Liver Disease

Fructose is converted to triglycerides by the liver, and excess fat accumulates within the cells of the liver, resulting in an unhealthy condition known as *non-alcoholic fatty liver disease (NAFLD)*. When the fatty liver becomes inflamed, the condition is known as *hepatitis*, which is generally followed by a progression to steatohepatitis that may lead to hepatocellular carcinoma (liver cancer).

Proteomic Analysis of Fructose-induced Fatty Liver in Hamsters
Metabolism. 2008 Aug;57(8):1115-24
http://www.ncbi.nlm.nih.gov/pubmed/18640390

Zhang L, Perdomo G, Kim DH, Qu S, Ringquist S, Trucco M, Dong HH.

Division of Immunogenetics, Department of Pediatrics, Children's Hospital of Pittsburgh, University of Pittsburgh School of Medicine, Rangos Research Center, Pittsburgh, PA 15213, USA.

"Abstract

High fructose consumption is associated with the development of fatty liver and dyslipidemia with poorly understood mechanisms. We used a matrix-assisted laser desorption/ionization-based proteomics approach to define the molecular events that link high fructose consumption to fatty liver in hamsters. Hamsters fed high-fructose diet for 8 weeks, as opposed to regular-chow-fed controls, developed hyperinsulinemia and hyperlipidemia. High-fructose-fed hamsters exhibited fat accumulation in liver. Hamsters were killed, and liver tissues were subjected to matrix-assisted laser desorption/ionization-based proteomics. This approach identified a number of proteins whose expression levels were altered by >2-fold in response to high fructose feeding. These proteins fall into 5 different categories including (1) functions in fatty acid metabolism such as fatty acid binding protein and carbamoyl-phosphate synthase; (2) proteins in cholesterol and triglyceride metabolism such as apolipoprotein A-1 and protein disulfide isomerase; (3) molecular chaperones such as GroEL, peroxiredoxin 2, and heat shock protein 70, whose functions are important for protein folding and antioxidation; (4) enzymes in fructose catabolism such as fructose-1,6-bisphosphatase and glycerol kinase; and (5) proteins with housekeeping functions such as albumin. These data provide insight into the molecular basis linking fructose-induced metabolic shift to the development of metabolic syndrome characterized by hepatic steatosis and dyslipidemia."

A medical clinic with the best reputation and highest credibility in the world **fails** to identify fructose as the primary contributor to fatty liver and liver cancer.

"Nonalcoholic fatty liver disease occurs when your liver has trouble breaking down fats, causing fat to build up in your liver tissue. Doctors aren't sure what causes this. The wide range of diseases and conditions linked to nonalcoholic fatty liver disease is so diverse that it's difficult to pinpoint any one cause."

Patients are advised to lose weight, exercise, and eat a healthy diet rich in fruits and vegetables.

"**Choose a healthy diet.** Eat a healthy diet that's rich in fruits and vegetables. Reduce the amount of saturated fat in your diet and instead select healthy unsaturated fats, such as those found in fish, olive oil and nuts."

Their advice is in stark contrast to the actual scientific cause of fatty liver disease—the low-fat diet and the high consumption of fructose. It's no wonder that they fail to identity the cause. This clinic will make your fatty liver disease worse and lead to inflammation, cirrhosis, scarring, liver failure, cancer, and a great risk of death. They are not alone. Your doctor is most likely to follow the same ill-conceived advice by recommending that you reduce your intake of saturated fat and consume more fruits and vegetables. If the most prestigious medical clinic in the world is wrong, the odds are that your doctor is also wrong. It is very difficult to find a physician who understands the science behind diet and human physiology.

Fruit juices plug the liver with fat.

Do dietary saturated fats cause a fatty liver? No! The high saturated fat diet in this book will cleanse the liver cells of fatty deposits within weeks, if not days. If you have been diagnosed with a fatty liver, will your physician or holistic practitioner recommend the high saturated fat diet that I present? Not one chance in 10 million. You will probably be told to drink lots of grape juice or orange juice as a liver cleanse. Fruit juices don't cleanse the liver. Fruits and fruit juices plug the liver with fat.

The body processes fructose from fruit in the same way that it processes fructose from soft drinks. There are no differences. Fructose is fructose no matter what the source. Fructose creates insulin resistance as scientific tests have proved. Fructose is highly addictive, and most people simply refuse to give up eating fruits no matter how sick they become. Fruit juices labeled "100% fruit" are very unhealthy because the fructose, sucrose, and glucose are concentrated. Watered-down fruit juices are less damaging, but it is best to avoid all of them.

Organic 100% fruit juices have the same amount of glucose and fructose as white table sugar.

Many diet gurus rage against white table sugar while they recommend a diet loaded with fruits and fruit juices. This logic is strange since the amount of fructose and glucose in fruits (55% and 45%) is the about same as in white table sugar (50% and 50%) and is exactly the same as high-fructose corn syrup used to sweeten soft drinks and other manufactured foods. A plant that processes white table sugar from sugar beets or sugar cane could just as easily produce bags of white sugar from truckloads of grapes, bananas, peaches, pears, pineapples, and mangos. They don't because fruits are more profitable when sold whole or made into juices. The sugar processing plant could also produce white table sugar from truckloads of honey. The plant would simply be doing the very same thing as the body does during the digestion of fruits and fruit juices.

One popular company that charges a membership fee to receive their dietary guidelines and weight-loss program is advising members that fruits are free and quantities are unrestricted. The members can eat all the fruits they want. This is called a healthy way of living. As a nutritional scientist, I am appalled that members are advised to eat as much as they desire of a food that has the same nutritional food count as white table sugar.

One advantage the company has by making this recommendation is the real possibility that the member will never reach his weight goal. If a member were to become skinny, he would discontinue his membership. Maybe this is why the paid programs for weight loss are such an utter failure for the general public. Some studies have estimated the failure rate on these programs to be 95%. Do weight-loss programs deliberately sabotage their members? Perhaps it's good business for them at the expense of poor health for you. Everyone seems to be on some sort of weight-loss program as the obesity rate continues to reach epidemic levels. A visit to the beach quickly reveals that weight-loss programs are total failures.

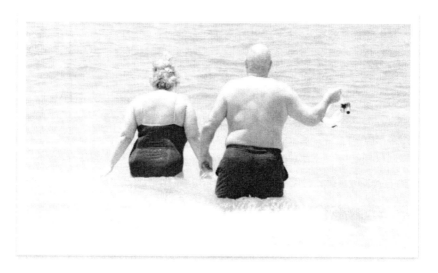

Low-Fat Diets Create Obese People

Fructose Causes Body Fat

We are told to eat lots of fruits and vegetables and to avoid fats (especially animal fats) and white table sugar. The vast majority of people swallow this rhetoric without a burp. Is this advice scientifically true? Let's look at the science of the metabolism of fruits and fruit juices. Fructose is a chemical molecule classified as a sugar with a name ending in "ose" as is common for sugars. When we eat fruits or drink fruit juices, the fructose immediately passes from the small intestine to the hepatic portal blood vein and is delivered directly to the liver. It does not flow out into the body as is the case with glucose, the other major sugar in fruits. Glucose is taken up in the small intestine and flows into the bloodstream where cells can use it as an energy source or store it as body fat.

The body can't metabolize fructose in the small intestine and use it for energy because humans lack the necessary fructokinase enzyme. Excess fructose from fruits such as peaches and pears or from pure refined fructose sugar is not absorbed well and leads to intestinal distress called *osmotic diarrhea* that is common in infants whose mothers overload them with too much fruit. Mothers tend to think fruits are the most wonderful foods for the baby. This is scientifically false. A trip down the baby food aisle in the supermarket gives the reason—shelf upon shelf of fruit, fruit, and more fruit. The old health adage, "An apple a day keeps the doctor away" is scientifically false.

The liver metabolizes the fructose in several steps and converts it into glycogen (a storage form of glucose) or a fatty acid in a process called *fructolysis*. The liver does not allow very much fructose to escape into the bloodstream. Neither does it allow the release of the fatty acid molecule directly into the blood because fatty acids are not water soluble. The liver also produces glycerol and combines glycerol and fatty acid molecules in a ratio of 1:3 to form a compound we call *triglycerides* that are then released into the blood to circulate throughout the body. The fat in your blood does not float to the top of the test tube as one prominent physician falsely claims. Triglycerides are water soluble, but the high levels of triglycerides in the blood present one of the most serious risks for cardiovascular disease. Now that we understand the true science of fructose metabolism, we can better understand why fruits and fruit juices are not the healthy dietary choices that people have been brainwashed to believe. Your blood test report will show a high level of triglycerides in the blood—hypertriglyceridemia. The professional nutritionists didn't tell you that fruits and fruit juices will give you hypertriglyceridemia? Surprise, surprise!

Low Fat, High Sugar Diets Prompt Production of Saturated Fats

http://runews.rockefeller.edu/index.php?page=engine&id=237

Hudgins, Hirsch, and Hellerstein of the Department of Nutritional Sciences at the University of California, Berkeley

"'Eating a low-fat diet may not always be as healthy as people wish. Results from a study, reported in the May 1 *The Journal of Clinical Investigation* by scientists at The Rockefeller University and the University of California, Berkeley, show that people on weight-maintenance diets low in fat but high in sugar increase their production of saturated fat.'

'Our study suggests that low-fat diets designed to maintain-- not lose--weight could be a hazard for people who also eat lots of simple carbohydrates, mostly sugars,' explains first author Lisa Cooper Hudgins, M.D., assistant professor in the Laboratory of Human Behavior and Metabolism at Rockefeller. 'Current public health recommendations suggest that people should reduce fat in their diets and increase their carbohydrates. However, too great a reduction in fats and too much of an increase in simple carbohydrates may prompt the body to make the sugar into saturated fats, which could harm the heart and blood vessels.'"

Fructose has other dark secrets. As many as 1 person per 20,000 of the world's population has hereditary fructose intolerance because the body lacks fructose-1-phosphate aldolase (aldolase B) that the liver needs to metabolize fructose. This leads to an accumulation of fructose-1-phosphate that inhibits glycogenolysis (breakdown of glycogen) and gluconeogenesis (building of glucose from protein or fats), resulting in an excessively low blood level of glucose called *hypoglycemia*. The condition can be life-threatening due to liver or kidney damage. Other outcomes are hyperuricemia (high uric acid), hepatomegaly (enlarged liver), hemorrhage, jaundice (yellowing of the skin caused by high levels of bilirubin in the blood), and vomiting. Is fruit a "free food" that you can eat in unlimited quantities? No!

Fruits are scientifically unhealthy.

Unhealthy High-Fructose Foods			
Oranges	Peaches	Grapes	Pineapples
Mangos	Apples	Apricots	Blackberries
Pears	Cherries	Plums	Raspberries
Bananas	Kiwis	Dates	Nectarines

Fructose Causes Strokes

Fructose raises the level of blood lipids in the form of triglycerides that have been proven to increase the risk for ischemic strokes. Standard blood tests only show the level of triglycerides after fasting, but the non-fasting triglycerides are much higher and present a greater health risk.

High non-fasting triglycerides increase the risk for stroke in both men and women. A Danish team followed 7,579 women and 6,372 men for 33 years in the Copenhagen City Heart Study. All of the participants were white and of Danish descent. The baseline measurements of non-fasting triglycerides and cholesterol were taken in the years 1976–1978.

Non-fasting Triglycerides, Cholesterol and Stroke in the General Population

Copenhagen University Hospital
Dr. Marianne Benn
February 18, 2011

Annals of Neurology; Published Online:
February 18, 2011 (DOI:10.1002/ana.22384).
http://doi.wiley.com/10.1002/ana.22384

"Abstract

Objective:

Current guidelines on stroke prevention have recommend-dations on desirable cholesterol levels, but not on nonfasting triglycerides. We compared stepwise increasing levels of nonfasting triglycerides and cholesterol for their association with risk of ischemic stroke in the general population.

Methods:

A total of 7,579 women and 6,372 men from the Copenhagen City Heart Study with measurements of nonfasting triglycerides and cholesterol at baseline in 1976–1978 were followed for up to 33 years; of these, 837 women and 837 men developed ischemic stroke during follow-up, which was 100% complete.

Results:

The fluctuation of nonfasting triglycerides and cholesterol over 15 years was similar. In both women and men, stepwise increasing levels of nonfasting triglycerides were associated with increased risk of ischemic stroke. Compared to women with triglycerides <1 mmol/liter, multivariate adjusted hazard ratios ranged from 1.2 (95% confidence interval [CI], 0.9–1.7) for triglyceride levels of 1.00–1.99 mmol/liter to 3.9 (95%CI, 1.3–11.1) for triglyceride levels ≥5 mmol/liter (trend: $p <$ 0.001); corresponding hazard ratios in men ranged from 1.2 (95%CI, 0.8–1.7) to 2.3 (95%CI, 1.2–4.3) (p = 0.001). Increasing cholesterol levels were not associated with risk of ischemic stroke except in men with cholesterol levels ≥9.00 mmol/liter vs <5.00 mmol/liter, with a hazard ratio of 4.4 (95%CI, 1.9–10.6).

Interpretation:

In women, stepwise increasing levels of nonfasting triglycerides were associated with increasing risk of ischemic stroke while increasing cholesterol levels were not. In men, these results were similar except that cholesterol ≥9.00 mmol/liter was associated with increased risk of ischemic stroke."

Stroke has become the third leading cause of death in the United States, 87% of which are ischemic stroke (blockage) and 13% are hemorrhagic stroke (leakage outside of the arteries and veins of the brain). Vegetarians appear to be at a higher risk than the general population when the diet is high in fruits and low in calories. Those who are particularly thin (a common condition that vegetarians wrongly believe to be exceedingly healthy) appear to have the highest risk.

High blood pressure is not the only cause of hemorrhagic strokes. The strength and health of the blood vessels are vitally important but often overlooked. Unhealthy blood vessels are why many people suffer hemorrhagic strokes even though they have normal or below normal blood pressure. The low-fat, low-protein, low-cholesterol vegetarian diet causes weak arteries that are a risk factor for hemorrhagic stroke. The low-carbohydrate diet with high levels of protein and natural animal fats provides the nutrition necessary to build strong, healthy blood vessels.

Fruit and vegetable juices will give you a stroke.

One raw food vegetarian became popular on the Internet because he lost 200 pounds on his special diet plan. He had become obese eating the high-carbohydrate diet as promoted by the *USDA Food Guide Pyramid* and decided to avoid all animal products in favor of a raw vegetarian diet with lots of fruits and vegetables. He promoted juicing raw fruits and vegetables using professional equipment.

His Internet videos claimed his new diet reversed his Type 2 diabetes and heart disease, but unfortunately, he nearly lost his brain to a stroke and apparently had a heart attack at about the same time. He was the darling of the of the raw food vegetarian diet gurus, but since his dreadful setback, many websites have deleted pages that flaunted him as the *Poster Boy of the Raw*

Vegetarian Diet. He has been dropped like a poisonous mushroom.

His raw vegetarian diet totally restricts animal protein and fats. It is also deficient in essential amino acids and essential fatty acids. Animal protein and fats build strong arteries and reduce triglycerides. As shown in the previously-cited studies, fruits and fruit juices increase triglycerides. This combination leaves the consumer at risk for ischemic and hemorrhagic strokes.

The big surprise is that the raw vegetarian diet did not result in death from colon or lung cancer like other cases I present in this book. I guess he simply had the heart attack and stroke first. A protein deficiency creates a weakened immune system and leads to cancer because all immune cells are made from amino acids.

The low-protein vegetarian diet causes strokes.

Societies in which the people have a low intake of animal protein and saturated fats have a higher risk for stroke and cancer. The incidences of stroke in Japan are two to three times higher than in the United States. Cancer is also higher in Japan. Both of these conditions are probably linked to the lower intake of animal protein.

Prospective study of fat and protein intake and risk of intraparenchymal hemorrhage in women

Circulation 2001 Feb 13;103(6):856-63

Iso H, Stampfer MJ, Manson JE, Rexrode K, Hu F, Hennekens CH, Colditz GA, Speizer FE, Willett WC.

Channing Laboratory, Division of Preventive Medicine, Department of Medicine, Brigham and Women's Hospital and Harvard Medical School, Boston, Massachusetts, USA

Chapter 3

"Background: Dietary animal fat and protein have been inversely associated with a risk of intraparenchymal hemorrhage in ecological studies.

Methods and results: In 1980, 85 764 women in the Nurses' Health Study cohort, who were 34 to 59 years old and free of diagnosed cardiovascular disease and cancer, completed dietary questionnaires. From these questionnaires, we calculated fat and protein intake. By 1994, after 1.16 million person-years of follow-up, 690 incident strokes, including 74 intraparenchymal hemorrhages, had been documented. Multivariate-adjusted risk of intraparenchymal hemorrhage was higher among women in the lowest quintile of energy-adjusted saturated fat intake than at all higher levels of intake (relative risk [RR], 2.36; 95% CI, 1.10 to 5.09; P:=0.03). For trans unsaturated fat, the corresponding RR was 2.50 (95% CI, 1.35 to 4.65; P:=0.004). Animal protein intake was inversely associated with risk (RR in the highest versus lowest quintiles, 0.32; 95% CI, 0.10 to 1.00; P:=0.04). The excess risk associated with low saturated fat intake was observed primarily among women with a history of hypertension (RR, 3.66; 95% CI, 1.09 to 12.3; P=0.04), but such an interaction was not seen for trans unsaturated fat or animal protein. These nutrients were not related to risk of other stroke subtypes. Dietary cholesterol and monounsaturated and polyunsaturated fat were not related to risk of any stroke subtype.

Conclusions: Low intake of saturated fat and animal protein was associated with an increased risk of intraparenchymal hemorrhage, which may help to explain the high rate of this stroke subtype in Asian countries. The increased risk with low intake of saturated fat and trans unsaturated fat is compatible with the reported association between low serum total cholesterol and risk."

Prestigious Health Organizations Ignore Fructose Science

Organizations that are considered to have the highest credibility and prestige always promote the same dietary guidelines that they call a healthy diet, and people have become so brainwashed that these dietary experts don't even bother to define what a healthy diet is. The public has been brainwashed to believe a healthy diet consists of eating lots of fruits, vegetables, and whole grains while avoiding meat, animal fats, and saturated fats from vegetable sources such as palm and coconut oils. These experts tell the public to eat a healthy diet as the epidemics of diabetes, obesity, cancer, and heart disease escalate. Maybe they should step back and look at the science of human anatomy and physiology.

Remember, this is a science book.

I see only very minor differences among government health organizations, vegetarian religious groups, highly credentialed medical clinics, medical specialty groups, and universities. Medical schools at the most prestigious universities are good examples of the current thinking about the dietary etiologies of various diseases. You will find that the top four medical schools consider to be the most respected and credible will all agree with the following representative school. The quotation that seeks to analyze the dietary cause of nonalcoholic fatty liver disease is from one of the most prominent university medical schools.

> "One leading theory is that the condition starts when muscle, fat, and liver cells stop responding normally to insulin. This so-called insulin resistance is a hallmark of obesity and diabetes. Insulin resistance also increases the amount of fat molecules circulating in the blood. The accumulation of these

molecules inside liver cells can lead to liver inflammation and damage. This is called nonalcoholic steatohepatitis (NASH)."

I will apply scientific truth to test the accuracy of the above statement.

- They did not make any connection to the scientific fact that the liver converts all dietary fructose into saturated and monounsaturated fats. The liver combines these fats with glycerol and discharges them into the blood as triglycerides. They also accumulate in the liver. This scientific fact is very important but the medical school ignored it.

- Fructose is not sent throughout the body as is glucose. The liver is forced to deal with fructose because it can't be metabolized directly by the cells as a source of energy. The liver also changes glucose into triglycerides, so this is a double hit for fat accumulation in the liver. The major sources of fructose and glucose are fruits, fruit juices, table sugar, pure refined fructose, high-fructose corn syrup, honey, and other sweeteners. If you want to die from fatty liver disease, eat a vegetarian breakfast of orange juice, a banana, low-fat yogurt with peaches, and a whole wheat bagel with honey on it.

- Yes, insulin resistance causes a fatty liver to become enlarged and inflamed resulting in cirrhosis, liver failure, and death; but the medical school did not warn that fructose is the primary cause of insulin resistance.

People question any claim that goes against the established medical community and certainly against the top four medical schools in the United States. Are these schools knowledgeable and unbiased beyond question? Certainly not! History has proved time and time again that popularity does not necessary equal truth. I cited this example in *Absolute Truth Exposed* –

Volume 1, but I will repeat the example because this book is a stand-alone volume.

U.S. President James A. Garfield's death in 1881 resulted from a pistol shot. He probably would have recovered had his team of Army doctors not treated him. Many people have recovered and healed very well with bullets lodged in their bodies. In the end, the doctors managed to take a 3" (75mm) wound and turn it into a 20" (500mm) canal that was heavily infected and oozed more pus with each passing day because they probed the bullet wound with unwashed hands and dirty instruments. This was one reason why bacterial infections were the leading cause of death throughout human history. Medicine had rejected the theory of bacterial infection even though bacteria had been discovered more than 200 years earlier. In 1676–1677, Antonie Philips van Leeuwenhoek, a Dutchman, was the first to record microscopic observations of bacteria and spermatozoa. Bacteria could be observed in infected flesh wounds, whereas fresh uninfected wounds were observed to be bacteria free. It seems ridiculous that highly-credentialed physicians could deny this simple truth for 200 years, but that's the nature of brainwashing. It's hard to imagine, but it's true. For ten generations, older physicians and medical schools brainwashed new students to reject the truth that invisible bacteria cause infections. Scientists, professors, and physicians are not immune to delusional thinking and false beliefs.

Physicians rejected the fact that bacteria cause infections for 200 years before accepting truth.

You will find that my beliefs and the scientific references I cite will clash time after time with established government health organizations, university medical schools, and professional nutritionists. I was able to reverse my heart disease quickly and in a very effective manner by rejecting health claims made by the major media and these prestigious health organizations. I doubt that you could do the same by following advice from the network staff physician on the evening news or your favorite heart disease organization. Millions of people are following their advice without success.

Let's look at the recommendations for reducing triglycerides made by the same university medical school.

> "Some forms of familial hypertriglyceridemia do not seem to increase the risk of developing heart disease, assuming that the rest of the person's cholesterol profile is normal and there are no other risk factors. Other factors that may cause high triglyceride levels include obesity, alcohol abuse, a diet high in saturated fats, or illnesses such as poorly controlled diabetes, chronic kidney disease, or liver disease."

> "Weight reduction and increased physical activity are an important part of treatment. The lifestyle changes that you can make to improve your triglyceride levels include losing weight, limiting alcohol to one drink a day, stopping smoking, and increasing your level of exercise."

> "Dietary changes can also help reduce high levels of triglyceride. Such changes include limiting your daily calorie intake as well as the amount of fat and carbohydrate in your diet."

The recommendations for weight reduction are to exercise, restrict calories, limit alcohol, stop smoking, and reduce dietary saturated fats and carbohydrates. They give a little hint that carbohydrates should be reduced but only in the context that lower calories will reverse fatty liver disease. They fail to make the direct connection between carbohydrates and fatty liver disease. Instead, they point the finger at dietary saturated fats as a contributing factor for fatty liver disease. Medical schools have a saturated fat phobia. Do dietary saturated fats increase triglycerides as measured in blood tests?

Medical schools have a saturated fat phobia.

My blood test results shown in this book prove the opposite. My diet of 70% fat, 30% of which is from saturated fats, results in an extremely low triglyceride level of 71 versus the normal recommended healthy limit of 150. My triglycerides are less than 50% of the recommended limit. My wife, Marti, eats a diet that is as high or higher in saturated fats, and her triglyceride level is only 45. So, what are the scientific proofs that dietary saturated fats raise triglycerides? There aren't any. The prestigious medical school is scientifically wrong, which you can easily prove by simply eating my diet yourself.

They mention nothing about reducing dietary fructose as a treatment for fatty liver disease even though the liver converts fructose directly into triglycerides. They claim high triglycerides can be caused by liver disease. Which is it? Do the high triglycerides cause liver disease or does the liver disease cause high triglycerides? The school has it backward. Carbohydrates alone cause nonalcoholic fatty liver disease, not dietary saturated fats.

Eating a high level of saturated fats along with a drastic elimination of all fructose and glucose reverses nonalcoholic fatty liver disease within weeks, if not days. If you are admitted to the hospital with advanced fatty liver disease, will your physician place you on a high-saturated fat diet and a 100% restriction of fruits and other carbohydrates? Probably not! Liver transplants are on the rise because of nonalcoholic fatty liver disease that physicians can't reverse.

Fructose causes nonalcoholic fatty liver disease.

The diet recommended by the medical school is still in the range of 50–60% carbohydrates, but they won't give a nutritional breakdown of their food pyramid because they are hiding the truth that it is a high-carbohydrate diet. They say:

> "Do not count the numbers."

> "A diet rich in vegetables and fruits has bountiful benefits. Among them: It can decrease the chances of having a heart attack or stroke; possibly protect against some types of cancers; lower blood pressure; help you avoid the painful intestinal ailment called diverticulitis; guard against cataract and macular degeneration, the major causes of vision loss among people over age 65; and add variety to your diet and wake up your palate."

Is it true that a diet rich in vegetables and fruits provides all of these health benefits? No! It's scientifically false. I have previously shown that fruits and vegetables increase triglycerides and glucose and lead to several eye diseases as is typical in diabetics. Fruits and vegetables will not lower your blood pressure and do not protect against cancer. Essential amino acids and fatty acids maintain healthy eyes and prevent macular degeneration. Amino acids are the building blocks for all of the immune cells that the body needs to destroy cancer cells. All of the calories in fruits and vegetables are converted into sugars, and sugars have been shown to feed cancer cells. The scientific evidence against fructose is overwhelming. Fructose will not build a strong, healthy body.

Fructose Causes Gout

Vegetarians spread misinformation about beef in the hope that you will panic and stop eating animals. One example is the common claim that protein causes gout. Many people are brainwashed to accept these lies. Gout is actually caused by carbohydrates in the diet and fructose is the prime suspect. Thus we see that science proves the vegetarian diet with its abundance of fruits and fruit juices is the primary cause of gout. Oh, you don't think so? Please read the results from the following study. Keep in mind that fruits and fruit juices consist of 55% fructose and 45% glucose, the same percentage of fructose in soft drinks sweetened with high-fructose corn syrup.

> **Gout Surge Blamed on Sweet Drinks**
> BBC NEWS – Health - February 1, 2008
> http://news.bbc.co.uk/2/hi/health/7219473.stm
>
> "Sugary drinks have been blamed for a surge in cases of the painful joint disease gout.
>
> Men who consume two or more sugary soft drinks a day have an 85% higher risk of gout compared with those who drink less than one a month, a study suggests.
>
> Cases in the US have doubled in recent decades and it seems fructose, a type of sugar, may be to blame, the British Medical Journal study reports.
>
> UK experts said those with gout would be advised to cut out sugary drinks."

Fructose is a very sinister sugar that is getting away with murder. We can see from this progression that fructose from table sugar, refined pure fructose sweetener, high-fructose corn syrup, honey, fruits, and fruit juices can lead to liver cancer, coronary artery disease, kidney artery disease, peripheral artery disease, stroke, gout, and most likely to Alzheimer's disease. Fructose also promotes liver cancer. Meanwhile, the professional nutritionists, professional health societies, physicians, universities, and government health departments strongly advise everyone to gorge themselves on fruits and fruit juices as obesity, cancer, heart disease, and diabetes escalate.

Fructose Causes Hyperuricemia and Metabolic Syndrome

Unlike other sugars, fructose produces hyperuricemia (high serum uric acid levels) that results in decreased nitric oxide (NO) in the endothelial layer of the arteries. Nitric oxide has been scientifically shown to increase blood flow by relaxing the arteries and to enhance the uptake of glucose throughout the body. These effects are very positive for good health and disease prevention. A reduction in nitric acid causes a reduction in the uptake of glucose by the cells and reduces the effectiveness of insulin. This condition is known as *insulin resistance* or *metabolic syndrome.*

It is a scientific fact that fructose causes insulin resistance, hyperuricemia, and metabolic syndrome that increase the risk for Alzheimer's disease, heart disease, high blood pressure, cancer, and diabetes. See the following study that proves fructose, as found in abundance in fruits and fruit juices, is one of the root causes of metabolic syndrome and hypertension. Metabolic syndrome is indicated by the following unhealthy readings on physical tests and blood tests:

- High triglycerides
- High LDL cholesterol
- Low HDL cholesterol
- High total cholesterol
- High glucose
- High uric acid
- High blood pressure
- Obesity
- Diabetes

Hypothesis: fructose-induced hyperuricemia as a causal mechanism for the epidemic of the metabolic syndrome
Nat Clin Pract Nephrol. 2005 Dec;1(2):80-6.
http://www.ncbi.nlm.nih.gov/pubmed/16932373?dopt=AbstractPlus

"Abstract

The increasing incidence of obesity and the metabolic syndrome over the past two decades has coincided with a marked increase in total fructose intake. Fructose--unlike other sugars--causes serum uric acid levels to rise rapidly. We recently reported that uric acid reduces levels of endothelial nitric oxide (NO), a key mediator of insulin action. NO increases blood flow to skeletal muscle and enhances glucose uptake. Animals deficient in endothelial NO develop insulin resistance and other features of the metabolic syndrome. As such, we propose that the epidemic of the metabolic syndrome is due in part to fructose-induced hyperuricemia that reduces endothelial NO levels and induces insulin resistance. Consistent with this hypothesis is the observation that changes in mean uric acid levels correlate with the increasing prevalence of metabolic syndrome in the US and developing countries. In addition, we observed that a serum uric acid level above 5.5 mg/dl independently predicted the development of hyperinsulinemia at both 6 and 12 months in nondiabetic patients with first-time myocardial infarction. Fructose-induced hyperuricemia results in endothelial dysfunction and insulin resistance, and might be a novel causal mechanism of the metabolic syndrome. Studies in humans should be performed to address whether lowering uric acid levels will help to prevent this condition."

Chapter 3

Triglycerides Cause Coronary Artery Disease

Elevated triglycerides are a primary risk factor for heart disease. Many people think high triglycerides are caused by eating fat because triglycerides are fat lipids in the blood, but this is not entirely correct. The body converts carbohydrates to blood glucose first and then converts the glucose to triglycerides. The liver converts fructose directly into triglycerides. The blood carries the triglycerides to the fat cells, where they are converted to body fat. Insulin is the prime motivator in this process since it deposits the triglycerides in the arteries. The low-fat diet actually promotes the production of triglycerides and promotes heart disease. Reducing dietary carbohydrates stops this deadly process. My low-carbohydrate, high-fat diet reduces triglycerides quickly and dramatically. The ratio of triglycerides (TR) to HDL cholesterol (TG/HDL) is one of the best indicators for heart disease risk.

Triglycerides are fats in the blood.

Triglycerides should be below 100 mg/dL, and HDL cholesterol should be above 50 mg/dL, for a ratio of 2.00. Improving the TG/HDL ratio will substantially reduce the heart disease risk. Some people are walking time bombs with a ratio of 6.00 or greater, and a ratio of 4.00 is very common. The ratio on my last blood test was (71/68) = 1.04, and my wife, Marti, had a ratio of (45/115) = 0.39. Our awesome results were obtained on a diet that is 70% fats on a calorie basis, 30% of which are saturated fats. Do dietary fats cause your blood lipids to increase? Absolutely not! The scientific truth is just the opposite. Eating animal fats will reduce your blood fats. Eating fruits and vegetables will increase your blood fats. Look at your report now to see how well you are doing on your present diet.

People on Internet message boards are totally perplexed and baffled when their blood tests reveal a very high level of triglycerides in the range of 200–500 or greater. They cannot understand how an ultra low-fat diet could result in blood lipids so high that their heart disease risk factors skyrocketed. In contrast, the high-fat diet I present in this book has been shown to lower triglycerides to 75 and reverse heart disease by reducing the size of arterial plaques. Yes, the low-fat, high-carbohydrate diet produces a high level of fats in the blood. People are either shocked, confused, or in denial when I tell them this scientific fact because low-fat diet books tell them just the opposite.

Recent Success Story from a Male Suffering from Outrageously High Triglycerides, Angina Heart Pain, Head Pain, Malaise, and a Stubborn Weight Plateau

"About 4 years ago was the last time I had a doctor check my cholesterol. My triglycerides were dangerously sitting at 1500 so I took his advice, stopped drinking so much pop, started eating what I thought was a healthy diet, and I eventually quit smoking. I'm 28 years old, and I had chest pains for at least 8 years. In the last few years, I started getting the same sharp pains in my head. At one point I even quit eating meat because of the chest pains, but they were always there.

One day, I ran into your website while searching for something that would clean blood clots, and from that day forward the sharp pains faded. It's been about 45 days on this diet, but the pains were completely gone within days. I honestly haven't felt them since that day when I ate a package of bacon and about 3 pounds of hamburger. I ate lots and lots of fatty meats, real butter, eggs, and green beans mixed with butter. I started feeling a lot more energetic and positive. My concentration increased by 10,000%. I always use to day dream in school, and now I know that was caused from sugar withdrawals. I am now sugar free. I've lost 15 pounds after years of being stuck at 195 no matter what I did.

I will always remember you as someone who saved and changed my life forever. Thank you very much."

Milk Causes Digestive Diseases and Heart Disease

People shun cows' milk for the wrong reason. The saturated animal fat phobia started by Dr. Ancel Benjamin Keys continues today as generation after generation is brainwashed to believe the false claim that saturated fat causes heart disease. I will talk more about Dr. Keys.

The milk industry has been its own worst enemy by supporting this claim. This doesn't mean that cows' milk is healthy food for people. It's not. The unhealthy macronutrient in milk is the sugar, not the fat. The lactose sugar in milk leads to many health problems. It has been estimated that 90% of oriental people are allergic to lactose. The symptoms appear as severe digestive problems that can lead to leaky gut syndrome, inflammatory bowel diseases, and many autoimmune diseases.

Babies can develop negative reactions to cows' milk at an alarming rate. This has prompted the baby food industry to develop alternative formulas from vegetable sources. Since these manufactured alternatives to natural mother's breast milk are unsatisfactory, health groups promote breast feeding rather than bottle feeding. Some groups have started milk banks so that women who are able to produce milk can supply those who cannot. Researchers have successfully spliced human mammary gland genes into cows that will enable them to produce the equivalent of human breast milk.

Milk causes many health problems.

The public has been severely brainwashed to believe that cows' milk and goats' milk are vital for growing children. They believe reduced-fat milk products advertised as 2%, 1%, or skim are healthier than natural whole milk. The high-lactose milk digests quickly as the lactose sugar is taken into the blood and immediately converted by the liver into triglycerides—one of the risk factors for heart disease. Milk from cows and goats also produces body fat weight gain and contributes to childhood obesity.

Nutrition Facts for 1% Low-fat Cows' Milk
Serving One Cup (244 g)

Nutrient	Amount, g	Calories	Percent Calories
Proteins	8	24	25.5
Fats	2	18	19.1
Carbohydrates	13	52	55.3

Note: Calories from 1% low-fat milk is 55% lactose sugar.

Chapter 3

Cholesterol in Atherosclerotic Plaque

The small, dense LDL_b cholesterol fraction or subfraction, classified as *pattern B LDL cholesterol*, is a strong heart disease risk (more atherogenic) in the presence of hyperglycemia and hyperinsulinemia. Cholesterol is a requirement in the healthy composition of the cell membranes, and LDL carries the cholesterol to all cells throughout the body. The cellular requirement for cholesterol as a membrane component is satisfied by being synthesized within the cell or delivered to the cell by LDLs. The primary plasma (blood) carriers of cholesterol for repair of vascular injuries are LDLs, but high levels of LDL_b are strongly linked to cardiovascular disease. My regimen drives the LDL cholesterol to very low levels and sharply decreases the pattern B small, dense LDL_b cholesterol fraction. The different LDL molecule fractions are not the same and do not present the same heart disease risk. You should ask your doctor to obtain a cholesterol blood test that differentiates the various fractions. Cardiovascular plaque cannot be removed from the arteries unless the cholesterol ranges and subfraction sizes match or exceed my actual test results shown in Chapter 4.

Cholesterol Subfraction and Characteristics		
Molecule	**Description**	**Risk Factor**
LDL_a	Largest	Less Atherogenic
LDL_{ab}	Medium	Atherogenic
LDL_b	Smallest	More Atherogenic
HDL_2	Large	Protective
HDL_3	Smaller, Dense	Less Protective

Blood Tests to Evaluate Heart Disease Risk

The commonly used blood tests to evaluate heart disease risks are almost worthless for truly determining those risks. Doctors will obtain a cholesterol test that measures only the total cholesterol (CT), high-density lipoprotein (HDL), and triglycerides (TR). These measurements are used to calculate the low-density lipoprotein (LDL), which then becomes the main focus. Medical authorities have set the limit for LDL lower and lower because cholesterol-lowering drugs have failed to have any positive effect on the rate of heart disease. The lower limit for LDL was 100, but people continued to develop heart disease at an increasing rate. Now the limit has been lowered to 70. This unreasonably low limit makes everyone in the world a prime candidate for cholesterol-lowering pharmaceutical drugs.

As a general rule, LDL cholesterol is not measured directly. The very-low-density lipoprotein (VLDL) is calculated by dividing the triglycerides by five. In most tests, the LDL is calculated according to the Friedewald Equation:

$$LDL = CT - HDL - VLDL, \text{ where } VLDL = TR/5$$

In order to accurately evaluate heart disease risk, a blood test is performed that includes the atherogenic risk factors. Unfortunately, most doctors will not request all of these tests, and insurance companies may be reluctant to pay for them as routine preventative diagnostic measurements. To make matters worse, many laboratories may lack the equipment and skills necessary to perform the tests. One blood test you can perform at home may be a more important indicator of your heart disease risk than the standard cholesterol test requested by your doctor. You can easily take your own blood glucose measurement with a simple, inexpensive glucose meter available at any pharmacy.

219

However some doctors neglect glucose as an important heart disease risk factor unless you are testing for symptoms of diabetes. The fasting glucose reading should be within the range of 70–110 mg/dL. The atherogenic factors below are believed to increase heart disease atherosclerotic plaque risk.

- Fasting insulin - Atherogenic - The number one risk factor, but doctors rarely measure it
- Fasting glucose - Atherogenic - The number two risk factor, but some doctors dismiss it as a heart disease risk
- Homocysteine - Atherogenic - An amino acid often wrongly considered to be the number one risk factor
- Triglycerides - Atherogenic - Fat in the blood that promotes plaque formation
- Fibrinogen - Atherogenic - Protein molecule that promotes clotting and thickens the blood
- LDL_b - Atherogenic - Low-density lipoprotein cholesterol

    Note: The total LDL reading is almost worthless as a risk factor. The LDL subfractions must be evaluated separately and consist of the following:

    - Lp(a) - Atherogenic - The protein shell of small, dense LDL that promotes plaque formation
    - IDL - Atherogenic - The intermediate-density lipoprotein
    - Pattern A LDL - Less atherogenic - The larger, less dense LDL cholesterol that is not a risk factor
    - Pattern A/B LDL - Atherogenic - Intermediate transitional size and density that is a medium risk factor
    - Pattern B LDL - More Atherogenic - The small, dense LDL cholesterol that is the highest risk factor

- VLDL - Atherogenic - Very-low-density lipoprotein cholesterol that consists of the following subfractions:

    - VLDL 1+2 - Less atherogenic
    - VLDL 3 - More atherogenic

- HDL - This is the favored, healthy, or good cholesterol. Values below 40 are an increased risk factor. Values above 50 are protective. High-density lipoprotein cholesterol consists of the following subfractions:

  - HDL_2 - Protective
  - HDL_3 - Less protective

- Total cholesterol - Not a risk factor because good HDL actually raises this value
- C-reactive protein (CRP) - An indicator that previous artery damage has occurred

In the following study, the results show that a reduction in total dietary fat and saturated fat had a negative effect by decreasing the good HDL cholesterol. In other words, the low-fat diet that most health authorities recommend actually increases coronary artery disease risks because the low-fat diet decreases both large (HDL_2 and HDL_{2b}) and small, dense (HDL_3) subpopulations. The HDL_2 and HDL_{2b} subfractions decreased the most. My scientific dietary regimen increases HDL cholesterol.

HDL-subpopulation patterns in response to reductions in dietary total and saturated fat intakes in healthy subjects
http://www.ajcn.org/content/70/6/992

"Background: Little information is available about HDL subpopulations during dietary changes.

Objective: The objective was to investigate the effect of reductions in total and saturated fat intakes on HDL subpopulations.

Design: Multiracial, young and elderly men and women (n = 103) participating in the double-blind, randomized DELTA (Dietary Effects on Lipoproteins and Thrombogenic Activities) Study consumed 3 different diets, each for 8 wk:

an average American diet (AAD: 34.3% total fat, 15.0% saturated fat), the American Heart Association Step I diet (28.6% total fat, 9.0% saturated fat), and a diet low in saturated fat (25.3% total fat, 6.1% saturated fat).

Results: HDL2-cholesterol concentrations, by differential precipitation, decreased ($P < 0.001$) in a stepwise fashion after the reduction of total and saturated fat: 0.58 ± 0.21, 0.53 ± 0.19, and 0.48 ± 0.18 mmol/L with the AAD, Step I, and low-fat diets, respectively. HDL3 cholesterol decreased ($P < 0.01$) less: 0.76 ± 0.13, 0.73 ± 0.12, and 0.72 ± 0.11 mmol/L with the AAD, Step I, and low-fat diets, respectively. As measured by nondenaturing gradient gel electrophoresis, the larger-size HDL2b subpopulation decreased with the reduction in dietary fat, and a corresponding relative increase was seen for the smaller-sized HDL3a, 3b, and 3c subpopulations ($P < 0.01$). HDL2-cholesterol concentrations correlated negatively with serum triacylglycerol concentrations on all 3 diets: $r = -0.46$, -0.37, and -0.45 with the AAD, Step I, and low-fat diets, respectively ($P < 0.0001$). A similar negative correlation was seen for HDL2b, whereas HDL3a, 3b, and 3c correlated positively with triacylglycerol concentrations. Diet-induced changes in serum triacylglycerol were negatively correlated with changes in HDL2 and HDL2b cholesterol.

Conclusions: A reduction in dietary total and saturated fat decreased both large (HDL2 and HDL2b) and small, dense HDL subpopulations, although decreases in HDL2 and HDL2b were most pronounced."

Cholesterol Test Ranges and Risk Factors

Blood test results usually give ranges that have been established as acceptable for the average person. These ranges may be fine for preventing heart disease in people without diabetes, hyperglycemia, hyperinsulinemia, or other health problems, but they are not suitable for reversing heart disease. The following are standard ranges for lipids in blood tests. LDL is calculated per the Friedewald Equation in which all concentrations are given in mg/dL, where < means less than and > means greater than.

Standard Cholesterol Test Ranges

- Total cholesterol, CT = HDL + LDL + VLDL.
- HDL is the high-density lipoprotein cholesterol.
- LDL is the low-density lipoprotein cholesterol.
- VLDL is the very-low-density lipoprotein cholesterol.
- TG is the triglycerides, blood lipids, or fatty acids.
- VLDL = TG / 5 based on a formula.
- LDL = CT - HDL − (TG / 5).
- CT < 200.
- CT / HDL > 3.0 and < 5.0, where the 3.0 should be ignored.
- HDL > 40 for men. Less than 40 increases coronary risk and above 60 is protective.
- HDL > 50 for women. Less than 50 increases coronary risk and above 60 is protective.
- LDL < 160, above increases risk.
- TG < 150, above increases risk.
- LDL / HDL < 3.0, above 3.0 increases coronary risk.
- TG / HDL < 3.0, above 3.0 increases coronary risk.
- Lp(a) < 30, lipoprotein (a).

Chapter 3

Cholesterol Test Ranges Needed to Reverse Heart Disease

Many factors relating to diet, hormones, and cholesterol levels must be driven to optimal extremes in order to reverse heart disease. Your physician may compliment you on your very good report based on the standard guidelines, but these are not nearly sufficient to reverse heart disease. The following cholesterol guidelines are based on my regimen that has reversed my heart disease. All concentrations are given in mg/dL, where < means less than and > means greater than.

- CT < 160, total cholesterol.
- HDL > 60, high-density lipoprotein.
- LDL < 80, low-density lipoprotein.
- TG < 80, triglycerides.
- CT / HDL < 2.5.
- TG / HDL < 1.1.
- Lp(a) < 15, lipoprotein (a).
- IDL < 10, intermediate-density lipoprotein.
- IDL + VLDL3 < 25, remnant lipoprotein.
- HDL-2 > 20, most protective HDL fraction.
- HDL-3 > 40, less protective HDL fraction.
- VLDL-3 < 10, small remnant, very-low-density lipoprotein.
- LDL-1 pattern A < 30, least dangerous LDL.
- LDL-2 pattern A < 25, less dangerous LDL.
- LDL-3 pattern B < 30, dangerous LDL.
- LDL-4 pattern B < 5, most dangerous LDL.

Lp(a) is determined by genetics and cannot be changed by diet or exercise. Supplemental niacin (vitamin B3) is the best way to reduce Lp(a), LDL cholesterol, and total cholesterol. Niacin rarely causes liver damage but can cause muscle damage as do prescription statin cholesterol-lowering drugs.

LDL Laboratory Results Are Wrong on the Low-Carb Diet

Blood testing laboratories do not perform a direct measurement of the LDL cholesterol that is shown on your report. The actual measurement of LDL is costly, time consuming, and requires the use of ultra-centrifugal equipment not readily available in some laboratories and certainly not available in your physician's office. The LDL value is calculated from other test measurements based on the following Friedewald (1972) Equations:

- Total cholesterol, CT = HDL + LDL + VLDL
- VLDL = Triglycerides (TG) / 5
- LDL = CT - HDL – (TG / 5)

This is an acceptable calculation for people who eat the standard high-carbohydrate diet, but it has been shown to be incorrect for those on a low-carbohydrate diet. My personal LDL blood test results are standard laboratory calculations. Actual laboratory measurements of the LDL were not taken. Therefore, my real LDL results are most likely lower than the laboratory reported value. In other words, my results are better than listed in the reports I received from the laboratories. The following Iranian study shows that the calculations using the Friedewald Equation above for LDL are inaccurate when triglycerides are less than 100. Actual measurements of LDL and total cholesterol are lower than shown by the Friedewald Equation.

> **The impact of low serum triglyceride on LDL-cholesterol estimation**
> Arch Iran Med. 2008 May;11(3):318-21.
> http://www.ncbi.nlm.nih.gov/pubmed/18426324
>
> Department of Pathology, Sina Hospital, Medical Sciences/ University of Tehran, Tehran, Iran. ahmadise@tums.ac.ir

Chapter 3

"Abstract

Most clinical laboratories directly measure serum triglyceride, total cholesterol, and high-density lipoprotein cholesterol. They indirectly calculate low-density lipoprotein cholesterol value using the Friedewald equation. Although high serum triglyceride (>400 mg/dL or 4.52 mmol/L) devaluates low-density lipoprotein cholesterol calculation by using this formula, effects of low serum triglyceride (<100 mg/dL or 1.13 mmol/L) on its accuracy is less defined. Two hundred thirty serum samples were assayed during a one-year period. In 115 samples, the triglyceride level was below 100 mg/dL and in 115 samples from age- and sex-matched patients the triglyceride level was 150 - 350 mg/dL (1.69 - 3.95 mmol/L). In both groups total cholesterol was above 250 mg/dL (6.46 mmol/L). On each sample, total cholesterol, high-density lipoprotein cholesterol, and triglyceride were directly measured in duplicate and low-density lipoprotein cholesterol measured directly and calculated with Friedewald equation as well. Statistical analysis showed that when triglyceride is <100 mg/dL, calculated low-density lipoprotein cholesterol is significantly overestimated (average: 12.17 mg/dL or 0.31 mmol/L), where as when triglyceride is between 150 and 300 mg/dL no significant difference between calculated and measured low-density lipoprotein cholesterol is observed. In patients with low serum triglyceride and undesirably high total cholesterol levels, Friedewald equation may overestimate low-density lipoprotein cholesterol concentration and it should be either directly assayed or be calculated by a modified Friedewald equation. Using linear regression modeling, we propose a modified equation."

Iranian (2008) LDL Formula:
$$LDL = TC / 1.19 + TG / 1.9 - HDL / 1.1 - 38 \ (mg/dL)$$

Typical Example
Iranian Cholesterol Equation vs Friedewald Equation

Actual Test Results	Friedewald Equation	Iranian Equation
Total Cholesterol	243	243
HDL	66	66
Triglycerides	58	58
LDL (calculated)	166	137
CT / HDL	3.7	3.7
LDL / HDL	2.5	2.1

Obtaining a Blood Test without a Physician's Prescription

Laboratory Corporation of America® and its affiliate, HealthCheckUSA®, will perform any of a large number of health screening tests without a doctor's prescription, and they provide a very detailed report of the results via the Internet and/or mail. You can elect to have a physician interpret the results at additional cost, or you can interpret the test results yourself from information on the report if you are self-trained. Websites and medical references provide information to assist you in understanding your test results. Any test result out of the normal range will be indicated and should be reviewed with greater concern.

HealthCheckUSA® provides an index of services on their website, including the VAP® Cholesterol Test that measures all of the cholesterol subfractions.

"The VAP™ cholesterol test is a comprehensive lipoprotein analysis. It provides a direct measurement of total cholesterol, LDL-C, HDL-C, VLDL-C, Lp(a), and triglycerides. Additional reported information includes the qualitative assessment of LDL particle size, HDL subfractions (HDL2-C and HDL3-C), and VLDL subfractions (VLDL 1+2-C, VLDL3-C, and IDL-C). The VAP™ cholesterol test is in compliance with current NCEP ATP III recommendations, and the additional information provided (beyond conventional lipoprotein profiles) relates to emerging risk factors and the metabolic syndrome as recognized in the report."

HealthCheckUSA® will also have a trained professional visit your home to take the necessary samples at an additional cost if desired, and you will receive the report with your results in the mail. All of this can be done without leaving your home.

An appointment and a 12-hour fast are required before the blood is drawn. Simply make the appointment in the early morning and eat breakfast afterward. Some services allow you to walk in without making an appointment after you have selected the tests and made payment via the Internet website.

HealthCheckUSA® affiliates have nearly 10,000 centers strategically located in all 50 states. Many doctors use these laboratories to conduct health screenings for their patients. Because HealthCheckUSA® helps hundreds of thousands of health-conscious consumers throughout the U.S., they can offer health screenings at some of the most affordable prices in the nation. Simply order your tests online and take the order to your nearest testing center.

Lifestyle Risk Factors

I am positive that the standard low-fat, high-carbohydrate diet is a high risk factor for diabetes, heart disease, and cancer. In all likelihood, this is the diet your cardiologist recommends if he complies with the guidelines of the American Heart Association®, *2010 USDA My Plate*, prestigious medical clinics, and medical schools at major universities.

People who are in the transition stage between hypoglycemia and early diabetes are at the highest risk because glucose, insulin, triglycerides, fibrinogen, and LDL_{3a} are all at lifetime highs. Diabetes is 100% preventable on the diet I present, but all English-speaking countries have raging epidemics of diabetes, heart disease, and cancer because health authorities promote the low-fat, high-carbohydrate diet.

The low-fat diet is a risk factor for heart disease.

Taking a statin cholesterol-lowering drug while eating the standard low-fat diet that causes surging glucose and insulin will not stop the advancement of heart disease, much less reverse it as the general public has clearly demonstrated. Don't expect statin drugs and the low-fat diet to prevent or reverse heart disease no matter how many recommendations you read from prestigious medical clinics, medical schools, professional health organizations, and government health departments that state otherwise. These groups have big microphones, numerous publications, and vast financial resources; but they don't have science to support their claims.

Chapter 3

Bacteria Causes Coronary Artery Disease

The evidence that bacteria can cause coronary artery disease is mounting daily. Fragments of bacteria have been found encased within coronary artery plaque, indicating they may have been initially involved. Statistical evidence has shown that people with a high level of bacteria in the mouth, bad breath, gum disease, bacteria in the nose, and other infections throughout the body have a higher incidence of coronary artery disease. Some of the typical bacterial infections that may place a person at risk for heart disease include:

- Helicobacter pylori - can cause stomach ulcers

- Chlamydia pneumoniae - can cause pneumonia

- Mycoplasma pneumoniae - another cause of pneumonia

- Hemophilus influenzae - bacteria that cause ear and upper respiratory infections

- Gum disease

The coronary artery plaque may have begun to form when bacteria invaded the lining of the artery. The body's typical response to the bacterial attack is to alarm the macrophages and patch up the damage with cholesterol. The evidence is strong that bacteria can and do cause coronary artery disease.

Systemic Diseases Caused by Oral Infection
Clinical Microbiology Reviews,
October 2000, p. 547-558, Vol. 13, No. 4
http://cmr.asm.org/cgi/content/full/13/4/547

"Recently, it has been recognized that oral infection, especially periodontitis, may affect the course and pathogenesis of a number of systemic diseases, such as cardiovascular disease, bacterial pneumonia, diabetes mellitus, and low birth weight. The purpose of this review is to evaluate the current status of oral infections, especially periodontitis, as a causal factor for systemic diseases. Three mechanisms or pathways linking oral infections to secondary systemic effects have been proposed: (i) metastatic spread of infection from the oral cavity as a result of transient bacteremia, (ii) metastatic injury from the effects of circulating oral microbial toxins, and (iii) metastatic inflammation caused by immunological injury induced by oral microorganisms. Periodontitis as a major oral infection may affect the host's susceptibility to systemic disease in three ways: by shared risk factors; subgingival biofilms acting as reservoirs of gram-negative bacteria; and the periodontium acting as a reservoir of inflammatory mediators. Proposed evidence and mechanisms of the above odontogenic systemic diseases are given."

Doctors have been treating infections of the heart muscle and blood vessels for decades. However, new studies in Germany and elsewhere have shown that bacterial infections can also cause the formation of arterial plaque. Parts of dead bacteria have been observed in arterial plaque since the early 1990s. The immune system fights the arterial infection by attacking the invader. The invader that has penetrated into the arterial wall is killed and encapsulated, resulting in inflammation and arterial plaque that restricts the blood flow in the artery. This condition can also occur in other arteries, including the carotid artery in the neck and the arteries in the legs. Plaque in these areas leads to stroke and peripheral artery disease.

A study in the Indian Journal of Medical Microbiology suggests that bacterial infection could cause coronary artery disease.

Infectious Aetiology in Acute Coronary Syndromes
Indian Journal of Medical Microbiology
Year 2002 | Volume : 20 | Issue : 2 | Page : 83-87

Chapter 3

"**Purpose:**

To ascertain the relationship between seropositivity to chronic infections with *Helicobacter pylori, Chlamydia pneumoniae* and *Cytomegalovirus* (CMV) and acute coronary syndromes and association of each of these infective agents with biochemical parameters and cardiovascular risk factors.

Methods:

The present study was a case-control study involving 117 patients [unstable angina (UA) n=101 and chronic stable angina (CSA) n = 16] attending cardiology clinic. The cases were aged 35-79 years and they were compared with age, sex and socio-economic status matched controls without evidence of coronary artery disease (CAD).

Results:

Fifty seven (58%) patients with UA and 9(56%) patients with CSA were seropositive for H. pylori. Sixty seven (66%) subjects with UA and 15(94%) patients with CSA subjects were seropositive for *C.pneumoniae*. Two (2%) patients with USA were seropositive for *Cytomegalovirus* (CMV). Seropositivity in normal subjects for H. pylori, *C. pneumoniae* and CMV was 7(43.25%), 10(62.5%) and 1(6.25%) respectively. In linear regression analysis seropositivity of CMV showed positive association with HDL-C (P< 0.05). No significant association of infective agents and coronary syndromes was observed.

Conclusions:

Higher levels of lipids, lipoproteins, C-reactive protein and higher percentage of coronary risk factors in patients seropositive for H. pylori in UA suggests the role of infective agents in pathogenesis of atherosclerosis."

232

Other studies have confirmed that bacterial infections may be a causal factor in the development of cardiovascular disease.

Infection's Role in Heart Disease
BBC News - January 8, 2002
http://news.bbc.co.uk/2/hi/health/1747507.stm

"Evidence suggesting that infections may contribute greatly to heart disease, has been reinforced by researchers.

While lifestyle and genetics are likely to play the greater role in the development of the killer illness, many doctors now accept there are other factors at work.

In particular, it is thought exposure to lingering infections may create the conditions necessary for heart arteries to narrow and harden, a process called atherosclerosis.

A study, published in the journal Circulation on Tuesday, has found a direct association between the number of infections to which a cardiac patient has been exposed, and the likelihood of death in the following three years.

Which came first?

However, it is still impossible to rule out the possibility that sicker cardiac patients fall prey to more infections because of their weakened condition, not the other way around.

A group of researchers from Johannes Gutenberg University in Mainz, Germany, looked at 572 heart patients.

They tested for antibodies in the bloodstream which would show that the immune system had at some stage been exposed to a variety of different viruses and bacteria.

These included herpes simplex 1 and 2, which cause cold sores and genital herpes, Epstein-Barr virus, which causes mononucleosis, Chlamydia, flu virus and Helicobacter pylori, which causes stomach ulcers.

Then they looked at the patients again three years later to see how many had survived.

The death rate was 3.1% in patients who tested positive for only a few of the viruses or bacteria, 9.8% for those with four or five, and 15% in those positive for six to eight.

Inflamed tissues

Among those who had the most advanced artery hardening, 20% of those exposed to between six and eight infections had died, compared to 7% of those with three or fewer.

Dr Hans Rupprecht said: "We showed a significant association between the number of infections to which a patient has been exposed and the extent of atherosclerosis in the arteries of the heart, neck and legs."

The reason behind the link is not totally clear, but most likely is the fact that some of the infections can cause inflammation in the body's tissues.

This can last for a long period while the immune system moves to eradicate the infection.

It has been suggested that this inflammation, when present in the lining of the arteries, can contribute to atherosclerosis.

Long-lasting infections

It is possible that aspirin, and cholesterol-lowering drugs, may work partly by reducing this inflammation.

Professor Juan Carlos Caski, from St George's Hospital in London, who specialises in the links between infections and heart disease, told BBC News Online: "It's now reasonable to assume that infections play a part in the development of atherosclerosis.

"This work is quite important because it endorses other results showing that there may be this link, and that it is not just a single infection, but more than one.

'It is likely to be chronic infections - chlamydia, for example, can persist for some time in circulating cells - which could be causing the problem.'"

Doctors and researchers in the United States seem to avoid investigating bacteria and viruses as causes of coronary artery disease. This may be due to their mantra that cholesterol, saturated fats, lack of exercise, overeating, and red meat produce heart disease. These excuses have been anchored in years of tradition that block all unbiased attempts to investigate other lifestyle or environmental factors as possible causes. Research has been suffocated.

Bacteria can cause cardiovascular disease.

Pharmaceutical companies that manufacture cholesterol-lowering drugs, carbohydrate food manufacturers, and vegetarian religious groups swamp the media with their false claims that cholesterol and saturated fat from feedlot steers and eggs cause heart disease. Representatives from these organizations infiltrate universities, medical societies, and government agencies in order to protect their sponsors. Medical schools fear losing research grants from the drug and food manufacturing companies who want to ensure that their products are not implicated in heart disease. True science has been blocked, and heart disease rages as the number two cause of death, having recently dropped behind cancer, which is now the number one cause of death in the United States.

Many news reporters, health organizations, and government health officials repeatedly downplay or deny the role that bacterial infection plays in coronary artery disease. They often state that taking antibiotics will not lower the risk. These are puzzling statements since many deadly bacteria can infect the heart, while others are known to produce lasting health problems. The extensive criticism of antibiotics has become so widespread that people with a known bacterial infection continue to suffer and refuse to take an antibiotic. In many cases, physicians refuse to prescribe antibiotics even though they know that the patient has a harmful bacterial infection or is most likely to have one.

Antibiotics can prevent cardiovascular disease.

Food poisoning kills 4,000 people each year in the United States. Even when the deadly bacteria Escherichia coli (E. coli) has been identified as triggering a widespread outbreak, many health organizations and physicians advise people to abstain from taking an antibiotic that could save their lives. Reporters, health practitioners, and biased organizations often try to deceive us by saying that taking antibiotics is more hazardous than the bacterial infection. Physicians often advise people with severe sore throats to go home and wait for a few days to see if it gets better or worse before they are willing to take a culture or prescribe an antibiotic. This approach can lead to heart diseases that can damage valves or begin the process of plaque formation in the coronary arteries.

For example, rheumatic fever is an inflammatory disease that often damages a heart valve and results in mitral valve prolapse. The Group A streptococcus bacterium cause an infection that is often diagnosed as strep throat or scarlet fever, but these can be treated with antibiotics and the heart disease prevented. In order to guard against heart disease, you should insist that an antibiotic be prescribed to anyone who has a sore throat. I have personally had a physician refuse to write a prescription for a drug because I would not submit to his high risk and expensive procedures. I procured the drug through another channel in order to resolve the issue. If your symptoms could possibly be the result of a bacterial infection, take an antibiotic. I take an antibiotic treatment at least once or twice every year simply as a cleansing treatment or preemptive strike against bacteria.

The entire medical establishment operates under the false premise that giving a patient an antibiotic will give the entire society drug-resistant bacteria. This unscientific phobia is based on the false assumption that antibiotics cause drug-resistant bacteria to evolve, but drug-resistant bacteria have always been around.

The deadly MRSA bacterium
was not created by patients who took antibiotics.

Methicillin-resistant Staphylococcus aureus (MRSA) is a bacterium that is classified as drug-resistant. Hospitals in the United Kingdom have struggled to eradicate this deadly infectious hazard with limited success. Many patients were admitted to the hospital for other health problems, but they contracted the bacterial infection and died. News reporters and health officials continue to claim that the MRSA bacterium evolved because of the overuse of antibiotics, but it has now been revealed that the oceans have been full of MRSA for eons. The theory that MRSA evolved from less deadly bacterial forms has at last been proven to be entirely bogus.

The claim has been made that patients who do not take their entire dose of antibiotic for the prescribed amount of time are allowing drug-resistant bacteria to live and become more virile and widespread. This claim is false for many reasons. Very few antibiotics are 100% effective against any particular bacterial infection and certainly not against all possible bacteria. This ineffectiveness is called *sensitivity* in the drug testing and research industry. So we see that even when a patient takes the prescribed dose for the full amount of time, complete eradication of the bacterial infection seldom occurs. The body's immune system is at work fighting the infection along with the antibiotic and hopefully will clean up the bacteria that remain. Resistant bacteria were always resistant even before the drug was administered. The drug did not create them.

The logic that antibiotics cause drug-resistant bacteria to evolve could also be made about the immune systems in humans and animals. Many humans and animals contract a deadly bacterial infection every year and die when the immune system fails to eradicate the disease. This allows the most resistant and robust bacteria to survive and spread. Does this mean that people and animals who succumb to a bacterial infection are manufacturers of immune system-resistant bacteria? No! Bacteria are not made more resistant by the immune system or by antibiotics. The more robust bacteria were always there and always had the potential to survive longer than the average in the statistical percentage that would resemble the Bell Curve.

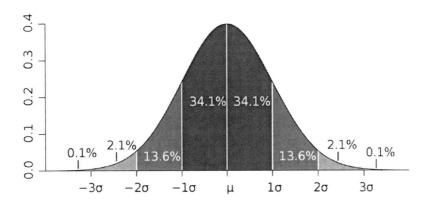

Bell Curve of Standard Deviation Diagram

We know that bacteria cultured from among the strongest survivors do not achieve higher and higher levels of resistance as claimed. If this were so, an evil bacteriologist operating a laboratory in his basement could make a bacterium that could destroy the world by culturing bacteria with higher and higher resistance to both antibiotics and the immune system. No! It just isn't so!

Physicians who refuse to give an antibiotic to a patient who has a sore throat or digestive distress from possible food poisoning are putting the patient at severe risk for a deadly bacterial infection. Why do doctors place the patient's life at risk? Most doctors have bought into the false theory that antibiotics create drug-resistant superbugs, and they accept the false reasoning that risking your life is worthwhile for the benefit of all mankind. They have been brainwashed to believe that you should be sacrificed for the good of society.

Take an antibiotic if you have a sore throat.

Pharmaceutical companies, carbohydrate food manufacturers, and vegetarian religious groups have swamped the media with false claims that feedlot steers create drug-resistant bacteria when they are given antibiotics. People are so brainwashed by this false claim that they ignore any contrary evidence or discussion. Vegetarians condemn feedlot steers because they have an agenda. They believe that brainwashing gullible people will discouraged them from eating beef, including outrageously expensive pasture fed beef. Why should vegetarians care if meat eaters consume feedlot steers or pasture fed cattle? It is a dishonest and clever ploy to trick naive and gullible people into restricting their consumption of animals.

Where are the superbugs that are created by giving antibiotics to farm animals or people? MRSA was not created this way because it has been scientifically proven that MRSA has always existed as a common bacterium of the oceans. Farm animals are not being overcome with deadly infections and wiped out by the imaginary drug-resistant bacteria. This is a science book, and I don't accept the science fiction antibiotic paranoia.

Feedlot steers do not create drug-resistant bacteria.

We know that antibiotics do not promote the evolution of super drug-resistant bacteria because the military has not developed a super-bacteria bomb. Military laboratories cannot propagate the most robust bacteria over and over until they have created a super-bacteria bomb. They may have the smallpox bacterium as a biological weapon, but they did not create the bacterium. In the same manner, lizards cannot be bred to selectively produce offspring that are bigger and stronger until the researcher has created a new Tyrannosaurus rex. The theory that antibiotics create drug-resistant bacteria is as much science fiction as the propagation of a lizard into a Tyrannosaurus rex.

There are several sources for newly discovered drug-resistant bacteria. Environmental researchers tromp through the deep jungles in Brazil, Borneo, and other countries where civilized men have never been. They discover many new animal and insect species before they fly back to New York City, carrying and spreading all of the exotic bacteria on their bodies, clothing, equipment, and luggage. The same is true of deep sea divers. NASA made little attempt to prevent spreading Earthly contamination to the Moon and Mars, and the efforts to prevent reverse contamination from the Moon were hardly effective. Thankfully, the Moon is sterile.

Reducing Your Risks for a Bacterial Infection

We should choose our antibiotic carefully to ensure it is the best choice for the bacterial threat and has the lowest side effects, but the general public has become so paranoid about antibiotics that they shudder at the thought of taking a drug even though their lives are at risk.

We are generally unaware that exposure to bacteria in the home and in public places can be extreme. Everything may appear to be clean when it is actually a cesspool of bacterial contamination. You may think you are cleaning the house, but you are actually spreading dangerous pathogenic bacteria. The following are some dangers:

Dirty Pets

Frankly, I do not recommend having any live pets in the house. These include cats, dogs, snakes, lizards, birds, insects, or anything else. Cats look cute as they groom themselves by licking their paws and washing their faces. Don't believe it. Cats carry staphylococcus aureus to which they are totally immune. The bacterium does not make the cat sick, but it will make you and your children sick. The staph bacterium is in the litter pan, transfers to the paws, and is tracked all over the house. I know a woman who had at least ten cats locked in a room. They were not allowed to roam the house, but everyone who entered the room to care for them tracked pathogens all over the house. She developed a serious infection in the area of the knee at the location where her knee contacted the floor when she knelt down. The drug she took caused a ruptured tendon and left her with a permanent disability. Yes, cats can cause you to die or become crippled for life.

Young children are highly susceptible to picking up pathogens on the floor because they crawl around on their hands and knees and place their fingers in their mouths.

Several years ago, a female patient in the United Kingdom was stricken with drug-resistant MRSA. The infection was eradicated after extensive treatment with a host of antibiotics. The infection returned a few weeks later and she was treated and cured again. Later it happened for the third time. The medical staff at the hospital launched an investigation and found that her cat was a carrier of the deadly MRSA bacterium. Yes, your cat can kill you. Bye, bye, kitty.

Household pets can cause your death.

Dogs are nearly as bad as cats at spreading germs. They lick everywhere and everyone. I see people on television who allow a dog to lick their mouths and noses. This is a totally irresponsible presentation since the viewers include children and childish adults.

Dirty Kitchen Dishcloths

Laboratory tests have shown that kitchen dishcloths are filthier than the toilet. Spilled food is wiped up into the fibers where it becomes food for a breeding culture of pathogenic bacteria. The moisture provides a perfect Petri dish. Change the cloth daily and wash it in a disinfectant such as chlorine bleach. Water with hydrogen peroxide (3% strength) is also a very good disinfectant. In addition to one of these cleaning steps, hang the clean cloth outside in the sun to dry. A normal washing machine and dryer are not good enough to disinfect laundry. Disinfectants such as chlorine bleach, quaternary, pine oil products like Pine-Sol®, or a phenolic product like Lysol®, are also good choices to add to the wash.

Another method for disinfecting kitchen dishcloths is to spread the cloth flat on a cookie sheet or baking dish. Prepare a mixture of 75% water and 25% hydrogen peroxide and fully cover the cloth with the mixture. Allow the cloth to remain for one hour, rinse, and dry in the sun.

Dirty Cutting Boards and Countertops

Cutting boards and countertops are susceptible to the accumulation of pathogenic bacteria. They should be cleaned daily with something other than a quick water wipe. A mixture of 75% water and 25% hydrogen peroxide (3% strength) can be used. Occasional contact with the hands and other skin is okay but use gloves for extended use.

Infants and Children

Infants and children are like little biohazards. They touch everything and everywhere, put their fingers in their mouths, get sick, and spread their germs to others. Daycare centers are like pathogenic bacteria and virus factories. This is why the children are sick so often.

Dirty Shopping Carts

Supermarkets have finally come to realize that the handle on the shopping cart is the filthiest thing you or your infant could touch. Many stores are providing sanitizing wipes at the entrance to clean your cart handle, although it is only marginally effective. Cross contamination is 100% because children hold onto the cart handles and then place their fingers in their mouths.

The infant seat on the cart should be called *Sewerville*. Fecal matter can escape from the infant's diaper and soil the seat. Shoppers often place food items in the seat area of the cart where they become contaminated. The carts are most likely never cleaned, and the little wipes at the entrance only spread the germs. Wash your hands well as soon as you get home.

Sneeze-Launched Airborne Bacteria and Viruses

Everyone backs up, turns away, or holds his breath when someone sneezes. I know I do. The cold medication aisle in the supermarket is the place to avoid during the flu season. I have seen tests and videos taken by high-speed cameras that show the slow motion spray of pathogen-ladened mist discharged by a sneeze. The mist from someone else's sneeze is extremely hazardous to your health.

Dirty Door Handles, ATM Buttons, and Public Computers

Anything that many people touch ranks high as a source of bacteria and viruses. People with bacterial or viral infections will pick their noses or touch their fingers to their mouths before touching door handles, handrails on stairways, safety guardrails, restaurant menus, pens and pencils, pointers at credit card signing stations, ATM buttons, public computer keyboards, and countertops.

Dirty Money

Money is one of the dirtiest things we touch and carry with us because it transfers pathogens from person to person. My favorite fast food restaurant has a policy that the employees do not touch a customer's cup when he returns for a coffee refill. Instead they fill a new cup and give it to the customer. This is fine, but the employee will also work the cash register, handle money, and fill orders at the same time. The cash register procedure violates the company policy intended to reduce the transfer of pathogens from person to person.

Medical Offices and Hospitals

We would like to think that medical offices and hospitals are clean and sterile, but the opposite is true. People with infections and contagious diseases who go to medical offices and hospitals for treatment will give their illness to someone else and pick up another ailment themselves.

A friend had quadruple heart artery bypass surgery. While he was recovering, the physician's assistant used her bare finger to touch and inspect the incision on his leg where a vein had been removed. You guessed it. He developed a severely resistant staph infection that required four weeks of treatment with multiple antibiotics.

Injury and Surgical Wound Infections

Water is not sterile unless it is specially treated, and it can easily carry bacteria to a wound or the site of a surgical incision where the bacteria quickly multiply. The best method of treatment is to keep the area completely dry after proper cleaning with boiled water that has been cooled or UV lamp-treated reverse osmosis water. Add hydrogen peroxide (3% mixture) in the ratio of 25% hydrogen peroxide to 75% water. Dry the wound with sterile gauze and apply the triple-antibiotic cream.

Surgical incisions that have been closed with sutures must be kept dry. The physician may tell you that taking a shower after three days is permitted, but don't do it. This is not a good idea because the sutures wick the water into the depth of the incision along with bacteria. The best treatment before taking a shower is to apply triple-antibiotic cream to the incision and sutures and cover the area with a plastic shield. Use a plastic sandwich bag or quart-size freezer bag and place tape along the bottom end and two sides. Position the bag upside down over the incision area with the tape at the top to shield the area like a shower curtain. Dry yourself completely before removing the shield. This protective procedure is well worth the effort.

Dirty Noses

The nasal passages harbor infectious bacteria that live on the surfaces of the nasal hair and skin. The immune system is not alerted because the infection is not blood borne. Patients in hospitals were found to have infected their own postoperative incisions by transferring pathogenic cultures from other areas of the body, particularly the nasal passages. Surgeons frequently swab the nasal passages with an antibiotic prior to surgery while the patient is sedated. The antibiotic I prefer for home use is ZYMAR® (gatifloxacin ophthalmic solution 0.3%) by Allergan that is generally prescribed as an antibiotic eye drop. It is available internationally from Magic Pharma at www.magicpharma.com.

Fungal and candida yeast infections in the nasal passages are common problems that persist for months or years if they are not treated by a physician or the patient. I describe the best treatment in more detail in Chapter 5. Grossman Breathe-ease XL is an over-the-counter product available on the Internet. This is an excellent product formulated and sold by Dr. Murray Grossman, M.D., an otolaryngologist (ear, nose, and throat medical specialist). Saline nasal spray is an alternative nasal moisturizer.

Bad Breath

Bad breath is a sure sign that the mouth, nasal passages, and colon have an infestation of undesirable bacteria. A stinging sensation upon urination is a sign that the infection has spread to the bladder and/or kidneys. Bad breath may be a sign of a systemic infection that should be treated as such.

Dirty Feet

Our feet get neglected unless they start to hurt. We wash our hands many times a day, but the feet may not be given a thorough washing even during the daily shower. Socks and heat cause the feet to sweat and provide a perfect environment for bacterial and fungal growth. The symptoms of bacterial colonies on the feet may not be obvious when open sores are not present, but a sure symptom is the feeling that the feet are abnormally hot. The body senses bacteria tying to invade the skin, which activates the immune system and raises the temperature.

The feet should be thoroughly washed with soap during the daily shower. Pour diluted hydrogen peroxide over each foot while in the shower on a monthly basis to kill the pathogens. Rub the feet with the hands to ensure a good cleaning and rinse with the shower water. Wash and rinse the feet daily.

Feet are very susceptible to fungal infections. An inexpensive but effective treatment is to add two tablespoons of sodium bicarbonate (common baking soda) to a pan of water. Soak the feet for ten minutes and rinse with clean water.

Food Poisoning Considerations

Food poisoning is very common. I recall being sickened at least nine times within the last ten years; once by rotten seafood, twice by a soft-serve ice cream sundae with chopped nuts, three times by dirty coffee, once by raw green peppers, once from an undercooked beef burger, and once by contaminated lamb ribs. I grilled the lamb ribs that had decorative diamond-pattern slices made by the butcher. Previously, I had grilled the same delicious lamb ribs without the slice pattern. Both of these ribs were cooked until medium rare. However, the ribs with diamond-pattern slices must have had bacterial contamination deep within the marks because I became ill a few hours later. I was prepared and quickly responded by taking 500 mg of Keflex® antibiotic. The treatment cured me within hours, but I continued the treatment for five days just to be certain it would not return. If you suspect that food has made you sick, take the antibiotics immediately. If your suspicions are correct, you will begin to recover quickly, but if you fail to treat food poisoning, your life could be in danger.

Take an antibiotic if you suspect food poisoning.

Restaurants have developed a scripted response to your complaint that their food made you sick. First, they ask you when you ate there. Suppose you answer by saying, "I ate at your restaurant and got sick five hours later." They will claim, "Oh, you couldn't have gotten sick from your meal at our restaurant. It takes three days for the symptoms to appear." No matter what time span you give, they always have an excuse that will nullify your claim. Food poisoning symptoms can actually appear within 30 minutes or less for some bacterial contaminations to as long as three days depending upon the pathogen.

Chapter 3

Vegetable salads are the most common source of deadly food poisoning because rinsing raw vegetables does not remove the pathogenic bacteria. Some pathogens are locked in the cells of the plant and can't be removed by washing in any manner. Four thousand people each year die in the United States from food poisoning and most from raw salads. The mass media will give headline news to anyone who becomes ill from eating meat but tend to hush up the story when the food poisoning is from vegetables. However, they have a more difficult time silencing a nationwide government recall of vegetables as occurred with contaminated spinach a couple of years ago. When multiple people die from the same contaminated source, the story is hard to hide.

> **E. coli infections kill 6, sicken hundreds in Germany, officials say**
> CNN News – May 30, 2011
> http://edition.cnn.com/2011/WORLD/europe/05/30/germany.e.coli/
>
> "(CNN) -- An E. coli outbreak linked to some raw vegetables has killed at least six people and sickened hundreds in Germany, national and global health authorities said Monday.
>
> The first investigation results released by the German federal unit responsible for disease control and prevention -- the Robert Koch Institute, under Germany's Ministry of Health -- indicated that the most recent infections were likely caused by consuming raw tomatoes, cucumbers and lettuce."

Food prepared for a large group should be avoided. Large containers of potato salad may have been placed in the refrigerator immediately after preparation, but the center of the container stays warm for a long period of time. The pathogens grow, multiply, thrive, and survive even though the container is refrigerated. The salad becomes deadly by the time it is transported, stored, and served at the gathering.

Food poisoning from coffee or tea occurs frequently since the current trend is to lower the brewing temperature so the customer cannot complain that a spill scalded him. Pots with rubber pumpers are a super high-risk design because the rubber is a breeding ground for pathogens and is difficult to clean. Spherical glass brewing pots are the best, particularly when the brewing water is kept near the boiling point.

Meat is not the source of deadly food poisoning as often as you are made to believe. Meat is very safe when it is thoroughly cooked. Grilled meat should be handled and turned with a clamp tool, not stabbed with a fork that pushes the pathogens from the external area of contamination into the center. Steaks cooked properly can safely be eaten with raw centers. The outside is seared to decontaminate the surface, and the untouched center is naturally clean. Eating raw meat (except pork or chicken) is perfectly safe when properly prepared. When in doubt, cook it thoroughly.

Keflex® (cephalexin) has now become my drug of choice for effectively treating food poisoning, although Flagyl® (metronidazole) is better for a broad spectrum of pathogenic and deadly bacteria and has been shown to be one of the drugs of choice for deadly Clostridium difficile (C. diff) and Escherichia coli (E. coli) infections in the colon. In another incident, I noticed that my beef burger was slightly pink in the center, but it was too late. I had eaten most of it and told Marti, my wife and editor of this book, that I would watch carefully to see if any negative symptoms developed. Sure enough, a few hours later, my stomach began to hurt. I immediately took one 500 mg capsule of Keflex. Later that day, I felt fine but took another capsule each day for two more days. Don't wait for food poisoning to get worse before taking action as many health clinics and physicians recommend. It could save your life in the near term and prevent heart disease in the long term.

Campylobacter jejuni is a bacterium that causes severely debilitating gastroenteritis. It is rarely fatal but is responsible for approximately 70% of the food poisoning worldwide. It is a Gram-negative, microaerophilic bacterium commonly found in mammal and bird feces, poorly prepared food, and raw milk. Symptoms include abdominal pain, fever, malaise, diarrhea, and bloody stools. Campylobacter jejuni can develop into Guillain-Barré syndrome (GBS), a disorder affecting the breathing muscles and peripheral nervous system, within two to three weeks after the initial illness. The drugs of choice are ciprofloxacin, moxifloxacin, levofloxacin, imipenem-cilastatin, meropenem, azithromycin, clarithromycin, and erythromycin. Treatment with ciprofloxacin is effective in 90% of cases and should included fluid and electrolyte replacement.

Cleanup of Undesirables and Pathogenic Bacteria

The diet I present in this book promotes a healthy immune system, and it does not contain the high levels of carbohydrates and fiber that encourage the proliferation of pathogens in the colon. A routine or annual colon cleanup with an antibiotic is recommended to clear the colon of bad bacteria that creep into the digestive tract. This is a healthy procedure when done correctly. Even those who show no sign of pathogenic bacteria in a stool analysis should take a treatment of antibiotics to eliminate these bacteria that could be continually disturbing digestion. Flagyl® (metronidazole) is the recommended prescription drug of choice for a broad spectrum of pathogenic and deadly bacteria and has been shown to be one of the drugs of choice for Clostridium difficile (C. diff) and Escherichia coli (E. coli) infections in the colon. An annual treatment should be considered to clear the digestive tract of pathogenic infections. Take 7.5 mg of Flagyl® per 2.2 pounds (1.0 kg) of body weight three times per day. A 150-pound person would take 500 mg three times per day for 10 days or as recommended by his doctor. Flagyl ER® (metronidazole extended release) is a good choice at 750 mg per day for 10 days or as recommended by your doctor.

An annual antibiotic treatment is a healthy practice.

Keflex® (cephalexin) is another generally well-tolerated drug to kill Escherichia coli bacteria as well as other pathogenic bacteria in the digestive tract, but it is not effective against Clostridium difficile. Take one 500 mg capsule three times per day for 5 days and reduce to one 500 mg capsule one time per day for 10 days or as recommended by your doctor.

Ciprofloxacin and ofloxacin have the undesirable side effect of possible tendon weakness, damage, or rupture, and they are not effective against Clostridium difficile infections in the colon. A visible side effect is marks or grooves in fingernails as they grow out. Do not take ciprofloxacin or ofloxacin in high doses or for an extended period of time because it can cause severely ruptured tendons. As an alternative, begin by taking 250 mg of ciprofloxacin two times per day with meals (breakfast and dinner) for the first two days, followed by 250 mg once per day with breakfast for five more days or as recommended by your doctor. As another alternative, take one 300 mg ofloxacin tablet with breakfast for five days. Doxycycline may have fewer side effects but is not as effective.

Chapter 3

Probiotics Replace Pathogenic Bacteria

Probiotics should also be taken at the same time when taking an antibiotic in order to replace the undesirable floras with these better choices. Take one each of the following two probiotics three times per day with meals for 10 days followed by one each per day with breakfast on a continuous basis. The daily supply of these good probiotics helps to prevent the growth of undesirable bacteria. Do not substitute other probiotics and don't take acidophilus because stomach acid simply kills the flora. Eating yogurt is not recommended.

- Bacillus Coagulans by Thorne Research are hearty and can be purchased and shipped without refrigeration.

- Multidophilus Lactic Flora by Solaray must be purchased locally from a refrigerated display case, taken directly home, and placed in the refrigerator as soon as possible.

People with the experience and training in self-administering drugs can purchase drugs for personal use online without a prescription on the following international websites. The drugs must be approved by the Food and Drug Administration (FDA) in the United States. The FDA does not prevent importation when the drugs are for personal use and do not appear to present a serious risk. Individuals can also travel to foreign countries for medical treatment, where drugs are prescribed by a doctor. The patients must continue to receive their drugs upon their return to the United States. Some foreign Internet companies provide a medical service by which a doctor can issue a prescription. The FDA can refuse importation of prescription and non-prescription drugs, and the U.S. Customs Service may return the shipment to the supplier.

Previous orders placed with the following pharmacies have been very satisfactory:

GenericDoctor.com
InternationalDrugMart.eu
Medformula.com
MedicinesMexico.com
Medrx-one.com
UnitedPharmacies.com

The following quotation from a USFDA manual addresses the topic of importation of prescription drugs for personal use. The law does not allow this practice, but the system in the United States has been overwhelmed by the volume of shipments. Some members of the U.S. House of Representatives and Senate have attempted to change the law without success. This is reminiscent of the 55-mph speed limit on the highways in the 1970s and 1980s when the average citizen refused to obey the unreasonable law. The pharmaceutical companies are fighting hard to keep people from buying lower-priced prescription drugs from foreign manufacturers. Health insurance companies should be pleased because people pay for the drugs themselves. The importation reduces government health care costs, but some bureaucrats go ballistic when they lose control over the citizens.

FDA - Regulatory Procedures Manual March 2008, Chapter 9 "Coverage of Personal Importations"

"PURPOSE

To provide guidance for the coverage of personal-use quantities of FDA-regulated imported products in baggage and mail and to gain the greatest degree of public protection with allocated resources.

BACKGROUND

Because the amount of merchandise imported into the United States in personal shipments is normally small, both in size and value, comprehensive coverage of these imports is normally not justified. This guidance clarifies how FDA may best protect consumers with a reasonable expenditure of resources.

There has always been a market in the United States for some foreign made products that are not available domestically. For example, individuals of differing ethnic backgrounds sometimes prefer products from their homeland or products labeled in their native language to products available in the United States. Other individuals seek medical treatments that are not available in this country. Drugs are sometimes mailed to this country in response to a prescription-like order to allow continuation of a therapy initiated abroad. With increasing international travel and world trade, we can anticipate that more people will purchase products abroad that may not be approved, may be health frauds or may be otherwise not legal for sale in the United States.

In addition, FDA must be alert to foreign and domestic businesses that promote or ship unapproved, fraudulent or otherwise illegal medical treatments into the United States or who encourage persons to order these products. Such treatments may be promoted to individuals who believe that treatments available abroad will be effective in the treatment of serious conditions such as AIDS or cancer. Because some countries do not regulate or restrict the exportation of products, people who mail order from these businesses may not be afforded the protection of either foreign or U.S. laws. In view of the potential scale of such operations, FDA has focused its enforcement resources more on products that are shipped commercially, including small shipments solicited by mail-order promotions, and less on those products that are personally carried, shipped by a personal non-commercial representative of a consignee, or shipped from foreign medical facility where a person has undergone treatment.

PERSONAL BAGGAGE

FDA personnel are not to examine personal baggage. This responsibility rests with the CBP. It is expected that a CBP officer will notify their local FDA district office when he or she has detected a shipment of an FDA-regulated article intended for commercial distribution (see GENERAL GUIDANCE below) an article that FDA has specifically requested be detained, or an FDA regulated article that appears to represent a health fraud or an unknown risk to health.

When items in personal baggage are brought to FDA's attention, the district office should use its discretion, on a case-by-case basis, in accordance with the guidance provided under GENERAL GUIDANCE below, in deciding whether to request a sample, detain the article, or take other appropriate action.

MAIL SHIPMENTS

FDA personnel are responsible for monitoring mail importations. It is expected that a CBP officer from the CBP Mail Division will examine a parcel and will set it aside if it appears to contain a drug, biologic, or device, an article that FDA has specifically requested be held, or an FDA-regulated article that appears to represent a health fraud or unknown risk to health. FDA should audit those parcels set aside by CBP in accordance with the guidance provided under GENERAL GUIDANCE below, using the following procedures:

Prepare a Collection Report for each parcel sampled. Generally, a physical sample is not required on mail importations because a documentary sample (for example, labeling, labels and inserts) will be sufficient for most regulatory purposes. If a physical sample is needed, collect only the minimum necessary for analysis by the laboratory. The remaining portion should not be removed from the custody of the CBP Mail Division. Importations detained in accordance with this guidance should be held by CBP until they are either released or refused entry. Attached as guidance are two specimen letters that may be sent with the Notice of Detention and Hearing when a parcel is detained. (See Exhibit 9-3 for use in general mail importations and Exhibit 9-4 for use in unapproved drug or device mail importations).

On occasion, products detained by FDA will be mixed with non-FDA-regulated products. When we refuse admission of the FDA-regulated portion, any request for the release of the non-FDA-regulated portion should be referred to the CBP Mail Division with a Notice of Refusal of Admission covering the detained article. Final disposition of all merchandise, including the destruction of detained merchandise, is the responsibility of CBP.

GENERAL GUIDANCE

The statements in this chapter are intended only to provide operating guidance for FDA personnel and are not intended to create or confer any rights, privileges, or benefits on or for any private person. FDA personnel may use their discretion to allow entry of shipments of violative FDA regulated products when the quantity and purpose are clearly for personal use, and the product does not present an unreasonable risk to the user. Even though all products that appear to be in violation of statutes administered by FDA are subject to refusal, FDA personnel may use their discretion to examine the background, risk, and purpose of the product before making a final decision. Although FDA may use discretion to allow admission of certain violative items, this should *not* be interpreted as a license to individuals to bring in such shipments."

Are Internet Drugs Safe?

Before purchasing drugs on the Internet, it is best to review the manufacturers' authenticity and standards by looking on their websites prior to placing orders. When the drugs are received, they should be sealed in special bubble-wrap packages with the manufacturer's name, drug name, and dosage clearly printed. The complexity of the package and the printing indicate that the drugs are genuine. Tablets or capsules that are packaged loose in a plain bottle or simple box are totally unacceptable. You can expect the package to have been opened by U.S. Postal Service employees for inspection.

Some of the above suppliers ship high-quality generic and name-brand drugs from multibillion dollar international pharmaceutical companies, such as Ranbaxy Laboratories® (India); GlaxoKlineSmith® (United Kingdom); CIPLA, Limited® (India); Sun Pharmaceuticals Industries, LTD.® (India); Surya Pharma® (India); Unichem Laboratories Limited® (India); Mega Fine Pharma® (India); Ind-Swift Limited® (India); Dr. Reddy's Pharmaceutical Company® (worldwide); and Stada Arzneimittel AG® (Germany). Avoid all drugs made in China. Ask your pharmacist if your current prescription drugs are made in China.

Are Prescription Drugs Bad for Us?

Some prescription drugs have been found to cause death, and the USFDA has pulled many off the market. Other drugs have serious negative side effects, but the bad drugs should not be used as a standard for labeling all drugs as unacceptable. Many drugs are awesome.

Scientific Causes of Cardiovascular Diseases

Viruses Cause Heart Disease

Viruses are strongly suspected to cause coronary artery disease in humans and have been proven to be the cause for atherosclerosis in chickens. The evidence that viruses cause coronary artery plaque is not easily detected because of their small size, unlike larger bacteria or bacteria body parts that have been found embedded in the plaque. The immune system is better able to engulf the viruses at the infection site and remove them from the body. However, healing of the site within the lining of the heart artery begins the process that builds a deposit of plaque, which contains cholesterol, protein scar tissue, calcium, and fats. The following viruses are the leading suspects linked to coronary artery disease.

- Herpes simplex 1 and 2
- Human Cytomegalovirus (HCMV), or Herpes-5 (HHV-5)
- Chlamydia pneumoniae
- Helicobacter pylori
- Epstein-Barr, which causes mononucleosis
- Coxsackie B_4
- Herpesviridae

A study in the *Indian Journal of Medical Microbiology* suggests that viral and bacterial infections could one of the causes of coronary artery disease.

Infectious aetiology in acute coronary syndromes
Indian Journal of Medical Microbiology
Year 2002 | Volume: 20 | Issue: 2 | Page: 83-87

"Inoculation of chicken with avian herpes virus produced arterial disease that resembled human atherosclerosis. Several authors have reported association of coronary artery disease (CAD) with gram negative bacteria (*Helicobacter pylori* and *Chlamydia pneumoniae*) and with certain herpes viruses (*Cytomegalovirus*). Endothelial injury or dysfunction, smooth muscle proliferation, local inflammation,7 chronic inflammation, cross reactive antibodies or changes in cardiovascular risk factors are proposed mechanisms for the reported associations between infections and CAD. The possible mechanisms by which *H. pylori, C. pneumoniae* and *Cytomegalovirus* may influence cardiovascular risk are unknown. *H. pylori* and *C. pneumoniae* contain hsp 60 like sub units."

Likewise, researchers in the United Kingdom also confirm that viral and bacterial infections are a likely cause of coronary artery disease. The Coxsackie B4 virus is known to cause Type 1 diabetes by triggering an autoimmune response that destroys the insulin-producing beta cells of the pancreas. The virus invades the beta cells and triggers the immune system to attack the site. In the process, the beta cells are also destroyed, and the pancreas can no longer produce insulin.

Infection and coronary heart disease
J Med Microbiology **46** (1997), 535-539; DOI:
10.1099/00222615-46-7-535
© 1997 Society for General Microbiology
ISSN 0022-2615

R. W. Ellis

Department of Clinical Bacteriology, University Hospital NHS Trust, Queen Elizabeth Medical Centre, Edgbaston, Birmingham B15 2TH

"A large body of evidence exists that implicates a number of microbial agents in the pathogenesis of coronary heart disease (CHD). This, if proven, may have far-reaching implications for the prevention and treatment of CHD and other atherosclerotic disease. The histopathology of atherosclerosis and its natural history suggest infectious causation at many points along the progression of disease, particularly with regard to CHD, and a number of pathogens have been the focus of study. Viral agents implicated include Coxsackie B_4 virus, for which tenuous sero-epidemiological associations exist, and the Herpesviridae. The animal herpesvirus causing Marek's disease in chickens causes atherosclerotic lesions in these animals. Herpes simplex virus I and II have been found in aortic smooth muscle and produce changes *in vitro* in smooth muscle that are similar to those seen at the beginning of atherosclerosis and which may also explain some of the features of atherosclerotic complications. Cytomegalovirus is implicated more strongly sero-epidemiologically by in-vivo detection in atherosclerotic lesions and by its links with post-cardiac transplant vasculopathy - a syndrome similar to atherosclerosis. Bacteria have also been shown to have links with CHD. *Chlamydia pneumoniae* and *Helicobacter pylori* have both been associated sero-epidemiologically with CHD, and these findings have been consolidated by recent work showing their presence in atherosclerotic lesions in adults. Bacterial infections in general lead to many changes in lipid, thrombic and other acute-phase protein metabolism, and some of these changes occur with both *C. pneumoniae* and *H. pylori* infections. The ubiquity and similar epidemiological features to CHD of all these microbial pathogens make the resolution of the causative issue impossible by retrospective means. All that can be shown at present are a variety of weak and strong links, the significance of which can only be determined by large and perhaps lifetime prospective studies."

The growth of viruses can be stimulated by some supplements. Arginine speeds the growth rate of viral infections, including Epstein-Barr (EBV), Human Cytomegalovirus (HCMV) or Herpes-5 (HHV-5), and Herpes Simplex I or II, all of which are strongly suspected to be causal factors in the development of coronary artery disease. Arginine should not be taken even though some references recommend it as a supplement for optimal cardiovascular health. It triggers insulin and glucagon release, which is undesirable for a healthy cardiovascular system since insulin is the primary cause of coronary artery disease. Arginine is another example of a dietary supplement that is incorrectly recommended for cardiovascular health. This is not to say that arginine is not beneficial in many ways, but I do not recommend supplemental arginine because of the negative effects.

However, I do recommend lysine because it lowers triglycerides and suppresses viruses, but it does not eradicate chronic viral infections. Lysine should be taken in the amount of 500 mg once or twice per day.

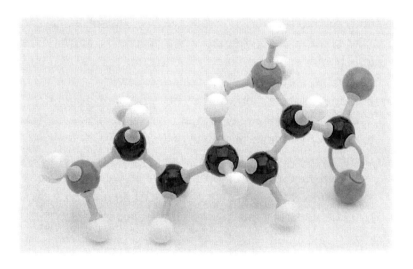

Lysine Amino Acid Molecule
May Prevent Viral Coronary Artery Disease

Omega-6 Vegetable Oils Cause Heart Disease

Vegetable oils contain a very high percentage of fatty acids called *omega-6 polyunsaturated fatty acids* that are extracted from grains, seeds, and nuts. These refined oils are sold worldwide in supermarkets and by wholesalers in bulk containers to restaurants, food manufacturing companies, and retailers. We obtain these fats in our diet from manufactured foods or from grains, seeds, and nuts. The liver can make saturated fats and monounsaturated fats but cannot make polyunsaturated fats.

Omega-6 polyunsaturated fatty acids from vegetable sources are more common in arterial plaque than saturated fats that we have been told to avoid. As a result of my scientific research, I have discovered the reasons why these fats are unhealthy.

Vegetable oils are bad fats.

The first clue that polyunsaturated fatty acids are unhealthy comes from the fact that they quickly turn rancid when left at room temperature. Polyunsaturated fatty acids are made from molecules that have empty electron bonds in the structure that attract and attach to oxygen and hazardous elements such as heavy metals and free radicals (any undesirable compound or molecule with a free electron looking for an empty site in which to bond) to form an unhealthy compound. This is the very same chemical process that occurs when we see iron combined with oxygen to form rust and corrosion. Polyunsaturated fatty acids have the ability to combine with glucose to form unhealthy glycated compounds that can be found in the arterial plaque. The evidence against polyunsaturated omega-6 fatty acids is overwhelming, but the major government health authorities continue to recommend these unhealthy fats as replacements for healthy saturated fatty acids.

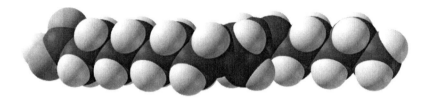

Linoleic Acid – Omega-6 Polyunsaturated Fatty Acid
Common source: Grain, nut, and seed oils

The edible oil industry produces omega-6 polyunsaturated vegetable, seed, and grain oils in vast quantities from maize (corn), soybeans, safflowers, sunflowers, peanuts, and cottonseeds. These oils are thought to be among the leading causes of heart disease and cancer, both of which increase in concert with increases of omega-6 fatty acids in the diet. Omega-6 fatty acids are pro-inflammatory and have been proven to cause or contribute to autoimmune diseases, such as rheumatoid arthritis, asthma, lupus, multiple sclerosis, Crohn's disease, fibromyalgia, irritable bowel syndrome, inflammatory bowel disease, and many others. Avoid these oils like a plague that they are.

Unhealthy Fatty Acid Foods		
Grain Oils	Seed Oils	Most Nut Oils
Vegetable Oils	Omega-6 Fats	Cottonseed Oil
Trans Fatty Acids	Soybean Oil	Corn Oil

Below are the percentages of unhealthy polyunsaturated omega-6 fatty acids contained in the most commonly consumed vegetable oils:

Safflower Oil	(80%)
Sunflower Oil	(68%)
Corn Oil	(57%)
Soybean Oil	(53%)
Cottonseed Oil	(53%)
Peanut Oil	(46%)

Omega-6 Polyunsaturated Vegetable Fats Are Inflammatory

Solid scientific research proves that polyunsaturated omega-6 vegetable fatty acids are highly inflammatory and should be strictly avoided by everyone in order to prevent heart disease, cancer, bowel disease, arthritis, or many other autoimmune diseases. Everyone should severely limit omega-6 fats, such as safflower oil, corn oil, soybean oil, cottonseed oil, peanut oil, and many others. Dr. Robert C. Atkins' book, *Age-Defying Diet Revolution,* and Dr. Michael Eades' book, *Protein Power Lifeplan,* have long sections that describe the unhealthy effects of these oils.

Linoleic acid (LA) is the primary fat in omega-6 fatty acids, and the body uses desaturation and elongation enzymes to change LA into arachidonic acid (AA), the most inflammatory fatty acid. For this reason, the following study warns against the consumption of vegetable oils.

"Dietary polyunsaturated fatty acids and inflammatory mediator production"
http://www.ncbi.nlm.nih.gov/pubmed/10617994?dopt=Abstract

"The pro-inflammatory eicosanoids prostaglandin E(2) (PGE(2)) and leukotriene B(4) (LTB(4)) are derived from the n-6 fatty acid arachidonic acid (AA), which is maintained at high cellular concentrations by the high n-6 and low n-3 polyunsaturated fatty acid content of the modern Western diet." Omega-6 fatty acids should be avoided. They are found in vegetable, seed, and nut oils such as safflower oil, corn oil, soybean oil, peanut oil, and others."

Much has been written recently on the topic of inflammatory and non-inflammatory foods. People are advised to avoid red meat and add more whole grains, nuts, and seeds to their diets. This recommendation is backward. Whole grains, nuts, and seeds are the very sources of the inflammatory omega-6 vegetable fatty acids. Meat is assaulted because it contains a small amount of omega-6 arachidonic polyunsaturated fatty acid (AA), but arachidonic fatty acid is the essential omega-6 fat required in small amounts for good health. Meat provides AA in a healthy ratio with the essential omega-3 fatty acids which are anti-inflammatory.

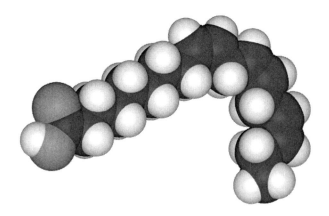

Alpha-linolenic Acid Molecule (ALA)
Healthy Omega-3 Essential Fatty Acid

Omega-3 Polyunsaturated Fatty Acids Lower CVD Risks

Omega-3 polyunsaturated fatty acids (fish oils) are the essential healthy fats that help to prevent cardiovascular disease. The three most nutritionally important omega-3 fatty acids are alpha-linolenic fatty acid (ALA), eicosapentaenoic acid (EPA), and docosahexaenoic fatty acid (DHA). Alpha-linolenic fatty acid is one of two fatty acids traditionally classified as *essential*. The other fatty acid traditionally viewed as essential is an omega-6 polyunsaturated fatty acid called *linoleic acid* (LA) that the body can use to make essential omega-6 arachidonic fatty acid. These fatty acids have traditionally been considered essential because the body is unable to manufacture them on its own and because they play a fundamental role in several physiological functions where deficiencies lead to diseases. As a result, we must be sure our diets contain sufficient amounts of both alpha-linolenic acid and linoleic acid.

Omega-3 fatty acids
lower cardiovascular disease risk.

Omega-3 fatty acids prevent and cure many diseases. They are contained in oils found in the flesh and skin of fish, liver of cod fish, and to a lesser extent in red meat and poultry. Omega-3 fatty acids improve the flexibility of red blood cell membranes, which allows blood to flow more easily to prevent clots. Omega-3 fatty acids are also highly anti-inflammatory. Everyone, including babies and children, should take Carlson's® Lemon Flavored Cod Liver Oil. Previous generations rightly considered cod liver oil to be medicinal even though much of the oil had a high degree of rancidity, which created the dreadful rotten fish taste. The product that I recommend is protected from rancidity and has a very mild flavor. Don't avoid it if you haven't tried it. When my granddaughter was three years old, she said, "More, Papa!" Children are eager to try it when they are told that it helps to keep them from getting sick. Children are more conscious about staying well than some parents believe.

Many highly-credentialed health experts fail to understand the great benefits of cod liver oil and strongly oppose it. They often comment that it contains dangerously high levels of vitamin D. Not true! One would have to eat 30 tablespoons per day for six months to approach a toxic level. I have found that the Carlson's cod liver oil may not contain the amount of vitamin D listed on the label. Therefore, I strongly recommend that you have your vitamin D level check as part of your blood test. Vitamin D is very important for a healthy cardiovascular system, and a deficiency in the general public is epidemic.

The number of diseases for which an omega-3 fatty acid deficiency is one of the causal factors is unlimited. Simply get out the medical dictionary and highlight all diseases. Omega-3 fatty acids perform very subtly, and a deficiency does not immediately jump up to make an announcement. Therefore, people and doctors tend to ignore this important dietary essential. Because breast-fed babies were always known to be healthier than formula-fed babies, omega-3 fatty acids have been added to commercial baby formula within the last few years. Omega-3 fatty acids are one of the reasons that breast-fed babies thrive, but not the only reason.

The Indians and Eskimos of North America lived in excellent health along the northern coasts on a diet of nearly 100% salmon containing very highs level of omega-3 fatty acids and low levels of saturated fats. Omega-3 fatty acids have no unhealthy side effects.

Heart Disease Risk Factors

Heart disease risk factors commonly listed as causal are generally not causes at all but rather symptoms of the true cause. Many of the risk factors are conjectures that have been repeated so many times that people simply assume they are backed by scientific studies. To paraphrase an old adage, "If a lie is repeated enough times, most people will eventually accept it as truth." Even the person or group that started the lie will brainwash themselves to believe the lie has become truth. This is the brainwashing tactic I discussed in *Absolute Truth Exposed – Volume 1.*

I will discuss some of the false claims about the causes and major risk factors for cardiovascular disease. This book presents scientific data that proves these claims are false, but you must study and read until you have deprogrammed yourself from a lifetime of brainwashing by the major media, professional nutritionists, physicians, medical and health associations, universities, government departments of health, and other highly-credentialed authorities. Remember, history has proved time and again that credentials do not necessarily equate to truth. In fact, it seems that the higher one goes on the leadership ladder, the less accurate the information becomes.

I will also discuss how cardiovascular disease can be prevented and reversed. This information must be studied carefully because it will be contrary to the conventional teaching most people have accepted. The information may appear to be confusing for those to have accepted the standard dietary and health risk factors. In fact, it may appear to be opposite to recommendations presented by the major media and numerous health organizations. This is the way I reversed my heart disease.

Chapter 3

Saturated Fats Do Not Cause Heart Disease

In the 1960s, Dr. Ancel Benjamin Keys (January 26, 1904 - November 20, 2004) began his attack on saturated animal fats in milk and meats that continues to this day. His studies and conclusions have since been criticized as unscientific and highly biased. It is now known that Dr. Keys plotted selected data from countries that made saturated fats appear to be linked to coronary artery disease. He ignored countries that would have given the opposite result. He would have discovered the truth had he made a graph of manufactured carbohydrate foods versus natural saturated fats. He should have concluded that carbohydrates cause coronary artery disease. His first study, *Six Country Study (1953)*, and his more famous second study, *Seven Country Study (1958 – 1964)*, gave us the lipid hypothesis for coronary artery disease. The hypothesis proclaims that saturated animal fats and cholesterol are the primary causes of coronary artery disease. The bogus results changed the eating habits in all English-speaking countries and led to millions of early deaths.

Dr. Keys also made the mistake of addressing all animal fats as saturated, when in fact the majority of fats in meats are monounsaturated fatty acids. His promotion of vegetable oils was a serious conflict of interest since the fast-growing vegetable oil industry at the time was funding the attack on animal fats.

The lipid hypothesis is the diet-cholesterol theory for coronary artery disease.

Dr. Keys began his attack when people in the United States were eating meat, eggs, and cheese for breakfast, lunch, and dinner. Cardiovascular diseases and diabetes were not the deadly killers we see today. Dr. Keys started the current dietary dogma that has people eating low-fat grain products, drinking low-fat milk, and stuffing themselves with fruit, fruit, and more fruit.

Dr. Ancel Keys promoted the body mass index (BMI) in an attempt to encourage people to become thinner by eating his low-fat diet that he promised was the optimal path to good health. People followed his dietary guidelines en-masse only to become fat and diabetic. His diet recommendations have since been compared with the data used in his studies and found to have little or no correlation. In other words, his recommendations were based on fraudulent interpretations of the data in order to fulfill his personal agenda.

He formulated the K-rations meals for U.S. soldiers during World War II that the men complained about constantly and avoided eating at every opportunity. The meals were named after Dr. Keys and packaged in a box made by the Cracker Jack Company®, but they were deficient in proper nutrition.

Dr. Ancel Keys retired to Pioppi, Italy, on the Mediterranean Sea, where he formulated and coined the Mediterranean diet. Ironically, he lived to the awesome age of almost 101, and the money he received from the vegetable oil industry for his fraudulent study served him well. But the low-fat, high-carbohydrate diet he thrust upon the world has been a health disaster for everyone else. His lipids hypothesis was bogus from the beginning.

Dr. Keys' assault on saturated animal fats was more than simply substituting animal fats for vegetable fats. It was much more far reaching and affected the dietary habits of all English-speaking people in three major categories.

First, refined omega-6 polyunsaturated vegetable oils did not appear in the human diet before the industrial revolution. Dr.

Keys could not analyze worldwide health results from the consumption of omega-6 vegetable oils because the consumption was minimal, and the oils were dispersed throughout the grains, nuts, or seeds. They were not separated and sold as bulk oils until the mid 1900s. People have been pressing and eating olive oil for thousands of years, but the primary fatty acid is an omega-9 fat, not an omega-6. We now have strong data that show omega-6 fatty acids may be involved in breast cancer, prostate cancer, cardiovascular disease, and other inflammatory diseases. This result was directly opposite to that which Dr. Ancel Keys had promised.

Second, avoiding saturated animal fats means avoiding animal products, red meats, game animals, poultry, fish, seafood, butter, and cheeses. The new diet consisted of vegetable products that are generally low in protein and essential omega-3 fatty acids, and high in carbohydrates. Animal products have a miniscule amount of carbohydrates except for the lactose in milk. This was a major shift from a low-carbohydrate diet to a high-carbohydrate diet.

Third, the vegetable oil industry that was supporting Dr. Keys' research had their eyes on a substitute for saturated animal fats that would be solid at room temperature. The goal was achieved by forcing hydrogen to bond with the vegetable oils in a process called *hydrogenation*. The new molecules that are rarely found in nature were created in a chemical processing plant. These new molecules should never have been considered a fatty acid food because they were actually a grease-like chemical.

Dr. Mary E. Enig, a world-renowned expert in edible oils and fats, warned that the new hydrogenated vegetable oils called *trans fats* should not be considered healthy food sources. Her warnings went unheeded because of massive pressure from the food manufacturing industry. These manufactured chemical fats have been shown to raise the bad LDL cholesterol and lower the good HDL cholesterol. The negative health effects of trans fats are well documented.

I remember my mother buying a large metal container of Crisco®. It looked just like a gallon of paint with a fancy label that said it was *shortening*, not a very descriptive term. It looked like pure white butter. I didn't understand why she needed to use it for frying and making pastry because the butter she used previously tasted better; besides, I churned the butter and it was free because we had a cow. Fully hydrogenated Crisco® is still sold in my neighborhood supermarket.

Thanks to Dr. Ancel Keys' attack on butter, margarine was heralded as the new healthy substitute about 50 years ago, but margarine was made from fully hydrogenated omega-6 vegetable oils with yellow-orange dye to make it look like butter. My mother also bought this product.

Mother's use of sugar in cooking and canning had very negative effects on the family's health. She died from cancer at age 50, and my father died from heart disease at age 56. The steel plant where he worked contributed to the deaths of many workers because they mounted salt tablet dispensers throughout the plant and strongly suggested that the men consume more salt. I believe the switch in the family diet away from animal fats had the worst effect, and I can confidently state that Dr. Ancel Keys killed my parents and nearly killed me.

The false claim that saturated fats cause arterial plaque, diabetes, cancers, and other diseases is repeated in nearly every article, news release, or broadcast concerning health. Because people have accepted this false allegation, it is literally impossible for them to erase it from the volume of brain cells it has implanted. They are unable to believe otherwise no matter how effectively the scientific truth is presented. Many people will read this entire book and summarily turn away saying, "I still think saturated fats cause heart disease." The brainwashing has been going on for decades, and any change in the public or experts' thinking is not in sight. It's so severe in some individuals that they've told me the thought of eating saturated fat, especially animal fat, makes them gag and practically vomit. They frown and scowl when they look at animal fats either raw or in the cooked meat. The degree of brainwashing is irreversible. They don't care about science. Their brains are locked up.

Books, literature, and websites are exploding with the statement, "Artery-clogging, long-chain saturated fats are derived from animals." This statement has one major scientific error. The fats found in clogged arteries are primarily polyunsaturated omega-6 fatty acids from whole grains, seeds, most nuts, and vegetable oils—not from red meat or other animal fats.

Studies of primitive people who were never brainwashed have shown that humans prefer eating animal flesh with a high fat content and also enjoy pure fat. I enjoy eating fat as found in meat, butter, cheese, or by itself. A chunk of fat is delicious.

The science behind saturated fatty acids as a causal factor for cardiovascular disease is completely nonexistent. Well documented studies have shown that people who ate the most saturated fat had the lowest weight and lowest incidence of heart disease. Saturated fats do raise LDLs slightly in some studies, but the larger increase in HDLs gives a higher ratio of HDL/LDL, which is an improvement in the risk factors for cardiovascular disease. The constant attack on saturated fats by professional nutritionists, physicians, health organizations, and government health agencies is based on pure emotional conjecture. In plain language, it's a big fat lie.

The U.S. government has funded study after study in an attempt to find a connection between dietary fat and coronary artery disease without success. These studies often entail fraudulent guidelines that the researchers hope can be twisted to condemn saturated fats. One tricky method is to place both the control and the test subjects on a high-carbohydrate diet similar to the *UDSA Food Guide Pyramid.* The saturated fats are increased in the test subjects in the attempt to prove saturated fats are unhealthy. The test only shows that carbohydrates and saturated fats are not a good combination. A test comparing a low-carbohydrate diet to a high-carbohydrate diet has always shown that carbohydrates increase cardiac risk factors, while saturated fats in the absence of carbohydrates reduce these risk factors.

Saturated animal fats do not cause heart disease.

The following study with postmenopausal women shows that a higher saturated fat intake is associated with less progression of coronary atherosclerosis, whereas a higher carbohydrate intake is associated with a greater progression. Women shun animal fats more so than men. Perhaps this is the reason heart disease has moved from second place to the number one cause of death in women.

Dietary fats, carbohydrate, and progression of coronary atherosclerosis in postmenopausal women
Dariush Mozaffarian, Eric B Rimm and David M Herrington
http://www.ajcn.org/content/80/5/1175.abstract

From the Channing Laboratory, Department of Medicine, Brigham and Women's Hospital and Harvard Medical School, and the Departments of Epidemiology and Nutrition, Harvard School of Public Health, Boston (DM and EBR); the Health Services Research and Development Program, Veterans Affairs Puget Sound Health Care System, Seattle (DM); the Cardiovascular Nutrition Laboratory, Jean Mayer US Department of Agriculture Human Nutrition Research Center on Aging at Tufts University, Boston (AHL and ATE); and the Section on Cardiology, Department of Internal Medicine, and the Department of Public Health Sciences, Wake Forest University, Winston-Salem, NC (DMH)

"**Background:** The influence of diet on atherosclerotic progression is not well established, particularly in postmenopausal women, in whom risk factors for progression may differ from those for men.

Objective: The objective was to investigate associations between dietary macronutrients and progression of coronary atherosclerosis among postmenopausal women.

Design: Quantitative coronary angiography was performed at baseline and after a mean follow-up of 3.1 y in 2243 coronary segments in 235 postmenopausal women with established coronary heart disease. Usual dietary intake was assessed at baseline.

Results: The mean (±SD) total fat intake was 25 ± 6% of energy. In multivariate analyses, a higher saturated fat intake was associated with a smaller decline in mean minimal coronary diameter ($P = 0.001$) and less progression of coronary stenosis ($P = 0.002$) during follow-up. Compared with a 0.22-mm decline in the lowest quartile of intake, there was a 0.10-mm decline in the second quartile ($P = 0.002$), a 0.07-mm decline in the third quartile ($P = 0.002$), and no decline in the fourth quartile ($P < 0.001$); P for trend = 0.001. This inverse association was more pronounced among women with lower monounsaturated fat (P for interaction = 0.04) and higher carbohydrate (P for interaction = 0.004) intakes and possibly lower total fat intake (P for interaction = 0.09). Carbohydrate intake was positively associated with atherosclerotic progression (P = 0.001), particularly when the glycemic index was high. Polyunsaturated fat intake was positively associated with progression when replacing other fats (P = 0.04) but not when replacing carbohydrate or protein. Monounsaturated and total fat intakes were not associated with progression.

Conclusions: In postmenopausal women with relatively low total fat intake, a greater saturated fat intake is associated with less progression of coronary atherosclerosis, whereas carbohydrate intake is associated with a greater progression."

Saturated fatty acids do not have any empty electron bonding site. This is the reason that coconut oil can be left on the counter for as long as one year without turning rancid. Coconut and palm oils are rare in the vegetable species because they are primarily saturated fats—not polyunsaturated fatty acids.

Saturated fatty acids do not attract heavy metals, free radicals, or glucose. They do not become oxygenated and do not stick to other molecules in the body where they are not intended to be. Saturated fatty acids are not found in coronary arterial plaque in the percentages we are led to believe. The consumption of saturated animal fats has decreased in the United States for the last 100 years as heart disease and the consumption of polyunsaturated vegetable oils have increased dramatically.

In the following study, the researchers concluded that saturated fat actually prevents coronary artery disease. This is directly contrary to the widely published advice from government health authorities that saturated fat should be kept below 10% of dietary calories.

Chapter 3

Saturated fat prevents coronary artery disease?
An American paradox

Robert H Knopp and Barbara M Retzlaff
http://www.ajcn.org/content/80/5/1102.full

Northwest Lipid Research Clinic, University of Washington School of Medicine, Seattle, Washington, USA

"It is an article of faith that saturated fat raises LDL cholesterol and accelerates coronary artery disease, whereas unsaturated fatty acids have the opposite effect (1, 2). One of the earliest and most convincing studies of the better efficacy of unsaturated than of saturated fat in reducing cholesterol and heart disease is the Finnish Mental Hospital Study conducted in the 12 y between 1959 and 1971. In this study, the usual high-saturated-fat institutional diet was compared with an equally high-fat diet in which the saturated fat in dairy products was replaced with soybean oil and soft margarine and polyunsaturated fats were used in cooking. Each diet was provided for 6 y and then the alternate diet was provided for the next 6 y (3). After a comparison of the effects of the 2 diets in both men and women, the incidence of coronary artery disease was lower by 50% and 65% after the consumption of polyunsaturated fat in the 2 hospitals.

In this issue of the Journal, Mozaffarian et al (4) report the opposite association. They found that a higher saturated fat intake is associated with less progression of coronary artery disease according to quantitative angiography. How can this paradox be explained? In food-frequency questionnaires, saturated fat intake is more precisely estimated than is total fat. If saturated fat is more precisely estimated, it will associate more strongly in statistical analyses with the outcome variable, even though other variables—such as total fat or carbohydrate—could be more relevant physiologically. We believe that these possibilities deserve a closer look.

278

Unlike the diet used in the Finnish Mental Hospital Study, the diet described by Mozaffarian et al was low in fat, averaging 25% of energy. The study subjects were women with coronary artery disease: most were hypertensive, many had diabetes (19–31%), their body mass index (kg/m^2) ranged from 29 to 30, and their lipid profile indicated combined hyperlipidemia (triacylglycerol concentration: 200 mg/dL; HDL-cholesterol concentration: 40–50 mg/dL; above-average LDL concentration: 135–141 mg/dL); these characteristics are consistent with the metabolic syndrome. In addition, two-thirds of these women were taking sex hormones. The importance of each of these points is addressed below.

What are the effects of a low-fat, high-carbohydrate diet in comparison with those of a higher-fat, lower-carbohydrate diet? The response differs by the 2 main types of hyperlipidemia: simple hypercholesterolemia and combined hyperlipidemia. In our studies of simple hypercholesterolemia in men, a fat intake <25% of energy and a carbohydrate intake >60% of energy was associated with a sustained increase in triacylglycerol of 40%, a decrease in HDL cholesterol of 3.5%, and no further decrease in LDL in comparison with higher fat intakes (5). In contrast, a low-fat diet in persons with combined hyperlipidemia caused no worsening of triacylglycerol or HDL, but intakes of fat >40% of energy and of carbohydrate <45% of energy for 2 y were associated with a lower triacylglycerol concentration at a stable weight (6). In the subjects of Mozaffarian et al, a greater saturated fat intake paralleled a total fat intake, which ranged from 18% to 32% of energy in the first to fourth quartiles. Modest favorable trends in triacylglycerol and HDL-cholesterol concentrations were observed with higher fat intakes.

Triacylglycerol and HDL-cholesterol concentrations are stronger predictors of coronary artery disease in women, whereas the LDL-cholesterol concentration is a stronger predictor in men (7). Because VLDL triacylglycerol secretion and removal rates in healthy women are double those of men (8), conditions impairing lipoprotein removal would be expected to exaggerate the hyperlipidemic response in women as compared with that in men (9). This sex difference is seen with the development of diabetes. The increment in lipids is greater in women than in men and is associated with a greater increment in coronary artery disease risk in women than in men (9). Similarly, the development of insulin resistance and obesity is associated with a greater lipoprotein increment in women than in men (10). The exaggerated decreases in HDL- and HDL_2-cholesterol concentrations observed with the consumption of a low-fat Step II diet in women but not in men appear to be another facet of this effect (11).

The failure of female sex hormones to prevent coronary artery disease has been a great disappointment (9). This effect might also be due to an estrogen-induced increase in lipoprotein entry against a fixed or impaired rate of lipoprotein removal, as might be expected in women with the metabolic syndrome and coronary artery disease.

Would saturated fat still be bad for anyone? Not necessarily. The effect of saturated fat and cholesterol ingestion in the form of 4 eggs/d for 1 mo in obese, insulin-resistant subjects is 33% of that seen in lean, insulin-sensitive subjects, likely because of diminished cholesterol absorption (12). Thus, the classic effects of saturated fat as compared with those of unsaturated fat seen in the Finnish Mental Hospital Study are likely blunted in the subjects of Mozaffarian et al, whereas the effects of low fat and high carbohydrate intakes on triacylglycerol and HDL-cholesterol concentrations appear to be exaggerated by the interactions of female sex, exogenous sex hormones, and the metabolic syndrome. A major effect on cardiovascular disease risk would be the result of hypertriglyceridemia and low HDL-cholesterol concentrations, which are attenuated by an increase in saturated fat intake itself or in total fat intake, for which saturated fat is a more statistically stable surrogate (4).

In conclusion, the hypothesis-generating report of Mozaffarian et al draws attention to the different effects of diet on lipoprotein physiology and cardiovascular disease risk. These effects include the paradox that a high-fat, high–saturated fat diet is associated with diminished coronary artery disease progression in women with the metabolic syndrome, a condition that is epidemic in the United States. This paradox presents a challenge to differentiate the effects of dietary fat on lipoproteins and cardiovascular disease risk in men and women, in the different lipid disorders, and in the metabolic syndrome."

See the full report for the numbered references.

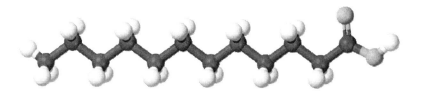

Lauric Acid - Saturated Fatty Acid
Common sources: Mothers' breast milk and coconut oil

Carbon atoms (dark) along the spine of the lauric acid molecule have hydrogen atoms (light) attached at all the electron bonding sites, hence the term *saturated*. Empty electron sites prevent harmful molecules from attaching. Saturated fats in cell membranes provide a stable shield against attack by heavy metals and oxygen molecules. This is why saturated fats have scientific support for their cancer prevention properties. Saturated fats do not coat the linings of the arteries, and they do not form atheromatous plaque as erroneously stated by many unscientific medical sources. Saturated fats are very healthy foods. The following study found that eating coconut oil reduced abdominal fat in women because it contains lauric acid, a medium chain saturated fat.

Effects of Dietary Coconut Oil on the Biochemical and Anthropometric Profiles of Women Presenting Abdominal Obesity

Monica L. Assunção, Haroldo S. Ferreira, Aldenir F. dos Santos, Cyro R. Cabral and Telma M. M. T. Florêncio
http://www.springerlink.com/content/02ngg2413wm2w630/

"Abstract

The effects of dietary supplementation with coconut oil on the biochemical and anthropometric profiles of women presenting waist circumferences (WC) >88 cm (abdominal obesity) were investigated. The randomised, double-blind, clinical trial involved 40 women aged 20–40 years. Groups received daily dietary supplements comprising 30 mL of either soy bean oil (group S; $n = 20$) or coconut oil (group C; $n = 20$) over a 12-week period, during which all subjects were instructed to follow a balanced hypocaloric diet and to walk for 50 min per day. Data were collected 1 week before (T1) and 1 week after (T2) dietary intervention. Energy intake and amount of carbohydrate ingested by both groups diminished over the trial, whereas the consumption of protein and fibre increased and lipid ingestion remained unchanged. At T1 there were no differences in biochemical or anthropometric characteristics between the groups, whereas at T2 group C presented a higher level of HDL (48.7 ± 2.4 vs. 45.00 ± 5.6; $P = 0.01$) and a lower LDL:HDL ratio (2.41 ± 0.8 vs. 3.1 ± 0.8; $P = 0.04$). Reductions in BMI were observed in both groups at T2 ($P < 0.05$), but only group C exhibited a reduction in WC ($P = 0.005$). Group S presented an increase ($P < 0.05$) in total cholesterol, LDL and LDL:HDL ratio, whilst

HDL diminished ($P = 0.03$). Such alterations were not observed in group C. It appears that dietetic supplementation with coconut oil does not cause dyslipidemia and seems to promote a reduction in abdominal obesity."

The North American Plains Indians lived in excellent health for centuries on a diet that was nearly 100% buffalo meat of which 75% was fat containing high levels of saturated fats. Both groups proved that vegetables, fruits, and grains are essential in a healthy diet, and animal fats in the diet at any level provide excellent health. The picture below was taken in 1892 at Ft. Washakie, Wyoming. It reveals the slender, rugged health of the elderly Shoshone Indians prior to being sent to a reservation. Chief Washakie extends his right arm as some of the Shoshones dance. The likelihood that the Plains Indians developed diabetes and coronary artery disease is negligible because they ate very few carbohydrates.

Today, September 18, 2011, I was listening to a radio program sponsored by the American Indians. They were announcing an upcoming meeting, a pow-wow where they sell hand-crafted products and enjoy native dance and music. Food will be provided, and Indian fry bread is the favorite. The host mentioned that fry bread was a "reservation food" that her people had not eaten prior to being placed on the reservation, where they were told to eat wheat instead of game animals. She called it "fried dough" and said, "What could be wrong with that?" The inference was that the fried dough is a wonderful food. How wrong she was. Fry bread may be the number one cause of the obesity, diabetes, cancer, and heart disease epidemics on the reservations today. The American Indians and Alaskan Inuits are 1.6 times as likely to be obese than Non-Hispanic whites. Much is wrong with fry bread.

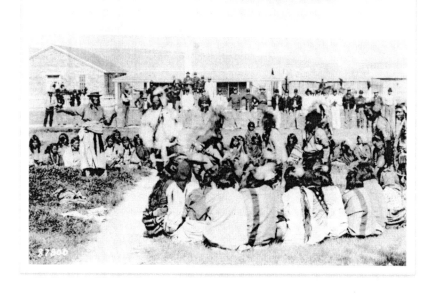

Shoshone Indians at Ft. Washakie, Wyoming, in 1892
Today they live in the beautiful Wind River Valley, Wyoming, but
have high levels of obesity, diabetes, and heart disease.

Saturated animal fats actually reversed my heart disease. My diet that I present in this book is extremely high in saturated animal fats with a total absence of vegetable fats and olive oil. The results are a reduction in heart artery plaque of 50% in only 25 months based on the analysis of two angiogram heart catheter procedures performed by a highly trained cardiologist with extensive experience. He has placed heart stents in approximately 2,000 patients.

Saturated animal fats are an important part of my diet regimen because they raise the level of good HDL cholesterol and change the harmful LDL cholesterol from the most hazardous LDL$_b$ subfraction to the less harmful LDL$_a$ subfraction as measured by Berkeley HeartLab, Inc. The HDL cholesterol is also changed to a high percentage of the most protective HDL subfraction and a lower percentage of the less protective HDL subfraction. In other words, everything moved in the right direction to reverse and prevent cardiovascular disease. The results are amazing, and I show my personal cholesterol test data in Chapter 4 directly from the laboratory reports.

Healthy Fatty Acid Foods		
Animal Fats	Arachidonic Acid	Saturated Fats
Fish Oils	EPA Omega-3	DHA Omega-3
Butter	Coconut Oil	Mono Fats
Palm Oils	Hard Cheeses	Eggs

The low-fat diet causes HDL cholesterol to plunge. HDL cholesterol cleans the arteries by capturing and removing LDL cholesterol from the arterial plaque deposits. Low HDL is a high risk factor, yet it is not listed as a risk factor at all in most heart disease literature patients receive in the doctor's office or find in literature racks in the hospital cardiac unit.

The low-fat diet also causes the LDL to shift from the less harmful LDL_b subfraction to the more hazardous LDL_a subfraction. The standard low-fat, high-carbohydrate diet recommended for diabetics causes the hazardous LDL_a cholesterol to skyrocket.

French women have the lowest rate of heart disease in the western world even though they consume high levels of butter, cheese, and animal fats. France is reported to have 265 brands of cheese that typically contain 65–70% fat on a calorie basis, and 45–50% of these fats are saturated. French women have been healthier because of their high levels of saturated fats and low levels of sugar and refined carbohydrates in the diet. The confused low-fat dietitians have come to know this high level of saturated fat and low heart disease rate as the French Paradox. Yes, it is a paradox to them because the false guidelines they follow are pure conjecture and prejudicial assumptions. Sadly, the French are beginning to turn away from their natural foods to manufactured high-carbohydrate foods.

French women prove that a diet high in saturated fats achieves the lowest rate of heart disease.

The Thai people are another paradox. They have a very low level of heart disease and diabetes, but they consume exceedingly high levels of saturated fats from coconut oil and pork lard.

The Greek Mediterranean Diet has been touted as healthy because it contains olive oil and fish. Indeed, fish is a healthy food, but the Greeks consume high levels of saturated fats in feta cheese, butter, lard, and poultry fats. Those who claim the Mediterranean Diet is low in saturated fats are simply wrong. The Italians eat a similar diet, and both consume high levels of carbohydrates in the form of pasta. Obesity, diabetes, cancer, and heart disease are worse than in the United States. The Italians were thinner and healthier 50 years ago, but today the Italian children are the most obese in Europe as the amount of saturated fats in the diet have decreased and carbohydrates have increased.

The Okinawans have earned the title *The Longest-Lived People on Earth*. Questionable claims have been made about the Okinawa diet, attributing their extra longevity to the consumption of seafood, fruits, and vegetables. The fact that the Okinawans consumed a lot of pork, lard, and saturated fats from coconut oil and swine has been hidden and distorted. The Okinawans also have a low incidence of coronary heart disease (CHD) as shown in the following table.

The Okinawa Centenarian Study			
Rank	Country	Life Expectancy	CHD
1	Okinawa	81.2	13
2	Japan	79.9	22
3	Hong Kong	79.1	40
3	Sweden	79.0	102
8	Italy	78.3	55
10	Greece	78.1	55
18	USA	76.8	100

http://www.okicent.org/
Sources: Sources: World Health Organization 1996;
Japan Ministry of Health and Welfare 1996

"**Makoto Suzuki MD PhD** is a cardiologist and geriatrician. He is Professor Emeritus and former Director of the Department of Community Medicine at the University of the Ryukyus in Okinawa, Japan. Currently, he is Director, Okinawa Research Center for Longevity Science, in Urasoe, Okinawa. He recently retired from his position as professor in the Department of Human Welfare at Okinawa International University. He is Principal Investigator of the Okinawa Centenarian Study, a Japan Ministry of Health-funded study of the world's healthiest and longest-lived people. The study is entering its 31st year and is the longest continuously running centenarian study in the world."

Okinawa is a small mountainous island only 60 miles (96.5 km) long and 9 miles (14.5 km) wide in the western Pacific Ocean south of Japan. It had not been heavily industrialized, and the economy and people were rather poor compared to the large industrialized nations.

The features aided in the longevity of the Okinawans for the following reasons:

- Their weather comes from the vast Pacific Ocean and provides clean, fresh air; and the country has relatively low industrial pollution.

- The ocean provides easy access to seafood.

- The mountain people raised pigs as the primary meat supply because pigs are the most productive farm animals, and their religion did not forbid the consumption of pork and saturated fats.

- The mountains prohibited the growing of vast areas of grains such as wheat, corn, and rice.

- The economy did not provide sufficient income for the people to import foreign foods such as sugar, grains, vegetable oils, fruits, fruit juices, and potatoes.

- The economy had very few food manufacturing plants that turn sugars, grains, and potatoes into boxes and bags of high-carbohydrate foods.

The Okinawians ate a diet of meat from pigs, chickens, and fresh seafood; and avoided high-carbohydrate, high-fiber foods, such as whole grains, legumes, starchy vegetables, and sugars. They also avoided bad omega-6 vegetable oils and consumed large quantities of fresh animal fats and coconut oil. Okinawans included pork and lard in almost every dish and were proud of the fact that they "used every part of the pig except the squeal."

The United States ranks 18th in the Okinawa Centenarian Study with a life expectancy of 76.8 years and a baseline coronary heart disease rating of 100. This is no surprise considering all the handicaps that Okinawa did not have.

The United States has the following disadvantages:

- Burdened with the USDA Food Guide Pyramid
- Highly industrialized with people living in large cities
- Expansive plains ideally suited for growing grains
- Expansive farmland ideally suited for growing potatoes
- Expansive farmland for growing sugar beets
- Mega food manufacturing plants
- Expensive seafood
- Inexpensive pork but the people are told to avoid it
- Medium-priced beef but the people are told to avoid it

The United States spends more on health care than any other country in the world, but the results are dismal. Even so, life expectancy continues to creep upward. The following tables show the life expectancy at birth for people in the United States for the years 1980 through 2007. This increase has been achieved by heroic efforts during the later years of life and the significant achievements in treating coronary artery disease with stents and open heart surgery as well as outstanding success in heart valve replacement. Heart surgery, diagnosis, and drug treatment have made amazing advancements in the last 20 years. Life expectancy in the United States between the years 1980 and 2007 rose from 77.4 years to 80.4 years for females and from 70.0 years to 75.4 years for males.

Whites have a considerably longer life expectancy than blacks in all categories. This can most likely be attributed to a lower standard of living and the consumption of inexpensive manufactured carbohydrate foods. They are also likely to consume less protein from meat, poultry, seafood, and fish. The result is an increased consumption of sugars that leads to obesity, diabetes, heart disease, and cancer. The lower average income prohibits them from obtaining the necessary medical care to treat their diet-related health problems.

Life Expectancy at Birth, United States, 1980–2007						
	All Races			Male		Female	
Year	All	Male	Female	White	Black	White	Black
1980	73.7	70.0	77.4	70.7	63.8	78.1	72.5
1990	75.4	71.8	78.8	72.7	64.5	79.4	73.6
2000	76.8	74.1	79.3	74.7	68.2	79.9	75.1
2007	77.9	75.4	80.4	75.9	70.0	80.8	76.8

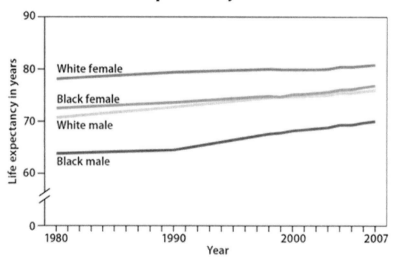

Life expectancy at birth

Respondent-reported lifetime heart disease prevalence

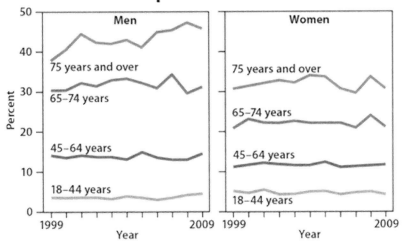

Source: CDC/NCHS, Health, United States, 2010, Figure 1
Data from the National Vital Statistics System

Heart disease was the leading cause of death in 2007 at 25%, followed closely by cancer at 23%. This trend shifted in 2010, and cancer is now becoming the leading cause of death with heart disease a close second. The heart disease death rate actually declined in those over age 65 but still accounted for 28% of the deaths in 2007. However, it still remained the leading cause of death among the elderly.

According to new longevity statistics prepared by the Organization for Economic Cooperation and Development (OECD) and released on November 25, 2011, longevity has increased in most countries. However, the United States and United Kingdom have not fared as well as others as shown in the following table. The media often blame the expensive medical systems in these two countries for the poor performances instead of pointing the finger at the real culprit—government dietary recommendations.

The medical establishment in the United States is among the best in the world. We have access to the finest pharmaceuticals, most advanced diagnostic and scanning technologies, and the most highly-trained surgeons; but these treatments cannot overcome the excessive carbohydrate consumption by those who follow the low-fat diet recommendations of the *USDA Food Guide Pyramid*.

In 1996, longevity in the United States was 76.8 years according the World Health Organization. In the same year, longevity in Japan was 79.9 years according to the Japan Ministry of Health and Welfare. The 2011 news report placed Japan at 86.4 years vs 80.6 years in the United States. The gap between the two countries is increasing, and the United States is moving lower and lower in the ranking against other countries in each subsequent survey. Okinawa is not listed in the most recent survey because it is one of Japan's southern prefectures, not an independent country.

OECD Longevity Data, November 25, 2011		
Rank	**Country**	**Life Expectancy**
1	Japan	86.4
2	Spain	84.9
3	Switzerland	84.6
4	France	84.4
5	Australia	83.9
6	Korea	83.8
7	Israel	83.5
23	United Kingdom	81.8
27	United States	80.6

http://stats.oecd.org/index.aspx?DataSetCode=HEALTH_STAT

Scientific Causes of Cardiovascular Diseases

We have hundreds of thousands of books, millions of web pages, dozens of universities, hundreds of medical clinics, numerous religious groups, and millions of physicians claiming that saturated fats cause heart disease. It's no wonder that 99.99 % of the world's population believe this most popular lie. Government health and human services in the United States have failed the people. The number of major health departments in the United States Department of Health and Human Services alone is staggering. Rather than helping, these government organizations actually contribute to the poor health and obesity epidemics. These departments are:

> Administration for Children and Families (ACF)
>> Administration for Children, Youth and Families (ACYF)
>
> Administration on Aging (AoA)
> Agency for Healthcare Research and Quality (AHRQ)
> Agency for Toxic Substances and Disease Registry (ATSDR)
> Centers for Disease Control and Prevention (CDC)
> Centers for Medicare and Medicaid Services
> Food and Drug Administration (FDA)
> Health Resources and Services Administration (HRSA)
> Indian Health Service (IHS)
> National Institutes of Health (NIH)
>> National Cancer Institute (NCI)
>
> Office of the Inspector General (OIG)
> Substance Abuse and Mental Health Services Administration (SAMHSA)

Those who proclaim that saturated fats cause heart disease continue to ignore the scientific truth. In doing so, they cause this dreaded disease to continue unabated. This type of mass brainwashing is very common throughout the history of mankind.

My wife and I were having dinner with another couple at a Chinese restaurant, and he was eating roast duck while avoiding

293

the skin and fat. I mentioned that the Chinese do not avoid the saturated fat as commonly believed and falsely stated in books, recipes, and website. He challenged my statement by calling the waiter to our table and asking him the question, "Do the Chinese avoid the fat in your personal diets?" He replied immediately, "No! We eat the fat. We also collect the extra fat for a special meal once a month. We eat only fat for this meal. We believe the fat purges the body and makes us clean."

The claim that saturated fats cause heart disease is the world's biggest lie.

Harvard University participated in several very large studies to gain insight into the effects of diet on health and disease. These major studies should certainly give us information needed to establish dietary recommendations based on scientific studies. I have voiced my opinion, but you may want to see the conclusion from an independent source. Carefully read the following quotation from Wikipedia about these studies:

Lipid
From Wikipedia, the free encyclopedia
http://en.wikipedia.org/wiki/Lipid#Metabolism

"A few studies have suggested that total dietary fat intake is linked to an increased risk of obesity and diabetes. However, a number of very large studies, including the Women's Health Initiative Dietary Modification Trial, an eight year study of 49,000 women, the Nurses' Health Study and the Health Professionals Follow-up Study, revealed no such links. None of these studies suggested any connection between percentage of calories from fat and risk of cancer, heart disease or weight gain. The Nutrition Source, a website maintained by the Department of Nutrition at the Harvard School of Public Health, summarizes the current evidence on the impact of dietary fat: "Detailed research—much of it done at Harvard—shows that the total amount of fat in the diet isn't really linked with weight or disease.""

The Nurses' Health Study
http://www.channing.harvard.edu/nhs/

Women's Health Initiative Dietary Modification Trial
http://www.nhlbi.nih.gov/whi/diet_mod.htm

Health Professional Follow-up Study
http://www.hsph.harvard.edu/hpfs/

What?
Harvard studies show the total amount of fat in the diet isn't really linked to weight or disease.

Harvard University was given millions of dollars by the United States Department of Health and Human Services to manage health studies. The Department of Nutrition at the Harvard School of Public Health has summarized the current evidence on the impact of dietary fat.

> "Detailed research—much of it done at Harvard—shows that the total amount of fat in the diet isn't really linked with weight or disease."

So what does Harvard Medical School now recommend regarding the amount of fat in the diet in the Harvard Health Publication, *Focus on Nutrition, Part 1 of 3,* February 20, 2011?

"Nutrition 101: Good eating for good health"

"Total fat: 25–35% of total calories"

"Saturated fat: Less than 7% of total calories"

Chapter 3

Harvard University's major studies show there are no links between the amount of dietary fat and weight or disease, yet they continue to recommend a very low-fat diet that would constitute a very high-carbohydrate intake directly associated with weight gain and disease. The studies were ignored, and recommendations were made that are directly opposite to the results of the three major studies.

The inconsistencies among dietary recommendations promoted by health studies, medical schools, professional dieticians, and government health organizations have left truth seekers confused and frustrated. Supporters can be found for any diet related health claim, but seeking the majority opinion is not the answer either. Out of frustration, patients often turn to their physicians for dietary recommendations without realizing that doctors receive very little nutritional training in medical schools. Factions have consolidated into diet-philosophy groups in which people are pressured into siding with one group or another. Those who opt out often say they simply eat a balanced diet.

Are you convinced that eating natural animal fat is healthy and will heal your body? If not, you most likely will not be able to reverse or prevent heart disease as I have done. Do you believe saturated animal fats plug the arteries as claimed by your physician, religion, health insurance provider, employer, family members, favorite books, or millions of websites? If so, you most likely will not be able to reverse or prevent heart disease. Do you squirm or gag when you eat a big chunk of white fat from the edge of ribeye steak or a big chunk of real butter on your veggies? If you do, you most likely will not be able to reverse or prevent heart disease as I have done.

Red Meat Does Not Cause Coronary Artery Disease

Eating fresh red meat does not contribute to heart disease in any way. Many health professionals attempt to label red meat as unhealthy because it contains saturated fat within the tissue that cannot be easily removed. Vegetarians label red meat as unhealthy simply because eating animal flesh is a religious issue. However, the science against eating fresh red meat does not exist. It is all conjecture or based on falsified studies. Some studies find fault with high-salt, high-sugar deli meats and attempt to apply these same faults to fresh red meat. These studies are fraudulent. Fresh red meat is an excellent food and very healthy. Eating fresh red meat provides complete nutrition for healing and building a strong body. Processed meats should be avoided. But because bacon is so delicious, I break the rule a few times each year to enjoy it. I buy the brands labeled "No Sugar Added" that usually have a lower salt content also.

Red meat does not contribute to heart disease.

All saturated fats have molecules with the electron bonds occupied. Because of this, saturated fats cannot be oxidized. Saturated fats cannot be attacked by other molecules or free radical ions and cannot be glycated. For these reasons, a saturated fat such as lauric fatty acid in coconut oil can be left on the kitchen counter for a full year without turning rancid or degrading. Beef fat cannot be left on the kitchen counter without refrigeration because the fat is only 30% saturated. The primary fatty acid in beef fat is monounsaturated. Monounsaturated fatty acids are considered much healthier than polyunsaturated fatty acids that have multiple free electron spaces for easy oxidation.

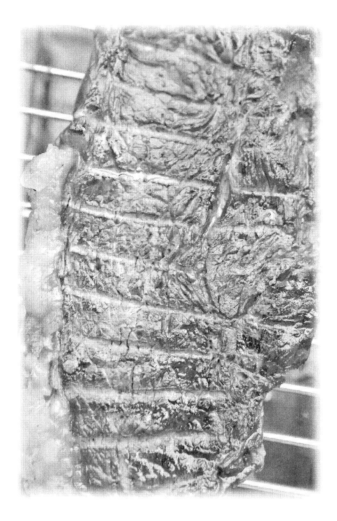

Beef Roast with Delicious Fat

Some studies claim that eating saturated fat increases the percentage of LDL in the blood and thereby increases the risk for heart disease. These studies fail to realize that eating saturated fat causes the LDL molecules to become the larger, less-dense variety that present the lowest heart disease risk. Eating saturated fats from animal or plant sources does not contribute to heart disease in any way.

The National Heart, Lung, and Blood Institute (NHLBI) conducted the Framingham Study over a period of 20 years beginning in 1948. According to NHLBI Director Dr. Claude Lenfant, "This study suggests that obesity is an important risk factor for heart failure in both women and men." The study found a small correlation between heart disease and elevated LDL cholesterol and total cholesterol. It also found that those who ate the most saturated fat, the most calories, and the most cholesterol were the most physically active. They also weighed the least and had the lowest levels of serum cholesterol. The people who ate the most saturated fat were the healthiest and had the lowest risk for heart disease.

> **NHLBI Framingham Heart Study**
> A Project of the National Heart, Lung and Blood Institute and Boston University
> http://www.framinghamheartstudy.org/
>
> "'In Framingham, Massachusetts, the more saturated fat one ate, the more cholesterol one ate, the more calories one ate, the lower people's serum cholesterol...we found that the people who ate the most cholesterol, ate the most saturated fat, ate the most calories weighed the least and were the most physically active.' Dr. William Castelli, Director of the Framingham study, 1992."

This quotation has become a major point of controversy because it has been used extensively, but it has neither been confirmed nor denied by recent directors of the Framington Heart Study. The study was started by Dr. Thomas Dawber, a Boston University physician, who stated that the initial results confirmed that dietary saturated animal fats were associated with a high incidence of coronary artery disease. However, it has been reported that Dr. Dawber gave excuses for not releasing the supporting data. Later, Dr. William Castelli became the new director and released the above statement reversing Dr. Dawber's claim.

United States government-funded nutrition studies cannot be trusted because accurate data is easily twisted, falsified, erased, or hidden.

The Framingham Heart Study proves that major health and nutrition studies funded by the United States government and costing hundreds of millions of dollars cannot be trusted. We do know there is a strong link between heart disease and obesity, but the cause of obesity is a now the major controversy. However, the statistical evidence has become overwhelming to anyone willing to face the facts. Obesity, diabetes, heart disease, cancer, and Alzheimer's disease continue to advance as the public is urged to conform to the *USDA Food Guide Pyramid* and the new *2010 USDA My Plate*. The study does confirm the link between obesity and heart failure, but that is of no benefit without knowing the cause of obesity. However, the study is correct in recognizing the escalation of the obesity problem. As stated below, "During the past two decades the prevalence of overweight has doubled among children and has almost tripled among adolescents."

Testimony and Success Story from a Person Suffering from Heart Disease, Obesity, and High Blood Pressure

"I find myself spending more and more time on your website! As I emailed a month or so ago, the "perfect diet-perfect nutrition" section of your site has really helped me a lot following a heart attack in 2004 and two more (clots in the right coronary artery) within the next year and a half. These were

fixed with stents (4 total), and when I was told in October 2005 that the next procedure would be a bypass, I decided to explore other health remedies. I had already stopped smoking, lost a lot of weight through calorie restriction (260 lbs down to 210 lbs) and did multiple vigorous cardio workouts each week after my first (June 2004) heart attack, but I was still eating low-fat and high-carb until October 2005 when my last blockage occurred (by the way, my last two attacks occurred after vigorous exercise). It was at this time that I discovered your website and tried the diet you recommend.

My cardiologist was supportive (except for the high-fat part, of course), and my blood work was awesome after a month on this diet, and I was allowed to discontinue two cholesterol medications, an anxiety medication and my beta blocker blood pressure medicine. I also believe the magnesium supplements, a reduction in hard cheese and the potassium chloride salt substitute have corrected my atria fibrillation. The last three medications that I would like to discontinue are the aspirin, Plavix and Coumadin — working with my cardiologist of course. I ordered some Carlson's Cod Liver Oil and some Co-Q10 to add to my current regimen of vitamin C, magnesium, and selenium supplements, but being on the Coumadin, I want to be cautious about the amount of cod liver oil I use, as my PT/INR is at about a 2.2 right now and beyond 6 is considered dangerous."

Notice that this gentlemen continued to suffer heart artery blockage even after following his doctor's recommendations to eat a low-fat, high-carbohydrate diet, quit smoking, lose weight, exercise, and take many drugs. It just didn't work. His health and blood test reports began to improve after he switched from a low-fat to a high-fat diet. His physician agreed that he could stop taking several of the drugs previously prescribed for his heart disease.

Although this patient's health and blood test results were greatly improved, his cardiologist did not recognize the reason for his awesome improvements and continued to recommend the low-fat diet that had failed. Too many cardiologists will not venture away from the diet recommendations of their medical societies, and too many patients are terrified at any suggestion that they deviate from their doctor's advice.

High HDL Cholesterol Reverses Heart Disease

This is one of the most important scientific facts for you to know in order to achieve optimal health. Without increasing HDL cholesterol, you cannot reverse heart disease. My regimen worked like a miracle to increase my HDL cholesterol. It's amazing.

High-density lipoprotein (HDL) cholesterol is called the *good cholesterol*. HDLs are synthesized in the liver and small intestine as primarily protein-rich, disc-shaped particles. These newly-formed HDLs are nearly devoid of any cholesterol and cholesteryl esters. Natural animal fats increase the level of HDL cholesterol in a highly desirable way. The HDL cholesterol molecules function like little scrub brushes to clean the LDL cholesterol, rancid polyunsaturated omega-6 fatty acids, plaque, and other deposits from the arterial walls. The cholesterol is carried within the protein shell of the HDL particle, making it swell into a spherical shape. The HDL cholesterol carries the LDL cholesterol, rancid polyunsaturated omega-6 fatty acids, and arterial plaque to the liver, where it is reprocessed and discarded in the intestines.

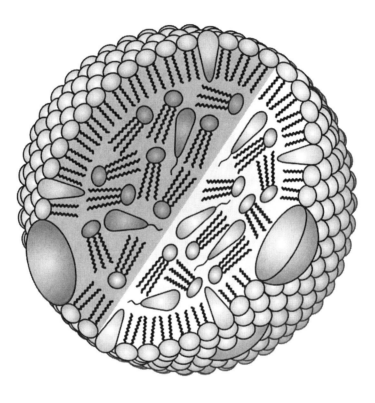

SURFACE COAT	LIPID CORE
unesterified cholesterol	cholesteryl esters
phospholipids	triglycerides
apolipoproteins	

Lipoprotein Cholesterol Molecule

The high-fat, high-protein, low-carbohydrate diet presented here reverses heart disease by removing deposits from the arteries. This occurs because the blood insulin level is kept at an absolute minimum. Insulin creates deposits in the arteries and prevents existing deposits from being removed by the HDL cholesterol. Therefore, it is imperative to eat a low-carbohydrate diet in order to prevent and reverse deposits in the arteries of the heart, neck, and legs. The low-carbohydrate diet reverses and prevents heart disease by removing and preventing these deposits.

High HDL cholesterol reverses heart disease.

The low-fat diet recommended by the *2004 USDA Food Guide Pyramid* and new *2010 USDA My Plate* raises glucose and insulin levels. Glucose and insulin contribute to coronary artery disease, strokes, and peripheral artery disease. The low-fat diet decreases good HDL cholesterol and causes bad LDL cholesterol to form the most dangerous LDL$_b$ fraction. These movements are all in the wrong direction.

Heart disease patients who are placed on the low-fat diet receive the bad news about their undesirable cholesterol readings each and every time they have a blood test. The low-fat diet also increases triglycerides, another risk factor for heart disease according to my scientific analysis. Because their physicians wrongly assume that they have not taken the recommendations to reduce dietary fat seriously, patients are often advised to decrease fat intake even more. When their cholesterol readings don't improve, they are advised to increase their exercise. The patients become scapegoats for the failure of the unscientific *USDA My Plate* dietary and exercise guidelines.

Low HDL Cholesterol Increases Heart Disease Risk

A low-fat diet reduces the level of good HDL cholesterol and increases heart disease risk. The high-fat diet I recommend raises the level of the good HDL cholesterol and reduces heart disease risk. HDL cholesterol acts as a vacuum cleaner in the arteries, removing plaque buildup one molecule at a time to prevent heart attacks. HDL removes cholesterol from the arteries and carries it back to the liver for reprocessing and discharge into the intestinal tract. An HDL level of 35 mg/dL is a dangerous heart disease risk. Many normal weight people with normal total cholesterol readings will develop plugged arteries and suffer a heart attack when the HDL cholesterol is precariously low. Fifty percent of the people who suffer a heart attack have a normal total cholesterol level. A blood test after a heart attack will generally show a low HDL cholesterol level and a high triglyceride level.

Low HDL cholesterol is a serious heart disease risk.

A reduction in HDL is a heart disease risk factor. The following study proves that eating saturated fats is healthy. The low-fat diet leads to a decrease in HDL cholesterol, while the low-carbohydrate diet along with a substantially high dietary intake of saturated animal fats is associated with an increase in HDL cholesterol. Reducing dietary saturated fats reduces the good HDL cholesterol fractions HDL_2 and HDL_{2b}. In other words, eating saturated animal fats increases the good HDL cholesterol as confirmed by my personal blood test reports shown in Chapter 4. It moves the HDL fraction in the most desirable direction.

Study Proves Reducing Saturated Fat Reduces Good HDL Cholesterol

HDL-subpopulation patterns in response to reductions in dietary total and saturated fat intakes in healthy subjects

American Journal of Clinical Nutrition, Vol. 70, No. 6, 992-1000, December 1999

"Background: Little information is available about HDL subpopulations during dietary changes.

Objective: The objective was to investigate the effect of reductions in total and saturated fat intakes on HDL subpopulations.

Design: Multiracial, young and elderly men and women (n = 103) participating in the double-blind, randomized DELTA (Dietary Effects on Lipoproteins and Thrombogenic Activities) Study consumed 3 different diets, each for 8 wk: an average American diet (AAD: 34.3% total fat,15.0% saturated fat), the American Heart Association Step I diet (28.6% total fat, 9.0% saturated fat), and a diet low in saturated fat (25.3% total fat, 6.1% saturated fat).

Results: HDL_2-cholesterol concentrations, by differential precipitation, decreased ($P < 0.001$) in a stepwise fashion after the reduction of total and saturated fat: 0.58 ± 0.21, 0.53 ± 0.19, and 0.48 ± 0.18 mmol/L with the AAD, Step I, and low-fat diets, respectively. HDL_3 cholesterol decreased ($P < 0.01$) less: 0.76 ± 0.13, 0.73 ± 0.12, and 0.72 ± 0.11 mmol/L with the AAD, Step I, and low-fat diets, respectively. As measured by nondenaturing gradient gel electrophoresis, the larger-size HDL_{2b} subpopulation decreased with the reduction in dietary fat, and a corresponding relative increase was seen for the smaller-sized $HDL_{3a,\ 3b,}$ and $_{3c}$ subpopulations ($P < 0.01$). HDL_2-cholesterol concentrations correlated negatively with serum triacylglycerol concentrations on all 3 diets: r = -0.46, -0.37, and -0.45 with the AAD, Step I, and low-fat diets, respectively (P < 0.0001). A similar negative correlation was seen for HDL_{2b}, whereas $HDL_{3a, 3b}$, and $_{3c}$ correlated positively with triacylglycerol concentrations. Diet-induced changes in serum triacylglycerol were negatively correlated with changes in HDL_2 and HDL_{2b} cholesterol.

Conclusions: A reduction in dietary total and saturated fat decreased both large (HDL_2 and HDL_{2b}) and small, dense HDL subpopulations, although decreases in HDL_2 and HDL_{2b} were most pronounced."

The following study shows that taking a statin drug in the presence of low HDLs does not improve coronary artery disease risk factors, does not prevent the development of further coronary artery disease, and does not prevent a future heart attack. This is why cholesterol-lowering drugs do not prevent future heart attacks in most people. This finding is in stark contrast to the prevalent claim that you will be protected from developing coronary disease simply by taking a statin drug and eating a low-fat diet.

Meta-analysis: Statin Therapy Does Not Alter the Association Between Low Levels of High-Density Lipoprotein Cholesterol and Increased Cardiovascular Risk
Annals of Internal Medicine, December 20, 2010

Haseeb Jafri, MD; Alawi A. Alsheikh-Ali, MD, MS; and Richard H. Karas, MD, PhD

"Abstract

Background: Low levels of high-density lipoprotein cholesterol (HDL-C) are associated with an increased risk for myocardial infarction (MI). Although statins reduce the risk for MI, most cardiovascular events still occur despite statin treatment.

Purpose: Using meta-analysis of large randomized, controlled trials (RCTs) of statins to determine whether statins alter the relationship between HDL-C level and MI.

Data Sources: MEDLINE search to February 2010, ClinicalTrials.gov, and reference lists from eligible studies.

Study Selection: English-language RCTs of statin-treated patients versus control participants with 1000 or more person-years of follow-up and reported HDL-C levels and MI.

Data Extraction: Two independent investigators extracted data from eligible RCTs.

Data Synthesis: Twenty eligible RCTs were identified (543 210 person-years of follow-up and 7838 MIs). After adjustment for on-treatment LDL-C levels, age, hypertension, diabetes, and tobacco use, there was a significant inverse association between HDL-C levels and risk for MI in statin-treated patients and control participants. In Poisson meta-regressions, every 0.26-mmol/L (10-mg/dL) decrease in HDL-C was associated with 7.1 (95% CI, 6.8 to 7.3) and 8.3 (CI, 8.1 to 8.5) more MIs per 1000 person-years in statin-treated patients and control participants, respectively. The inverse association between HDL-C levels and MI did not differ between statin-treated patients and control participants ($P = 0.57$).

Limitation: The observed associations may be explained by unmeasured confounding and do not imply causality in the relationship between HDL-C level and cardiovascular risk.

Conclusion: Statins do not alter the relationship between HDL-C level and cardiovascular risk, such that low levels of HDL-C remain significantly and independently associated with increased risk despite statin treatment. The remaining risk seen in statin-treated patients may be partly explained by low HDL-C levels or other factors associated with low levels of HDL-C."

High LDL Cholesterol Increases Heart Disease Risk

High LDL cholesterol in the presence of low HDL cholesterol increases heart disease risk. The ratio is very important because a ratio of LDL/HDL above 3 is a risk factor. Many organizations are insisting that everyone be put on cholesterol-lowering drugs if the LDL level is greater than 100, but what does the drug manufacturer say?

Zocor® (generic name simvastatin) Data Sheet

"Why is this drug prescribed: Zocor is a cholesterol-lowering drug. Your doctor may prescribe Zocor in addition to a cholesterol-lowering diet if your blood cholesterol level is too high, and if you have been unable to lower it by diet alone. For people at high risk of heart disease, current guidelines call for considering drug therapy when LDL levels reach 130. For people at lower risk, the cut-off is 160. For those at little or no risk, it's 190. In people with high cholesterol and heart disease, Zocor reduces the risk of heart attack, stroke and "mini-stroke" (transient ischemic attack) and can stave off the need for bypass surgery or angioplasty to clear clogged arteries."

High LDL cholesterol is a heart disease risk, but it is not independent from other blood chemistry factors. LDL cholesterol, triglycerides, insulin, and glucose are risk factors for heart disease, and they each multiply the severity of the risk. Avoiding coronary artery plaque when all of these factors are elevated is almost impossible, and reducing the plaque requires all of these factors to be extremely low and HDL cholesterol to be high.

All LDL cholesterol molecules are not the same. The LDL cholesterol has a spectrum of sizes called *fractions* or *subfractions* that are divided into three groups with separate risk factors. The three classifications are called *A*, *A/B*, and *B*, or may be identified as LDL$_a$, LDL$_{a/b}$, and LDL$_b$. The LDL$_a$ subfraction cholesterol is larger, more buoyant, and presents the lowest risk. The LDL$_{a/b}$ subfraction has an intermediate size and density. The LDL$_b$ subfraction has the smallest size, highest density, and presents a threefold increase in heart disease risk. This is the LDL cholesterol to avoid.

LDL$_b$ cholesterol is the highest heart disease risk.

Unfortunately, the low-fat, high-carbohydrate diet recommend by the *USDA Food Guide Pyramid* causes an increase in the dangerous LDL$_b$ subfraction, triglycerides, glucose, and insulin. Taking a statin cholesterol-lowering drug really does not reduce the risk as the previous study has shown. This is why several people I know have had a continuing progression of heart disease even though they followed the low-fat guidelines and took the prescribed statin drug. It didn't work for them, and it didn't work for President Bill Clinton.

People who are pre-diabetic or in an early stage of Type 2 diabetes will have all of these risk factors when they continue on the low-fat, high-carbohydrate diet recommended by the American Diabetes Association®. The pre-diabetic enters a stage in which glucose and insulin soar because of increasing insulin resistance, and the LDL$_b$ subfraction is very high. Heart disease is almost guaranteed. He is now in the Rieske Instant Atherosclerosis Cycle (IAC).

I shudder at the foods recommended for diabetics. I have seen people progress from hypoglycemia to pre-diabetes and Type 2 diabetes on a very predictable timetable when they followed the recommended low-fat, high-carbohydrate diet. They could have prevented diabetes 100% of the time by simply switching to a high-fat, low-carbohydrate diet when they were hypoglycemic, but they are erroneously told that carbohydrates are necessary for energy and that fats will give them heart disease. They are told the high-fat diet puts them at risk for heart disease when actually the low-fat diet is the culprit.

You may have received a good report from your physician based on the standard cholesterol measurements and still be at risk for plugging your heart arteries from one side to the other. Most likely your physician did not order the comprehensive cholesterol test that measures the subfractions of LDL and HDL cholesterol. Your physician may not know your insulin level because it is usually neglected on the standard tests. These solid predictors of heart disease risk have been neglected, leaving you unsuspectingly exposed to instant atherosclerosis.

What are your measurements for
LDL subfractions and insulin?

My high-fat diet in combination with the vitamin and drug therapy has achieved the impossible by reducing my coronary artery plaque. Reversing coronary heart disease requires a completely different approach than preventing it. The error many physicians and patients make is to assume that a statin drug in combination with a low-fat diet can prevent coronary artery disease and possibly reverse it. It can't do either one.

Insist that your cardiologist measure your LDL and HDL subfractions in order to fully evaluate your cardiac risk factors. Insulin must be measured as well but is often ignored. Glucose and triglycerides are commonly included in blood tests and must be considered in the final analysis.

Obesity Is a Symptom of Other Heart Disease Risks

Obesity does not cause heart disease. Both are symptoms of excessive carbohydrate consumption. Obesity is a symptom, not a causal factor. We see the story on television about the morbidly obese man who weighed 700 pounds (315 kg) but did not have heart disease, yet I know a man who is very thin, exercised, ran 10 km races, ate the recommended low-fat diet, and plugged all four of his major heart arteries. The millions of thin people who have had quadruple heart artery bypasses prove it is not simply a weight problem. Why doesn't the man who can't walk because of morbid obesity get heart disease? I will answer this question.

The morbidly obese tend to have little insulin resistance in their adipose (body fat) tissue. Dietary carbohydrates are digested as glucose, fructose, and other sugars before being converted into triglycerides by the liver. The triglycerides are transported in the form of chylomicrons (large lipoprotein particles that allow fats to be carried within the water-based bloodstream) or carried by VLDL to all areas of the body. To a lesser degree, triglycerides are carried by LDL and HDL and are used by cells as fuel or deposited in the adipose tissue with the assistance of insulin. Because the morbidly obese have low insulin resistance in the adipose tissue, body fat easily increases without a surge in insulin. As I have previously discussed, insulin is the major culprit that causes coronary artery plaque.

Fasting insulin should be less than 25 (microU/mg) to prevent and reverse coronary artery disease.

312

Thinness Is Not a Shield Against Heart Disease

Thin people can have a high degree of insulin resistance in their adipose tissue that makes it resist fat deposits. They eat a high-carbohydrate diet without gaining weight and are tricked into a false sense of security that they could never have a heart attack because they are thin. Their skinny profiles hide the fact that insulin is packing their heart arteries with plaque. They have been brainwashed to think their low-fat, high-carbohydrate diet and ultra-low body mass index is protecting them from cardiovascular disease (CVD). Thin people get coronary artery plaque, heart attacks, and require multiple bypass surgeries in order to save their lives. Don't fall for the false promise that maintaining your weight or being underweight will shield you from developing coronary artery plaque that could cause a heart attack and death.

Thinness does not ensure lowest CVD death rate.

We often hear the comment about the obese being "a heart attack waiting to happen," but the cardiac unit at the local hospital has many thin patients. Thinness has been hyped as the ultimate expression of good health, but the following study shows this assertion to be false propaganda. People classified as overweight are the longevity champions—not the skinny models.

The results of a study released in *The Journal of the American Medical Association*® (JAMA), November 7, 2007, shows that overweight people have a lowest death rate from all causes. Those classified as overweight with a body mass index (BMI) of 25–30 have the lowest deaths from coronary artery disease as well. The following gives the surprising results:

Death Rates from Coronary Heart Disease
Thousands of Excess Deaths in 2004

Underweight	BMI less than 18.5	**+ 2,000** deaths
Normal weight	BMI 18.5 to 25	**Baseline**
Overweight	BMI 25 to 30	**- 12,000** deaths
Obese	BMI 30 or greater	**+ 45,000** deaths

Source: JAMA, Cause-Specific Excess Deaths Associated With Underweight, Overweight, and Obesity
http://jama.ama-assn.org/content/298/17/2028.full

Body Mass Index (BMI) formula:

Metric Units BMI = Weight (kg) / Height^2 (meters^2) or

English Units BMI = Weight (lbs) x 703 / Height^2 (inches^2)

We see from this data that overweight people had 12,000 fewer deaths from coronary heart disease than those of normal weight and 14,000 fewer deaths than underweight people. Contrary to the popular myth, skinny folks have a higher death rate from coronary heart disease than do the normal weight and much higher than those who are classified as overweight. Only the obese have a higher death rate than the underweight group.

Being skinny increases your heart disease risk.

Another shocking statistic shows that people who were underweight had an equal or higher death rate than normal weight persons in every death measurement category. The overweight had a much lower death rate than normal weight people in many categories and a slightly higher rate in only 2 out of 10 categories.

The same trend continues for overall death rates, with the overweight being the champions with the lowest death rate. Normal weight people were second, the underweight third, and the obese had the highest death rate. The obese suffered much more than those of other groups, racking up high death rates in the categories of cancer, coronary heart disease, other cardiovascular diseases, diabetes, and kidney disease.

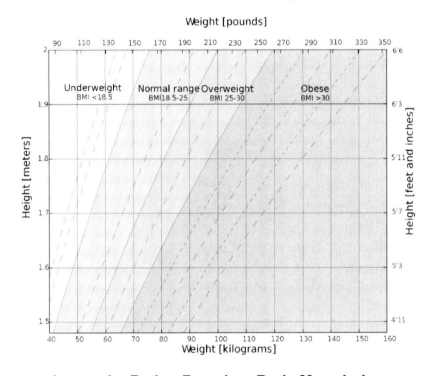

Longevity Rating Based on Body Mass Index

No. 1 Champions are those who are overweight.

No. 2 Runner-ups are those who are normal weight.

No. 3 Third place are those who are underweight.

No. 4 Last place are those who are obese.

I have nicknamed JAMA, "King of Prestige Medical Journals," so it's surprising that the above study showed results starkly contrary to the false body-weight versus heart-disease agenda widely published by other organizations. Let's see what the American Heart Association® (AHA) says about weight versus heart disease:

> "Many obese and overweight people may have difficulty losing weight. But by losing even as few as 10 pounds, you can lower your heart disease risk."

Is this quotation scientifically correct according to the JAMA study published more than three years earlier? No! It is half right, half wrong, and neglects to cover other weight categories. Yes, the obese could lower their heart disease risk by losing weight, but people in the overweight category are already the champions with the lowest death rate from heart disease. Overweight people would not benefit from weight loss because those of normal weight have a higher death rate. The AHA failed to mention that underweight people have a higher death rate from coronary heart disease and other cardiovascular diseases than the normal and overweight. The AMA should encourage skinny and underweight people to eat my diet and gain weight as a method of reducing heart disease risks.

Body fat is constantly being railed against as a major heart disease risk factor. Normal weight people are made to feel that they should be skinny in order to have the lowest cardiac disease risk. These misconceptions have been promoted for several decades until most people accept them without a second thought. Statistics show that being slightly overweight is the healthiest body type, and body mass index recommendations are wrong.

Sleep Apnea Does Not Cause Heart Disease

Most health authorities claim that sleep apnea can lead to heart disease. I believe this analysis is backward. Sleep apnea is caused by existing heart disease. A weakened cardiovascular system results in a reduced amount of oxygen in the blood that manifests as apnea during deep sleep. The blood with reduced oxygen reaches the brain, where it causes the sufferer to wake up gasping for air and breathing heavily. A person with sleep apnea should be checked for heart disease.

Homocysteine Increases Heart Disease Risk

Homocysteine is an amino acid that has a positive effect on the heart but has been implicated as a possible risk factor for cardiovascular diseases. For this reason, it is commonly included in blood test measurements. Homocysteine is required for the body to operate properly, but too much homocysteine can be destructive to the heart and artery walls. Homocysteine is known to damage blood vessels by injuring the endothelial cells that line arteries and stimulating the growth of smooth muscle cells. Homocysteine can also interfere with the normal blood clotting mechanism and increase the risk for clots that can cause a stroke or heart attack.

Concern about homocysteine as a cardiovascular risk factor dates back to 1969, when Dr. Kilmer S. McCully discovered that children born with a genetic metabolic error called *homocystinuria* occasionally died at a very young age from advanced arterial disease. Homocystinuria is the term used for abnormally high homocysteine levels. Although homocysteine is an amino acid, high levels of homocysteine are not caused by eating meat. High levels of homocysteine are more likely caused by deficiencies of protein, vitamins, and minerals. Homocysteine can be reduced by taking high levels of vitamins B6, B12, and folic acid. Vegetarians may be at higher risk for heart disease because of protein and vitamin B12 deficiencies and the fact that they are frequently underweight.

Caution:

Do not supplement the diet with methionine amino acid. The metabolism of methionine produces homocysteine, which is a sulfur-containing amino acid. It exists at a critical biochemical juncture between methionine metabolism and the biosynthesis of the amino acids cysteine and taurine. Homocysteine is used to build and repair tissues, but an excess of homocysteine has been shown to be a major factor in hardening and obstruction of the arteries that leads to full-blown heart disease.

C-Reactive Protein (CRP) and Serum Amyloid A (SAA)

Elevated levels of C-reactive protein (CRP) and serum amyloid A (SAA) are inflammatory markers that have been associated with increased cardiovascular disease risk. They are symptoms of heart disease, not causes. CRP is commonly included in blood test measurements. CRP and SAA levels do not change with a low-fat diet, but both CRP and SAA levels decrease with a low-carbohydrate diet, indicating a high-fat, low-carbohydrate diet lowers heart disease risk. These are additional measurements that prove the diet regimen I present is the correct approach to preventing and reversing heart disease.

Cholesterol Risks Are Lower on the Low-Carb Diet

People on the low-carbohydrate diet should be less concerned with the cholesterol risk factors commonly associated with heart disease because cholesterol is not the primary cause of coronary artery disease. Dr. Michael DeBakey, the famous heart surgeon who performed the world's first heart transplant, spoke against blaming cholesterol for coronary artery disease.

> **Anthropological Research Reveals Human Dietary Requirements for Optimal Health**
> **H. Leon Abrams, Jr., MA, EDS**
> Associate Professor Emeritus of Anthropology, ECJC, University System of Georgia, Swainsboro, Georgia.
> Journal of Applied Nutrition, 1982, 16:1:38-45
>
> "Michael DeBakey, world renowned heart surgeon from Houston, who has devoted extensive research into the cholesterol coronary disease theory, states that out of every ten people in the United States who have atherosclerotic heart disease, only three or four of these ten have high cholesterol levels; this is approximately the identical rate of elevated cholesterol found in the general population. (10) His comment: "If you say cholesterol is the cause, how do you explain the other 60 percent to 70 percent with heart disease who don't have a high cholesterol?" In 1964 DeBakey made an analysis of cholesterol levels from usual hospital laboratory testing of 1,700 patients with atherosclerotic disease and found there was no positive or definitive relationship or correlation between serum cholesterol levels and the extent or nature of atherosclerotic disease."
>
> (10) De Bakey, Michael, *JAMA*, 189:655-659, (1964).

Cholesterol does not have a connection to heart disease on the low-carbohydrate diet because the foundational cause of diabetes and heart disease is a high intake of dietary carbohydrates that leads to high levels of insulin and glucose in the blood—not cholesterol. The low-fat, high-carbohydrate diet recommended by the *USDA Food Guide Pyramid* and the American Heart Association® causes glucose and insulin to skyrocket. These chain reactions cause plaque buildup in arteries and lead to a heart attack. Polyunsaturated vegetable oils and hydrogenated vegetable oils (trans fats) are also prime contributors to plugged coronary arteries. These vegetable oils are highly inflammatory and contribute to heart disease, intestinal diseases, and cancer.

The LDL cholesterol levels on the low-carbohydrate diet I present are not serious risk factors because of the absence of hyperglycemia and hyperinsulinemia. The diet, supplements, and drug therapy that I used to reverse my heart disease lower LDL cholesterol drastically and cause the good HDL cholesterol to soar. This combination results in a very low LDL/HDL ratio that is scientifically necessary in order to remove coronary artery plaque. Low glucose and insulin will prevent the formation of arterial plaques but will not remove existing deposits. Arterial plaque is removed by HDL in the absence of hyperglycemia and hyperinsulinemia.

On the other hand, a low LDL level in the presence of hyperglycemia and hyperinsulinemia gives no protection whatsoever. Cholesterol-lowering drugs are worthless when glucose and insulin levels are high. This is the reason why 65% of diabetics die from coronary artery disease. The percentage would be higher if some did not die sooner from other causes, such as accidents, cancer, or stroke. Diabetics who switch to the low-carbohydrate diet can escape this horrible fate.

The low-carbohydrate, high-fat, high-protein diet promotes the formation of larger, less dense LDL_a subfraction cholesterol and discourages the formation of the more dense LDL_b subfraction cholesterol. HDL cholesterol is increased while triglycerides, glucose, and insulin are reduced. All of these factors move in the right direction to prevent and reverse coronary artery disease. The American Heart Association's® low-fat diet actually promotes heart disease as demonstrated by the current epidemic.

For many centuries, primitive Eskimos lived in igloos eight months of the year on the frozen Arctic Ocean north of the Canadian Yukon Territory. Their diet of seal meat and blubber was 80% fat and 20% protein with zero carbohydrates. The women and children huddled in the igloo with a small oil fire for months on end. They did not have any signs of heart disease, cancer, or diabetes whatsoever; but when they moved to the white man's settlements these diseases escalated.

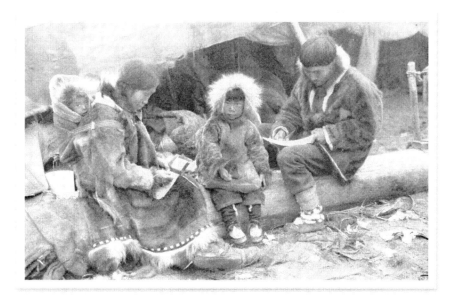

Inuit (Eskimo) Family
National Geographic Magazine, volume 31 (1917), page 564
Public domain. Copyright has expired.

Chapter 3

Hypertension Does Not Cause Coronary Artery Disease

Hypertension is always listed as a risk factor for coronary artery disease, and everyone seems to accept this claim without a second thought. Actually, hypertension is more likely to be a symptom of cardiovascular disease. A restriction in any artery can initiate bodily reactions and result in hypertension as the body attempts to increase the blood supply to the affected area.

However, hypertension caused by other factors, such as endocrine disorders, hormone deficiencies or excesses, cancers or tumors, kidney disease, or diabetes, can eventually lead to cardiovascular problems. Many organs and glands produce hormones that can affect blood pressure.

- Pineal gland in the brain
- Pituitary gland in the brain
- Thyroid gland in the neck
- Thymus gland in the central chest area
- Adrenal gland on the top of the kidneys
- Pancreas near the stomach and the duodenum
- Ovaries in women
- Testes in men

High blood pressure can and does damage the arteries and lead to hemorrhage and sudden death. Ruptures of the aorta near the heart or of arteries in the head are the most common arterial failures that result from hypertension. Blood pressure consistently higher than normal overloads the heart muscles and leads to cardiomegaly (an enlarged heart), heart muscle weakness, and congestive heart failure.

Kidney malfunction often causes high blood pressure because the kidneys excrete an enzyme that regulates the renin-angiotensin system (RAS) that in turn can affect extracellular fluid volumes of the blood plasma, interstitial fluid, and the lymphatic system. The RAS produces powerful arterial vasoconstricting hormones that are the primary regulators of the body's arterial blood pressure. Drugs such as diuretics may reduce the extracellular fluid volume and thereby reduce blood pressure, but they are not dealing with the primary cause, which could be excess renin production by the kidneys. Drugs classified as *beta blockers* can reduce the heart rate and thereby reduce blood pressure, but they too are not dealing with the primary cause when the kidneys are producing excess renin. Drugs classified as *renin blockers* can be very effective at controlling blood pressure with few side effects when the primary cause is excess renin production.

Nanobacteria Do Not Cause Coronary Artery Disease

Nanobacteria do not cause arterial plaque or heart disease. Some researchers claim that small crystalline molecules are in fact miniature bacteria 100 times smaller than regular bacteria. They claim nanobacteria are living organisms that cause plaque to accumulate in heart arteries. These claims are false. Nanobacteria do not exist. The crystalline formations are simply calcium phosphate crystals that can form in bodily organs. These crystals tend to propagate, not reproduce. Products sold to treat or rid the body of nanobacteria are a fraud.

Chapter 3

Lifestyle Guidelines That Don't Prevent Heart Disease

The major media are awash with lifestyle recommendations for preventing heart disease, most of which are totally false. The vast majority of medical associations, diet gurus, professional nutritionists, professional health trainers, universities, medical clinics, and physicians flaunt ineffective lifestyle guidelines. Much of the advice contributes to heart disease, not the reverse. I will present a few of the most prominent erroneous recommendations.

The following is a direct quotation from one of the most prestigious medical schools in the United States. The "five white knights" are based on conjecture, false assumptions, sideline issues, and inherited dogma that has locked them into history. I established my recommendations on a hard, critical evaluation based on science and human physiology. I will address the recommendations in the following quotation one at a time.

> "Count on these five white knights to protect your heart, your arteries, and the rest of you. They will make you look better and feel better. And it's never too late to start.
>
> 1. ***Avoid tobacco.*** Smoke from cigarettes, cigars, and pipes is as bad for the heart and arteries as it is for the lungs. If you smoke, quitting is the biggest gift of health you can give yourself. Secondhand smoke is also toxic, so avoid it whenever possible.
>
> 2. ***Be active.*** Exercise and physical activity are about the closest things you have to magic bullets against heart disease and other chronic conditions. Any amount of activity is better than none; at least 30 minutes a day is best.

3. ***Aim for a healthy weight.*** Carrying extra pounds, especially around the belly, strains the heart and tips you toward diabetes. If you are overweight, losing just 5% to 10% of your starting weight can make a big difference in your blood pressure and blood sugar.

4. ***Enliven your diet.*** Add fruits and vegetables, whole grains, unsaturated fat, good protein (from beans, nuts, fish, and poultry), and herbs and spices. Subtract processed foods, salt, rapidly digested carbohydrates (from white bread, white rice, potatoes, and the like), red meat, and soda or other sugar-sweetened beverages.

5. ***Drink alcohol in moderation (if at all).*** If you drink alcohol, limit your intake — one to two drinks a day for men, no more than one a day for women."

I will give the source some credit for recommendations 1 and 5. Smoking introduces chemical compounds (free radicals) into the body that can contribute to heart disease and cancer. Definitely avoid smoking.

Drinking alcohol in moderation is a good recommendation, but drinking less than the amount suggested is a better approach. Many people have a genetic predisposition to alcoholism and therefore must totally abstain.

Exercise Does Not Prevent Heart Disease

Claim Number 2 states,

> **"Be active.** Exercise and physical activity are about the closest things you have to magic bullets against heart disease and other chronic conditions. Any amount of activity is better than none; at least 30 minutes a day is best."

Chapter 3

The claim is made that activity and exercise are the "closest things you have to magic bullets against heart disease and other chronic conditions." This is scientifically false. Insulin is so powerful that it can blow past any exercise and plug your arteries in less than one year. Many people are brainwashed to think exercise can protect them from coronary artery disease. The story about President Bill Clinton is a good example.

Exercise does not prevent heart disease.

Running for hours day after day does not prevent heart disease. This false claim is so prevalent that I felt compelled to devote an entire chapter to the subject even though I would need an entire book to attempt to adequately squelch the brainwashing that the mass media broadcast. Chapter 7 goes beyond proof that exercise does not prevent heart disease. It gives solid scientific proof that excessive exercise can kill you.

I know a man who contracted polio as a youngster that left him with a severe disability. He has difficulty walking even with the aid of a four-point walker. He is now about 70 years old and has trouble moving from the walker to a sitting position, but he has never had a heart attack. This is surprising because his diet is not the best by any standard. To my knowledge, his total inactivity did not cause him to develop heart disease. He has certainly outlived many marathon and triathlon competitors as well as weekend exercise addicts.

More than likely, excessive exercise increases the heart attack risk. Runners tend to eat a high-carbohydrate diet, thinking they need extra glucose for energy. This is not the healthiest approach because the glucose causes insulin resistance and raises the blood insulin level, which by itself is a heart disease risk. The heart muscles burn fatty acids and ketone bodies for energy, not glucose. The following two marathon runners are prime examples of those who exercised excessively but still developed heart disease at a relatively young age.

James F. Fixx wrote two books on the health benefits of exercise and running, but while on a daily run in 1984, he died in his running shoes from a heart attack at the young age of 52,. Many try to cover the facts by blaming it on heredity or his smoking, which he quit nine years earlier, but Fixx developed severe atherosclerosis during his running years. One coronary artery was almost totally restricted, and another was 80% restricted. There was also evidence of a recent heart attack. In addition, his heart was somewhat enlarged, a condition doctors call *hypertrophic cardiomyopathy*. This occurs when the heart muscles become thick and make it more difficult for the heart to work. His exercise and underweight body mass index did not prevent the progression of coronary artery disease.

The disastrous effects of his diet caused his heart disease, and exercise did little or nothing to stop it. James F. Fixx bought into the myth that fat in the diet is unhealthy, when in fact it is essential to life. He also became a vegetarian and refrained from eating meat. Fixx bought into the philosophy (relatively new at the time) that runners need carbohydrates in their diets as the primary source for muscle energy. He ate a low-calorie diet to keep from gaining weight, but the percentage of carbohydrates was high. He failed to take any vitamins, minerals, or other supplements on the false premise that his vegetarian diet could provide them. He undoubtedly suffered from essential amino acid and fatty acid deficiencies that were compounded by his refusal to supplement with vitamins and minerals. Amino acids from protein are the building blocks of life, and it's difficult to obtain all of the essential amino acids from the diet without eating meat, fowl, fish, or seafood. The effects of these deficiencies can take several years to manifest themselves, and the resulting diseases can be numerous. This is why it is extremely difficult to pinpoint the cause and effect of a low-fat, low-protein diet on health.

The vegetarian diet does not prevent heart disease.

Marathon runner and PowerBar® founder, Brian Maxwell, collapsed and died at 51 years of age on March 20, 2004, in San Anselmo, California. He reportedly collapsed in a post office, and emergency personnel were unable to resuscitate him. His exercise, diet, and energy bars did not provide the awesome health as is commonly expected and may have contributed to his early death. PowerBar® had become a multimillion-dollar empire since Maxwell and his wife founded it in 1986. They began selling the popular energy bars out of their kitchen, and over the next 10 years the company grew to $150 million in sales. In March 2000, the couple sold the company to Nestle SA® for a reported $375 million. Maxwell conceived the idea for PowerBar® while running a 26.2-mile marathon. He had to stop the race after 21 miles, the point at which experts say the body stops burning carbohydrates and starts to burn muscle tissue. In 1977, *Track and Field News®* ranked Maxwell No. 3 runner in the world, and in 1980, he was part of the Olympic team that boycotted the games in Moscow. He frequently represented Canada in international competitions as a long-distance runner.

Maxwell has proved once again that exercise does not prevent heart disease and that the high-carbohydrate diet is the true cause. His wife was a professional nutritionist and co-developer of the PowerBar® high-carbohydrate snack. Most of the ingredients become simple sugars upon digestion.

- High fructose corn syrup
- Grape and pear juice concentrate
- Maltodextrin
- Brown rice
- Glycerin (sweetener that does not raise insulin levels)

After a number of years, marathon runners develop plugged heart arteries on the high-carbohydrate diet. Athletes binge on complex carbohydrates (carb-loading) because the method is thought to give the best performance. The body becomes insulin resistant over time and the blood insulin level rises. The runner can stay perfectly thin while the insulin level approaches that of a person with hypoglycemia. Insulin packs the glucose into cells for energy, but it also packs omega-6 vegetable fatty acids and LDL cholesterol into the heart artery walls and leads to coronary artery disease. Athletes should live and train on the low-carbohydrate diet in order to prevent insulin resistance, but carbohydrates can be eaten before races if desired. Even so, carb loading only lasts through half of a marathon race, and the body is forced to burn stored fat for energy. Burning dietary fat and stored body fat is the healthier way to live and compete.

Weight Loss Will Not Prevent Heart Disease

Claim Number 3 states,

*"**Aim for a healthy weight.** Carrying extra pounds, especially around the belly, strains the heart and tips you toward diabetes. If you are overweight, losing just 5% to 10% of your starting weight can make a big difference in your blood pressure and blood sugar."*

This statement has validity only for the obese. I have already established that underweight people have a higher incidence of heart disease than those who are normal weight or overweight. According to the previously-cited study in *The Journal of the American Medical Association*® (JAMA), November 7, 2007, weight loss for an overweight or normal weight person will actually increase heart disease risk.

Low-fat, Balanced Diet Does Not Prevent Heart Disease

The prestigious medical school above says you can prevent heart disease by adopting the following diet:

"Add fruits and vegetables, whole grains, unsaturated fat, good protein (from beans, nuts, fish, and poultry), and herbs and spices. Subtract processed foods, salt, rapidly digested carbohydrates (from white bread, white rice, potatoes, and the like), red meat, and soda or other sugar-sweetened beverages."

Is this claim true? No! It is scientifically false. I certainly recommend that you avoid white bread, white rice, and potatoes, but whole grain bread, fruits, and unsaturated fats are the cause of coronary artery disease, not the magic bullet for awesome health. Whole grain bread contains as much glucose in the form of complex carbohydrates per serving as white bread. All the calories in fruits are fructose and glucose that spike insulin and are converted by the liver into blood triglycerides and body fat. Again, they totally miss the cause of heart disease by ignoring the primary causal factor— insulin. The prestigious medical school recommends that you "subtract red meat" from your diet. Is this good advice? No! Absolute not! Red meat and natural animal fats do not cause heart disease, but the medical school mistakenly thinks they do.

Chelation Does Not Remove Coronary Arterial Plaque

Chelation is a process in which a chemical compound is introduced into the body for the purpose of removing undesirable elements. The chemical, called a *chelator,* has physical properties that cause it to be attracted to elements such as heavy metals, minerals, and radioactive nuclear isotopes. The process is very effective when a chelator is created specifically for certain elements. Chelators are used in hospitals worldwide to remove lead, mercury, cadmium, uranium, arsenic, and other elements from contaminated individuals.

Many physicians and chelation salesmen claim that it can remove plaque from the arteries and reverse cardiovascular disease, but the proof is weak and the science misleading. Chelation will not remove or shrink coronary artery plaque because it is not effective in removing embedded cholesterol and rancid omega-6 polyunsaturated fatty acids. It may be somewhat effective in removing calcium from the arteries but not from arterial plaque, where it is embedded below a layer of cholesterol and fatty acids. Chelation of arterial plaque has not been proven by scientific studies or a scientific analysis of the chemical processes. Don't waste your money on intravenous or oral chelation as a treatment to remove plaque. Use the regimen in this book that reduced my arterial plaque by 50% in only 25 months.

Chelation Removes Heavy Metals That Can Cause Heart Disease

Heavy metal contamination is a general term used to describe a condition in which people have abnormally high levels of toxic metals such as mercury, lead, cadmium, and arsenic in the body. This contamination can be very real, detrimental to health, and deadly. Unfortunately, sales people are propagating myths and distortions about heavy metal contamination as scare tactics to sell fraudulent or partially effective products to treat the supposed contamination.

Heavy metals are subtle, silent, stalking killers. They can enter the body from a wide variety of sources, including foods, drinks, contaminated air, skin, vaccines, injections, and surgical implants. They slowly accumulate in the kidneys, liver, pancreas, bones, central nervous system, and brain, where they subtly and silently degrade health. Heavy metals can and do cause cancer without ever being implicated in the diagnosis. Because they allow the body to retain sodium, heavy metals cause high blood pressure. They can and do cause heart disease and mental retardation. Everyone is contaminated with heavy metals, some seriously without their knowledge.

Avoid heavy metal testing and treatment scams.

Those who sell treatments and products would like you to believe that everyone is suffering severe health problems from toxic heavy metal contamination. These claims are false. Very few people have problems that result from toxic heavy metal contamination. These fanatical sales people create panic and heavy metal paranoia. Care should be taken to avoid nutrition and health-care practitioners who perform heavy metal testing and offer treatments or products as cures. Test reports and treatments can be easily faked to show amazing successes. Always obtain heavy metal testing from an independent laboratory. Testing is advisable even when the symptoms are mild because heavy metal contamination can be very elusive. The following table provides a summary of the symptoms and diseases caused by heavy metal contamination.

Summary of Heavy Metal Contamination, Symptoms, and Disease Pathology	
Common Heavy Metal Contamination	**Symptoms and Pathology**
Mercury	Paresthesia skin disorders Dysarthria speech disorders Visual disorders Deafness Teeth problems Kidney disorders Liver disorders Gastrointestinal disorders Cognitive and nerve damage
Lead	Central nervous system disorders Peripheral nerve disorders Kidney disorders Cardiovascular disease Decreased fertility Accumulation in the bones Gastrointestinal disorders
Arsenic	Central nervous system disorders Peripheral nerve disorders Kidney disorders Painful urination Cardiovascular disease Gastrointestinal disorders
Cadmium	Flu like symptoms Bronchitis and pulmonary edema Kidney disorders Liver disorders Cancer

Nickel	Cardiac arrest Dermatitis Asthma Respiratory disorders Lung and nasal cancer
Iron	Cardiovascular disease Gastrointestinal disorders Death

Vegetarians want you to believe that eating fish, red meat, fowl, and cheese greatly increases the risk for heavy metal contamination. They cite examples such as mercury in ocean fish or cows that eat grass contaminated by agricultural chemicals. They often cite pesticide and herbicide ingestion as the source of heavy metals in supermarket meats. This is not the case. For proven scientific reasons, vegetarians are much more likely to be contaminated with heavy metals. Fruits, vegetables, legumes, nuts, and seeds commonly eaten by vegetarians can easily become tainted with heavy metals that occur naturally in the soil and air. We'll see that vegetarians are at higher risk because their diet contains fewer natural chelators than the diet of meat eaters. Whole grains and other high-carbohydrate foods hold toxic metal ions and release them within the body. High levels of carbohydrates in the diet result in a heavy load of glucose and insulin, and glucose has no chelating properties. The anabolic nature of insulin opposes the catabolic nature of chelators. Eating meat detoxifies heavy metals from the body naturally using amino acids, but eating fruits and whole grains causes the accumulation of heavy metals and prevents their discharge. Hair testing laboratories frequently find heavy metal contamination in vegetarians.

Metallothioneins (MTs) are a family of cysteine-rich, low molecular-weight, metal-binding proteins that are naturally synthesized within the cells of the body. MTs regulate the levels of zinc, copper, and selenium and bind to or detoxify cadmium, mercury, platinum, and silver. MTs prevent free radical ions like heavy metals from attacking the cell membrane lipids or mitochondrial DNA and damaging the ATP (energy generating) structure of the cell. The damaged cells are called *reactive oxygen species (ROS)*. The free radicals can enter the body and easily bond to healthy molecules in a process often referred to *oxidative stress.* Cancer can occur when the free radicals attack the cells' DNA.

The production of MTs depends on the availability of dietary minerals such as zinc, copper, selenium, and the amino acids histidine and cysteine. A deficiency of these minerals and amino acids results in a deficiency of metallothioneins and the accumulation of heavy metals. The vegetarian diet is naturally deficient in zinc and amino acids. This leads to a deficiency of protective metallothioneins, which allows heavy metals to accumulate. At a conference in 2002, Dr. Dietrich Klinghardt made the following comments in his presentation.

> "Proteins provide the important precursors to the endogenous metal detox and shuttle agents, such as coeruloplasmin, metallothioneine, glutathione and others. The branched-chain amino acids in cow and goat whey have valuable independent detox effects. Amino acid supplements, especially those with a concentration of branched-chain amino acids, are valuable."

Nonessential heavy metal ions promote aging in addition to serious diseases and death. People who are otherwise very healthy will age faster because these ions cross-link between normal molecules in the body. This cross-linking has been identified in diseases such as hardening of the arteries, skin ailments, carpal tunnel syndrome, degeneration of organs, nerve damage, etc. Therefore, detoxing heavy metals from the body is a good anti-aging step even in people who appear to be perfectly healthy. Vitamins, minerals, and supplements that have an affinity for heavy metal ions are called *antioxidants* because they attach to and remove free radicals from the body. Aging rubber is a good example of cross-linking. The rubber molecules are cross-linked with oxygen atoms that cause the rubber to lose elasticity and crack. People age in a similar manner as a result of free radical attacks on bodily tissues.

Toxic heavy metal poisoning can be manifested as mental retardation in children, dementia in adults, central nervous system (CNS) disorders, kidney (renal) diseases, liver (hepatic) diseases, insomnia, personality changes, emotional instability, depression, panic attacks, memory loss, headaches, vision disturbances including peripheral neuropathy, excess salivation, excess sweating, and lack of coordination (ataxia). Death is often caused by encephalopathy (degenerative diseases of the brain) or cardiovascular diseases. Heavy metal toxicity can cause the blood pH to become acidic, and the body buffers this acidity by extracting calcium from the bones. The calcium (not a heavy metal) tends to accumulate in the soft tissue of the arteries, causing hardening of the arteries. It is extremely difficult to remove calcium from soft tissue, but the regimen I present may help to reduce hardening of the arteries as well as remove the toxic heavy metals.

Even though dental amalgam fillings are the primary source of mercury in the body, older people who have a large number of these fillings suffer no observable health problems. According to health authorities, it is better to leave them in place because removal could actually increase the amount of mercury in the body.

Mercury in some fish has been a problem, but supermarket fish is safe to eat. Shark, swordfish, king mackerel, and tile fish are the species most likely to contain elevated levels of methylmercury, an organic form of mercury. In the past, mercury contamination has come from broken thermometers, contact lens solutions, disinfectants, vaccines, and injections.

Lead contamination can come from old lead water pipes, lead-based paint, lead-acid batteries, and lead-contaminated cookware. Other sources of exposure are lead-based candle wicks, unglazed ceramic pottery, being shot with lead pellets or bullets, or employment in the chemical, electronic, or mining industries.

Cadmium contamination can come from cadmium batteries, industrial processes, mining, etc. Arsenic is used in rodentcides as poison. Arsenic-laced (chromated copper arsenate, or CCA) pressure-treated lumber was common before regulations forbade the manufacture after January 1, 2004. Utility poles and railroad ties are also common hazards. Contamination from cutting the wood with power saws or touching it with the hands is common. Never use old pressure-treated lumber, poles, or ties. Play sets and patio decks made from arsenic pressure-treated lumber are very dangerous for children. Touching the wood with bare hands or bare feet can cause toxic arsenic poisoning.

In addition those listed above, a wide assortment of heavy metal contaminations can come from many sources, including untested water wells and untested natural spring water. Other sources are industrial exposure, manufacturing, paints and dyes, jewelry, mining, soils, criminal intent, research exposure, unapproved chemicals, and the misapplication of approved chemicals.

Bodily symptoms give the first clue that contamination has occurred, and they help to identify the contaminant. Many people who are asymtomatic or have mild symptoms suffer a general malaise and declining health without ever knowing about heavy metal toxicity. Others have been hospitalized, and some have died from heavy metal poisoning without ever knowing the cause. Cadavers have been exhumed during homicide investigations only to find that death resulted from poisoning, not from the condition reported on the death certificate.

Many laboratories test for heavy metal contamination, but even with testing, the diagnosis can be difficult in mild cases. The final diagnosis generally includes an analysis of the physical symptoms and laboratory results. Hair testing is used to determine the long-term history because the heavy metals have become locked in the hair. The following company provides hair tissue mineral analysis without a physician's prescription.

> **Analytical Research Labs, Inc.**
> 2225 West Alice Avenue, Phoenix, Arizona 85021, USA
> http://www.arltma.com/index.html
>
> "Analytical Research Labs specializes in nutrition and the science of balancing body chemistry through hair tissue mineral analysis."

Genova Diagnostics listed below is one of the popular laboratories that physicians use, and they can perform tests on feces, urine, blood, and hair samples to check for contamination.

Genova Diagnostics
63 Zillicoa Street, Asheville, NC 28801, USA
http://www.genovadiagnostics.com/

"Genova Diagnostics is a fully accredited medical laboratory, certified in the areas of clinical chemistry, bacteriology, mycology, parasitology, virology, microbiology, non-syphilis serology, general immunology, hematology, toxicology, as well as molecular genetics by six separate health agencies including the Centers for Medicare & Medicaid Services which oversees clinical labs in the United States under the federal Clinical Laboratory Improvement Amendment (CLIA)."

Chelating compounds, agents, or molecules have the ability to bond metal ions with two or more of the atoms of the chelating agent. The resulting bond is stronger than the existing bond of the metal ion in the body. The chelator pulls the metal ion away from the body molecules and carries it off. Another important feature of a chelating agent is its ability to hold the metal ion while it is discharged by the liver into the digestive tract or the kidneys and into the urine. Heavy metal ions can become captured within the body where they cause damage, or they can be carried in the blood to the liver or kidneys where they are discharged. Those ions discharged by the liver into the intestinal tract are often picked up again and recycled back into the blood. Some of the ions can remain in the urine and feces and can be measured by the laboratory. Heavy metal ions can be discharged from the body in feces, urine, hair, sweat, and discarded skin cells.

Toxic heavy metal chelation can be accomplished with the use of intravenous chelators, oral chelators or by chelating vitamins, minerals, and supplements. The following are the popular pharmaceutical chelators as mentioned by Dietrich Klinghardt,

M.D., Ph.D. of the Jean Piaget Department at the University of Geneva in Switzerland. Dr. Klinghardt described the following chelators in a presentation titled, *A Comprehensive Review of Heavy Metal Detoxification and Clinical Pearls from 30 Years of Medical Practice,* at a conference held in October 2002 for physicians and dentists from Europe, Israel, several Arab countries, and Asia.

"Dimercaprol, British Anti-Lewisite - BAL or dimercapto-propanol, was developed by the British during World War II as a chelation agent for arsenic (Lewisite arsenic poison used by the British and Germans) during trench warfare in World War I. It is administered via deep IM injections only for chelation of arsenic, mercury and lead. About 50% is rapidly metabolized to inactive metabolites."

"DMSA, Dimercapto Succinic Acid or Succimer, is available in intravenous (IV) form or oral form. Succimer is available in oral form as *Chemet®*. DMSA is used to chelate heavy metals such as mercury, lead, and arsenic for removal from the body. It is not effective for other heavy metals. DMSA has the ability to cross the blood-brain barrier, and thus can remove heavy metals from the brain. DMSA can be used by people with existing amalgam fillings to remove mercury from the body tissue and should be used after any dental work related to amalgam (silver-mercury) fillings. Periodic treatments can be repeated as the existing amalgam fillings continue to leach mercury into the body."

"DMPS, 2,3-Dimercapto-1-propanesulfonic acid, was developed in the Soviet Union in 1956 for the purpose of removing radioactive polonium 210 from contaminated workers in the nuclear industry. DMPS is also related to another chelating agent, Dimercaprol, listed above. DMPS is rarely used in the practice of medicine since the development of oral DMSA for the chelation of mercury, arsenic, and lead."

Desferal®, Deferoxamine or Desferrioxamine, is a subcutaneous detox agent for the removal of aluminum and excess iron from the body. *Desferal*® binds to free iron in the bloodstream for elimination in the urine. Excess iron can damage various organs of the body, including the liver, and has been implicated in coronary artery disease."

"Na-EDTA or EDTA, Edetate Disodium, forms chelates with polyvalent metals, especially calcium, thus increasing their urinary excretion. EDTA is commonly used to chelate calcium from the arterial system and thereby reduce hardening of the arteries, but the claims are controversial. It has also been found effective for the removal of aluminum and other metals. One possible disadvantage is the redistribution of toxic heavy metals to other areas of the body rather than completely removing them. Disodium EDTA has been used to increase nitric oxide in the arteries of diseased heart muscle. EDTA is not effective in the removal of mercury. Oral DMSA is used for mercury chelation."

"Ca-EDTA, Edetate calcium disodium, exchanges the calcium atom with a heavy metal atom to form stable EDTA complexes that are excreted in urine. Ca-EDTA is therefore ineffective in the removal of calcium from the arterial system. Disodium EDTA should be used to treat hardening of the arteries."

"Intravenous Vitamin C has been used by dentists to detoxify mercury from within the colon during amalgam removal. It is also used to detoxify lead and aluminum. Oral vitamin C is less effective because bowel tolerance reduces the amount that can be taken."

"Penicillamine, *Cuprimine*® or Depen, is a chelating drug primarily used to treat Wilson's disease (an inherited disorder affecting copper metabolism, causing cirrhosis of the liver as well as brain and eye problems) and rheumatoid arthritis. It removes excess copper and also binds to and removes iron. Penicillamine is normally only available with a doctor's prescription."

I have taken oral DMSA and LipoPhos EDTA (Disodium EDTA plus Essential Phospholipids) as a general preventative self treatment without any heavy metal laboratory testing either before or after the treatment. The effectiveness is unknown.

Anti-Inflammatory Diet Does Not Prevent Heart Disease

Much has been written lately about inflammation within the body caused by the foods we eat, and this has become a hot topic. For example, one author suggests limiting foods from animal sources because he believes they cause inflammation. These authors have common guidelines because they falsely believe that red meat, saturated animal fats, cheese, and eggs are unhealthy. The following represent some of their typical recommendations:

> **Limits Per Week:** One egg, three ounces (0.08 kg) of skinless chicken, two ounces of cheese, and eight ounces of other dairy products.
>
> **Quality Guidelines:** Omega-3 fatty acid-enriched eggs, skinless chicken, natural cheese, and natural yogurt.
>
> **General Guidelines:** Reduce the consumption of food derived from animal sources. If eaten, chicken should be raised in an organic, free-range environment, and eggs should be from free-range hens fed meal from vegetarian sources only and enriched with ground flax seeds.

These strict recommendations are not based on a shred of scientific evidence. The limit of one egg and three ounces (0.08

342

kg) of skinless chicken per week is ridiculous. If eggs and chicken are inflammatory, don't eat them at all. It sounds like advising someone to eat a limited amount of arsenic. If you eat only one egg per week, the remainder in the carton would spoil before they could be eaten, and the amount of omega-3 fatty acid in one egg is totally insignificant. Today I bought five dozen factory eggs for only 10% more than the cost of 18 brown, cage-free, omega-3 enriched eggs. Don't fall for the inflammatory attacks against eggs, and don't waste your money on omega-3 enriched eggs.

I reversed my heart disease while eating at least two regular large eggs each day and occasionally as many as six eggs per day. Chicken is one of my favorite meals—one thigh and one drumstick with all of the skin. Animal fats are not inflammatory, and meat reduces inflammation. A high-protein diet boosts healthy antioxidant levels, but a low-protein diet induces oxidative stress. This means that a high-protein diet prevents undesirable atoms and ions from attaching to healthy body cells and causing disease.

Mind Control Does Not Prevent or Reverse Heart Disease

A philosophy of mind control over the body has been touted as a way to prevent and reverse heart disease by adjusting attitude, mood, feelings, outlook, and anger. This philosophy is scientifically false. The brain does not deposit or remove atherosclerotic plaque from the arteries of the heart, brain, or legs. People with very positive attitudes and calm personalities can develop coronary artery disease as easily as people who are negative and doubtful. It is true that controlling anxiety and stress can reduce excitatory hormones and reduce blood pressure by relaxing arteries as I will discuss in Chapter 5.

Low LDL Cholesterol Reverses Coronary Artery Disease

The diet, supplement, and drug regimen I present in Chapter 4 lowered my LDL cholesterol level 100 points, which is necessary to reverse coronary artery disease. Low LDL cholesterol reduces the work that HDL cholesterol must do to clean the arteries. This makes the HDL more productive and efficient. The LDL/HDL cholesterol ratio is one of the most important blood chemistry measurements for determining coronary artery disease risk.

However, reversing coronary artery disease and removing arterial plaque involves more than having good cholesterol readings. Although my recommended nutritional supplements and drugs make a major improvement in the LDL/HDL ratio, these numbers must be accompanied by other good blood chemistry measurements, the most important of which is the fasting insulin level. Unfortunately, most people have never had a fasting insulin measurement. Many patients have a heart attack followed by stent placement or heart artery bypasses without ever having fasting insulin measured either before surgery or in follow-up treatment. High insulin is the stealth executioner that will eventually kill you. Fasting insulin should be less than 25 (microU/mg) with a preferred goal less than 10 and the insulin measurement on my last test was 7.

High insulin is the stealth executioner.

I will give detailed information in Chapter 4 about blood testing that will provide the measurements you need to determine if your program is working. You won't be able to trick these measurements. You can't reverse heart disease if your measurements are not in accordance with my excellent results.

Removing Arterial Plaque from the Legs

The arteries in the legs are the second most common location for arterial plaque formation, where the deposit can restrict or block the blood flow. The effect is the same as in the heart, but the victim does not immediately die from the restriction. This condition is called *peripheral artery disease (PAD)*. The first symptom may be leg pain during activity or exercise. The pain is the result of the leg muscles being deprived of oxygen, and the symptoms become more severe as the restriction increases.

The body responds to a restriction in a leg artery by allowing greater blood flow to adjacent branches. The severity of the restriction or blockage depends on the location. For example, major arteries in the upper leg cause a much more severe reaction because the area of oxygen-deprived muscle is large.

I expect that the treatment I used to reverse my coronary artery disease will prevent and reverse arterial plaque throughout the body. I have had many positive improvements in health that show this to be true. My legs are stronger as I hike in the mountains or ride my bike, and this is an indication that my leg muscles are receiving a greater amount of blood flow.

Removing Arterial Plaque from the Neck and Brain

Arterial plaque in the arteries of the neck and brain can be life-threatening just as it is in the heart. The plaque restricts or blocks blood flow to the brain, resulting in an ischemic stroke. The plaque can build up slowly over time, or the deposit can rupture in the same manner as in a heart artery. This rupture forms a blood clot that quickly slows the flow to a trickle or stops it completely, and stroke occurs immediately.

Chapter 3

The first symptoms of reduced blood flow to the brain can go almost unnoticed. Cognition becomes slower and the memory weaker, which friends, relatives, or a physician may incorrectly diagnose as the onset of Alzheimer's disease. This reduction in mental capacity is thought to be irreversible. However, it is not irreversible if the cause is arterial plaque because my treatment regimen could very likely reverse the restriction and restore normal brain function.

Strokes can be prevented.

In order to have excellent mental health, the arterioles, metarterioles, and capillaries in the brain must have unrestricted blood flow. Alzheimer's disease could very well be caused by a disruption of the blood flow in these micro arteries. Diabetics have higher incidences of Alzheimer's disease, and their high glucose, triglyceride, and insulin levels are three of the major causes of arterial disease. I believe that my diet, supplements, and drug therapy presented in this book could very well prevent Alzheimer's disease.

The major difficulty with reduced blood flow to the brain is the inability of the victim to diagnose the condition himself. He is doomed unless someone else takes the initiative to seek help and effective treatment. The victim can't read this book with clear understanding if the blood flow to his brain is being restricted. Only a close friend or relative can read it and proceed to take corrective steps. Of course, all of this must be done with the assistance of a physician who has the knowledge and willingness to implement the procedure presented here. This has a small chance for success because most physicians either don't know how to reverse artery disease or insist on using standard methods that are ineffective.

Another major symptom of blood flow restriction to the brain is loss of bodily functions and consciousness. At this stage, the victim is in serious danger and a high percentage die without the problem being resolved. A fast-responding medical team can clear a blockage caused by a blood clot at the site of arterial plaque or a clot flowing from the neck or heart by administering a drug called *plasminogen activator (tPA),* nicknamed *clot buster.* The procedure is called *thrombolytic therapy.* Many people have had brain damage remarkably reduced when a physician responds quickly with this treatment.

Removing Arterial Plaque from the Kidneys

The arteries leading to the kidneys and within the kidneys are subject to the blockage of blood flow in the same way as the heart, legs, and brain. I expect that my therapy will reverse and prevent the formation of arterial plaque in the kidneys.

Removing Arterial Plaque from the Lungs

The medical community may deny that arterial plaque can form within the lungs because a restriction does not produce immediate symptoms as it does in the heart, legs, and brain. The lungs have no nerves to sense pain and the victim feels nothing. The lungs receive oxygen directly from the air and provide the oxygen to the blood, which is the reverse of that which occurs in other organs and throughout the body. It is my belief that a victim may have an arterial restriction in the lungs and die from another cause without ever being aware that the restriction existed. The first symptom could be shortness of breath, but this could be incorrectly diagnosed as a heart condition, not a lung problem. The lungs are also greatly oversized in order to handle high levels of activity, so reduction in blood flow to a section of one lung would not be noticed during normal daily activity.

Chapter 3

Removing Facial Wrinkles and Reversing Skin Aging

Reduced blood flow in small arterioles, metarterioles, and capillaries throughout the body can easily go unnoticed because the symptoms are mistakenly diagnosed as aging. The skin is a prime organ of the body for this condition without anyone being the wiser. I've noticed a big improvement in the appearance of my skin since I began the therapy I present in this book. Facial wrinkles have been reduced and my skin feels tighter and healthier. People often comment that I don't look as old as my birth date indicates. I attribute this improvement to the abundance of essential fatty acids and the removal of cholesterol in capillaries.

Healthy skin also results from the avoidance of free radicals and the body's ability to eliminate them. Smokers are known to have noticeably wrinkled skin. My diet, supplement, and drug program promote the removal of free radicals. Astaxanthin, a naturally derived carotenoid in the larger class of phytochemicals, is the most powerful antioxidant available to visibly improve the skin. It gives the natural red color to salmon. Astaxanthin is very safe to take as a supplement and is not converted to vitamin A. I recommend 4 mg twice a day with a meal.

Preventing Arterial Disease of the Eye

I believe it is possible to prevent eye disease by following my diet and drug regimen. Reversing existing disease may not be possible, but curtailing the advancement of the disease would be a big achievement. Diabetics are highly susceptible to eye diseases caused by high levels of glucose and insulin, and 45% have damage to the blood vessels in the retina (retinopathy) that results in degeneration.

Diabetic retinopathy and macular degeneration are caused by unhealthy arteries that leak, plug, or fail to properly provide oxygenated blood to the cells. My diet and supplement program provides all of the nutrients necessary to build strong, healthy arteries in the eyes and throughout the body. The blood-thinning therapy presented in Chapter 4 prevents micro blood clots from forming and causing leakage or rerouting of the arteries. My cholesterol therapy prevents and removes arterial plaque and cholesterol that disturb healthy blood flow within the eye.

U.S. National School Lunch Program Is Killing the Kids

As a society, we are clearly in a state of nutritional crisis and in need of radical remedies. The statistics are sobering. After 30 years of seemingly solid advice aimed at lowering dietary fat, Americans are collectively growing fatter than ever. Today more than 60% of adults in the U.S. are classified as overweight or obese. So many children have become obese that pediatricians are now facing epidemics of Type 2 diabetes and hypertension— diseases that were unheard of among youngsters just a generation ago.

U.S. government health officials are calling for schools to increase the students' exercise as the remedy for the exploding obesity and Type 2 diabetes epidemics in teenagers, who had been lean and healthy for centuries. The officials continue to increase the carbohydrate loading in the school lunches. Professional nutritionists in the school districts are dictating lunch menus that emphasize fruits, fruit juices, and complex carbohydrates from whole grain products. A piece of meat can't be found with a search warrant in the new lunch programs at public schools.

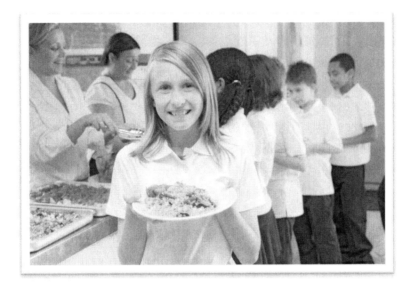

The United States Department of Agriculture has issued the 2011 National School Lunch Program as they have done every year since 1946. However, none of the students were fat or had adolescent Type 2 diabetes in 1946.

"The National School Lunch Program (NSLP) is a federally assisted meal program operating in public and nonprofit private schools and residential child care institutions. It provides nutritionally balanced, low-cost or free lunches to children each school day. The program was established under the National School Lunch Act, signed by President Harry Truman in 1946."

The program gives the following nutritional requirements for school lunches:

"School lunches must meet the applicable recommendations of the Dietary Guidelines for Americans, which recommend that no more than 30 percent of an individual's calories come from fat, and less than 10 percent from saturated fat. Regulations also establish a standard for school lunches to provide one-third of the Recommended Dietary Allowances

> of protein, Vitamin A, Vitamin C, iron, calcium, and calories. School lunches must meet Federal nutrition requirements, but decisions about what specific foods to serve and how they are prepared are made by local school food authorities."

This is called a "nutritionally balanced" lunch even though the carbohydrate content is at least 55% and could go as high as 80% depending upon the foods students throw away. Keep in mind that the scientific requirement for carbohydrates in the diet is zero. This outrageously high carbohydrate diet is giving the school children diabetes.

Carbohydrates are causing the diabetes epidemic.

These professionals and officials with advanced university degrees and the highest credentials are causing the current obesity and diabetes epidemics because they have embraced a nutritional dogma that is scientifically false. The students were thin, active, and healthy in 1946 before the government began dictating the school lunch program. Now we have obesity and Type 2 diabetes epidemics in school children. The school lunch program does not make children healthier because it was formulated by government employees with political and religious motivations, not by scientists like I am.

The following menu and food count was published by a high school in Florida on February 12, 2011.

- Italian Pasta
- Peas & Carrots
- Fresh Vegetable Cup or Tossed Salad
- Fresh Fruit
- Chilled 100% Fruit Juice
- Choice of Flavored & Unflavored Low Fat Milk

Food Name	Amount	Calories	Fat (g)	Carbs (g)	Protein (g)
Italian Pasta Pesto Sauce	1 cup	384	25.7	28.7	11.3
Peas and Carrots	1 cup	109	4.4	16.2	4.9
Fresh Vegetables	1 cup	147	3.9	23.2	5.1
Fresh Fruit	1 cup	73	0.3	18.8	0.9
100% Fruit Juice	1 cup	115	0.3	27.8	1.0
Chocolate Low-Fat Milk	½ pint	158	2.5	26.1	8.1
Total		986	36.9	140.8	31.3

Component	Grams	Calories	% of Calories
Fat, total	36.9	321	33%
Saturated	7.7	68	7%
Polyunsaturated	9.0	77	8%
Monounsaturated	17.0	149	15%
Carbohydrates	140.8	539	55%
Dietary Fiber	19.5	0	0
Protein	31.3	125	13%
Total		986	

The total percentage of fat is nearly within the 30% limit set by the USDA School Lunch Program, and the saturated fat is well within the 10% limit. The professional nutritionists are thrilled with the menu they have created for the students.

Where are the essential fatty acids and essential amino acids in the "nutritionally balanced" high school lunch? The pasta and milk contain a few amino acids but they are inadequate to build strong, healthy bodies. The meal contains very little if any of the essential fatty acids—omega-3 alpha-linolenic acid (ALA) and omega-6 linoleic acid (LA). The body uses alpha-linolenic fatty acid to make eicosapentaenoic acid (EPA) and docosahexaenoic fatty acid (DHA), often referred to as fish oils. The preferred diet should include EPA and DHA fatty acids directly because some people do not make the conversion easily or in insufficient amounts. The body uses linoleic acid to make arachidonic fatty acid (ARA) that is also abundant in meat. Again, it is better to obtain the ARA directly from the diet without depending on the body to convert it from LA. The school lunch fails miserably in the essential fat category. This is typical of a lacto vegetarian diet that has no fish, eggs, or meat but allows milk. The children must eat the food or go hungry.

Schools are forcing students
to eat a lacto vegetarian diet or go hungry.

The school lunches prepared under the guidance of the USDA School Lunch Program are inherently very protein deficient. The professional nutritionists claim that 10% protein in the diet is adequate, but this claim is false. It should be twice this amount for everyone, especially growing students.

The milk is essentially a chocolate sugar drink with the fat removed. The primary calories in the school low-fat milk come from galactose (from the Greek word *galaktos*, meaning *milk*), glucose, fructose, and lactose—all sugars. (Remember, the food components whose names end in "ose" are all sugars.) Hard cheese or eggs would have been a much better choice because they provide all of the essential amino acids and no sugars.

The nutritionists don't care that essential fatty acids are not included in the USDA School Lunch Program and neither do the government health authorities who formulated the program's requirements. The nutrients that are scientifically essential in the human diet have been left out of the high school lunch program, and carbohydrates that are scientifically nonessential constitute the majority of the calories. This school lunch is actually 55% sugars. The USDA School Lunch Program and the school professional nutritionists are killing the kids.

Parents, do something!
The high school lunch program is killing the kids.

Now that the nutritionists have stuffed the kids with glucose, fructose, galactose, and lactose, they will send them to physical education class, where the teacher attempts to make them burn off the excessive load of carbohydrates. Look at our high school kids. They are either so fat they will nearly die if they run, or they are pathetically thin *stick kids* who have hyperactive metabolisms from sugar overload.

The nutritionists insist that the program include high-fiber foods because some of the kids are suffering from diarrhea. This is the new dogma for dealing with lactose intolerance.

Unhealthy High-Fiber Foods			
Bran Cereals	Oats	Rice	Soybeans
Legumes	Split Peas	Lentils	Apples
Broccoli	Potatoes	Grapefruits	Pears

The high school students who have classes other than physical education after lunch are crammed full of glucose, fructose, galactose, and lactose that either put them to sleep or hype them to the ceiling like a metabolic supercharger. Now they are diagnosed with Attention Deficit Hyperactivity Disorder (ADHD). These students are easy to spot because they have the following physical, mental, and emotional characteristics:

- ADHD kids are usually skinny and have poor muscle tone.
- They can't sit still.
- They kick their legs and wiggle their feet while sitting.
- Their hands are always moving, tapping, or fidgeting.
- ADHD kids can't stop talking.
- They require constant discipline.
- ADHD kids talk to themselves when alone.
- They can't maintain an attention span beyond seconds unless they are engaged in a fast-action video game or television.
- ADHD kids are always moving their eyes.

The high school nurse gets involved because the nutrition program has created students with elevated blood glucose and ADHD. What solution does the school district employ to bring the students back down to Earth? Give them drugs:

- Methylphenidate (Ritalin, Concerta, Daytrana)
- Dextroamphetamine-amphetamine (Adderall)
- Dextroamphetamine (Dexedrine, Dextrostat)

Chapter 3

Drugs are given to students to combat the glucose high from the school lunch program.

They are more like zombies now, but at least they are not hyperactive. The teacher will allow them to sleep or stare glassy-eyed out the windows.

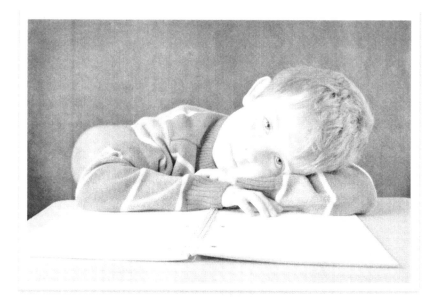

Now what are the students complaining about? Oh, the side effects of the drugs. The nurse records the side effects based on the students' complaints but insists these are nothing to worry about:

- Decreased appetite
- Weight loss
- Sleep problems
- Irritability as the effect of the medication tapers off
- Twitching, grimaces, and jerky muscle movements
- Reduced growth rate
- Increased risk of suicide
- Heart-related death

The high school counselor is then called in to deal with the negative side effects by talking to the students and their parents. These professional psychologists believe that talking to the students and parents will resolve the negative side effects of the pharmaceuticals and the high-carbohydrate school lunch program. They think words will make the students normal.

The high sugar load in the school lunch program has a completely different effect on the obese kids. These students show the same poor muscle tone under a layer of body fat. The sugar load produces completely different results in these kids because they suffer from insulin resistance. The sugar isn't pushed into their cells and therefore does not hype them up like it does the stick kids. The sugar is turned into body fat in the students who have insulin resistant muscle cells, and they develop the following physical, mental, and psychological characteristics:

- Obese kids are lethargic.
- They sit around, exerting the minimum amount of energy.
- They usually don't talk much and rarely disturb others.
- Obese kids cannot be made to run or exercise beyond a minimal effort.
- They fall asleep or into an inattentive trance.
- They are not interested in class participation.

The next day, the school will again stuff the kids with glucose, fructose, galactose, and lactose by giving them the government approved "nutritionally balanced diet."

The fat school children are told they're obese because they won't exercise and are lazy. The school administration doesn't recognize the scientific truth that the children are lethargic and fat because they are insulin resistant. Their muscle cells are resistant to the glucose and the cells can't produce energy. The fat is deposited because of insulin resistance as well. This all started before they were born when Mommy ate according to the *USDA Food Guide Pyramid*. The insulin rush made the fetus insulin resistant. The diet made Mommy fat and now the child is fat. It's not genetic at all.

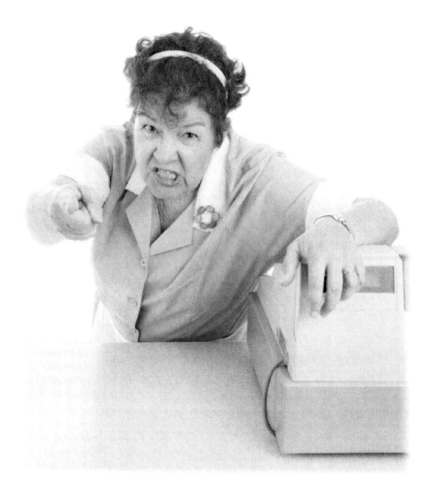

School Professional Nutrition Counselor
"No! You can't have red meat. Eat your carbs."

Scientific Causes of Cardiovascular Diseases

In February 2011, the high-carbohydrate diet for school children become law in Chicago, Illinois. The Little Village Academy on Chicago's West Side passed rules that force students to eat the food served in the cafeteria or go hungry unless they have a medical excuse signed by a doctor. Students are not allowed to bring lunches or snacks from home regardless of the parents' wishes. They must eat grains, fruit, and low-fat milk comprised primarily of glucose, fructose, and lactose—all sugars. The diet police have arrived on the school campus.

Diet police have arrived in Smile, Texas, to photograph the school children in order to make sure they eat all of their carbohydrates (aka sugars). The big unanswered question is, "What will the diet police do when a child throws away his peach or pear?"

In Texas schools, a picture's worth 1,000 calories

By PAUL J. WEBER, Associated Press – Wed May 11, 3:54 pm ET

"SAN ANTONIO – Smile, Texas schoolchildren. You're on calorie camera."

"That's the idea behind a $2 million project being unveiled Wednesday in the lunchroom of a San Antonio elementary school, where high-tech cameras installed in the cafeteria will begin photographing what foods children pile onto their trays — and later capture what they don't finish eating.

Digital imaging analysis of the snapshots will then calculate how many calories each student scarfed down. Local health officials said the program, funded by a U.S. Department of Agriculture grant, is the first of its kind in a U.S. school, and will be so precise that the technology can identify a half-eaten pear left on a lunch tray.

"This is very sophisticated," said Dr. Roberto Trevino, director of the San Antonio-based Social & Health Research Center, which will oversee the program."

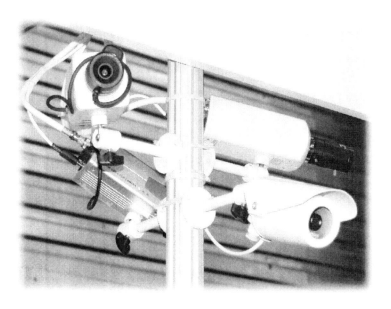

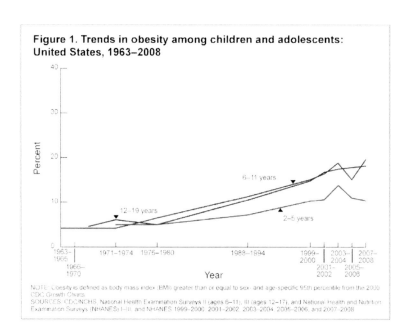

Figure 1. Trends in obesity among children and adolescents: United States, 1963–2008

NOTE: Obesity is defined as body mass index (BMI) greater than or equal to sex- and age-specific 95th percentile from the 2000 CDC Growth Charts.

SOURCES: CDC/NCHS, National Health Examination Surveys II (ages 6–11), III (ages 12–17), and National Health and Nutrition Examination Surveys (NHANES) I–III, and NHANES 1999–2000, 2001–2002, 2003–2004, 2005–2006, and 2007–2008.

Summary of Coronary Artery Disease Pathology

The following table compares two different hypotheses for the pathology of coronary artery disease. The column on the left contains the causes for coronary artery disease according to the United States Department of Health and Human Services and most diet and health organizations. This lipids hypothesis is obviously fictitious because it has been propagated for 50 years, and obesity and heart disease continue to escalate. The column on the right contains the scientific causes for coronary artery disease according to my research and personal experience. My research is obviously correct because it has reversed my heart disease.

Summary of Coronary Artery Disease Pathology	
Causes according to the United States Department of Health & Human Services	Causes According to My Scientific Research
Eating Saturated Fats	Eating Carbohydrates
Eating Cholesterol	Insulin
Eating Red Meat	Insulin Resistance
Eating Diary Products	Glucose
Eating Eggs	Triglycerides
Lack of Exercise	Bacterial Infections
Genetic	Viral Infections

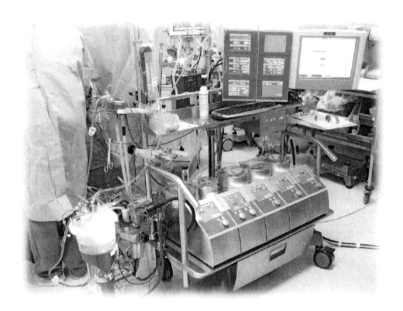

**Heart-Lung Machine
Used During Open Heart Surgery**

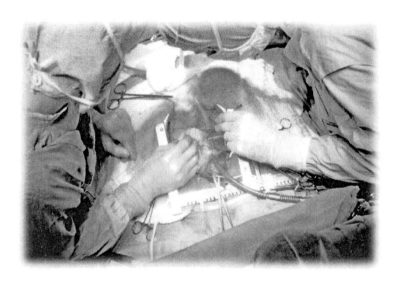

Coronary Bypass Surgery

Reversing Heart Disease and Preventing Diabetes

Chapter 4

Reverse and Prevent Heart Disease, Lower LDL Cholesterol 100 Points, and Reduce Arterial Plaque

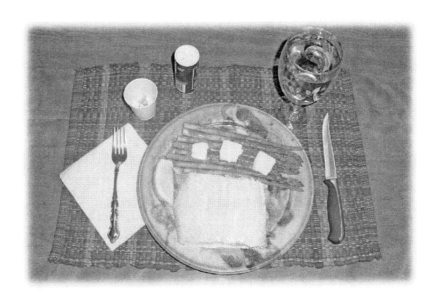

This chapter will present my diet regimen that reversed my coronary artery disease. My cardiologist performed an angiogram in 2009 and informed me that the two small areas of arterial plaque he saw in 2007 had been reduced to half the original size in only 25 months. In 2007, the plaque was causing 40% and 50% restrictions that were not enough to be symptomatic even during a treadmill test. During my most recent visit, he said, "Stay on your program and come see me again in one year."

I discussed my low-carbohydrate diet with my cardiologist after my heart attack in 2007 when he inserted a stent in the upper portion of one of the major heart arteries. This portion of the artery is large, and plaque in this location has been nicknamed *widow maker* because a total blockage results in death. I missed the bullet by a pinhole 1/8" (4mm) or smaller. Fortunately, the pinhole provided enough blood to the heart muscle to prevent any long-term serious damage. The heart enzymes that are produced when heart cells die were fairly low but still enough to confirm that I had suffered a heart attack.

My detailed regimen covers four major categories:

Diet Therapy to
Reverse Heart Disease

Drug Therapy to Prevent and Reverse
Cardiovascular Blood Clots

Vitamin and Drug Therapy to Prevent and Reverse
Cardiovascular Disease

Supplement Nutritional Therapy

I will cover the diet therapy first. Prepare yourself for recommendations that may be opposite to those recommended by most cardiologists, medical societies, medical schools, prestigious medical clinics, and government health agencies.

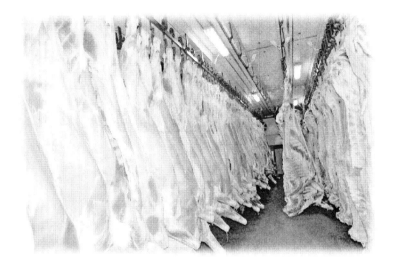

Beef Half Sides Ready to Ship to Market

Diet Therapy to
Reverse Heart Disease

Proper Diet Summary

After several years of searching scientific medical, health, and nutritional studies, I developed the diet program that has reversed my heart disease. Because many studies reach opposite conclusions, the key is to selectively reject those studies that have biased agendas. Since I had the advantage of seeing blood tests from other people, I moved forward with confidence based on nutritional science and human physiology rightly interpreted. I brushed aside the naysayers who told me that imminent death was just beyond the next high-fat prime rib dinner. People with heart disease have written to me stating that their cardiologists were outraged because they were eating a high-fat, low-carbohydrate diet. Fortunately I have a physician who insisted I stay on this diet. There are differences among physicians. If your doctor wants you to pump your blood full of glucose and triglycerides from eating fruits and vegetables, strongly consider finding another doctor.

My diet program avoids those foods that I have identified as contributing to cardiovascular diseases. I have identified the **Forbidden Foods** as those that increase blood sugars, insulin, and triglycerides, and that drive cholesterol subfractions in the wrong direction. High-carbohydrate foods are always on the **Forbidden Foods** list—period.

My diet program reduces your cancer risk because all of the amino acids are available in abundance to build a super-strong immune system. All immune cells are made from polypeptides—complex amino acid molecules. Cancer thrives in an environment of high glucose and high insulin. My diet program has neither. Don't believe people who tell you that whole grains, fruits, and vegetables build a strong immune system. Science does not support that claim.

Hemorrhagic stroke is common in people who consume a protein-limited diet because the deficiency of amino acids weakens the arteries in the head. If you are skinny, the walls in your arteries are skinny as well. My four-pronged program minimizes the risk for ischemic stroke because diet, supplements, and prescription drugs guard against the formation of blood clots.

The following recommendations may totally shock you. If so, you may experience strange mental feelings such as insecurity, puzzlement, and confusion as your brain attempts to reconcile two opposing views, both of which it thinks are true. You will either move forward into scientific truth or revert back into your previous state of dietary brainwashing.

The most difficult part of this diet is the mental anguish encountered when attempting to conquer the long string of myths and false information that clouds the mind. It is extremely difficult for people to believe that whole grains, bagels, 7-grain muesli cereal, pasta, bread, brown rice, nuts, legumes, milk, yogurt, organic fruit, honey, potatoes, soybeans, and vegetable oils are making them sick. They have always been taught that eating red meat and saturated fat is unhealthy. Intense study of this diet regimen is necessary for you to overcome past erroneous thinking. The previous chapters were written in an attempt to help you overcome the massive nutritional brainwashing that has taken place in the last 50 years. Nearly everyone has been brainwashed to believe dietary and medical propaganda that makes us sick and prevents our recovery. We have soaring rates of obesity, diabetes, heart disease, and cancer because of this brainwashing.

Your First Step
Acknowledge that the foods you have been eating made you sick and be willing to change your diet.

You will be eating red meats, fish, fowl, and seafood with their natural fats and a small amount of specially selected vegetables. Avoid all deli meats, such as ham, sausage, and hot dogs, because they can contain hidden carbohydrates in the form of sugars and starches and are always loaded with salt and additives that are not permitted on this diet. Ground meat must be viewed with suspicion since it can contain fillers, flavor enhancers, and other undesirable additives. If the label indicates any additives whatsoever, don't buy it. Meat labeled "100% ground beef" is probably okay, but don't buy any meat, chicken, turkey, or fish that has a flavor-enhancing additive of any kind—period.

Healthy High-Protein and High-Fat Foods		
All Fresh Meat	Beef	Lamb
Pork	Chicken	Turkey
Wild Game	Fish	Seafood
Shell Fish	Hard Cheeses	Coconut Oil
Butter	Organ Meats	Eggs

I reversed my heart disease while eating lots of red meat, fowl, fish, seafood, animal fats, eggs, cheese, butter, and coconut oil. You will be on the wrong path if you try to avoid fats because by doing so, your desire for carbohydrates will soar.

Beef and other red meats are some of the healthy foods you will be eating on my diet therapy. These meats are naturally loaded with essential vitamins, minerals, enzymes, and a multitude of other dietary nutrients needed for optimal health. Red meat is rich in heme-bound iron, the natural form of essential iron. People who avoid red meat and vegetarians can be iron deficient. Vegetarians cannot comply with my diet regimen—period. The body can also eliminate excess heme iron naturally, unlike elemental iron from supplements that can reach toxic levels. High levels of elemental iron have been identified as a heart disease risk. Diet and nutrition books typically underplay or ignore the broad spectrum of nutritional elements in red meat.

You may be shocked to see the percentage of fat in my diet therapy. These percentages were obtained from highly accurate food count internet sources and books. Hard boiled eggs are 62% fat and 35% protein on a calorie basis. Hard cheeses are 64% fat and 30% protein on a calories basis. So you can easily see that butter and other fats easily make this diet 70% fat.

Anti-Aging Metabolic Diet

The following is an anti-aging metabolic diet that reversed my heart disease. It heals the body and prevents premature aging. A good measure of metabolic aging is the appearance of the skin and the ability to balance easily. Premature aging is often seen in people who need a four-point walker to maintain their balance.

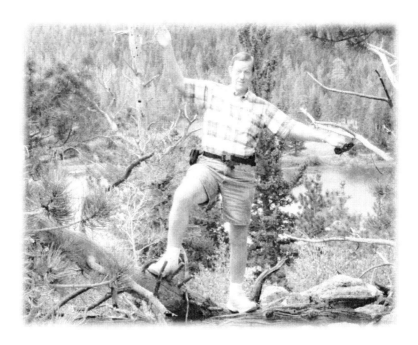

Kent at Lily Lake, Rocky Mountain National Park
August 2, 2011, climbing on fallen trees

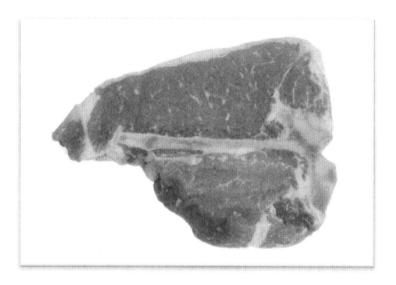

This book will prove that the healthiest diet for humans is:

70% total fat on a calorie basis
  31% saturated fat
  7% polyunsaturated fat
  25% monounsaturated fat
  7% other fats
27% protein
3% carbohydrates (20 gm of which 3 gm or less is fiber)

One thing is certain. People do not have cardiovascular diseases, diabetes, cancer, degenerative disc disease, inflammatory bowel diseases, and strokes because they eat too many Porterhouse steaks as pictured above. Red meat and saturated animal fats do not cause these diseases. Amino acids in meat build a strong heart. People have these diseases because their diets consist primarily of high-fiber, high-carbohydrate foods such as whole grain breads, bagels, cereals, pasta, rice, legumes, fruits, fruit juices, and potatoes. Refined sugar adds to the problem.

The claims that supermarket beef contains harmful antibiotics, hormones, insecticides, toxins, diseases, and bad fats are simply not true. These falsehoods have been propagated by vegetarians, grass-fed beef salesmen, and carbohydrate food manufacturing companies.

Amino acids in meat build a strong heart.

Antibiotics and hormones given to animals are withheld for a period of time before the animals are slaughtered. This waiting period allows the animals to clear the antibiotics and hormones from their bodies. Supermarket meat from feedlot steers does not contain any harmful antibiotics or hormones. This is one rare area in which the U.S. Department of Agriculture's regulations are helping to make our food supply healthier.

Insecticides are sometimes sprayed on farm animals and feedlot steers to rid them of biting and infectious insects. Insecticides that enter the animals through their hides are allowed to clear from their bodies before they are slaughtered. Supermarket meat does not contain unhealthy levels of insecticides. Don't believe the propaganda of the animal rights terrorists.

Because genetically modified grains and fodder fed to animals are broken down into individual amino acid and fatty acid molecules, the risk for GM contamination in the meat is reduced. Eating grains, fruits, and vegetables directly presents a higher risk; therefore, I consider meat to be a superior food.

Chapter 4

Don't Shop the Supermarket Aisles

We have become accustomed to shopping for food by pushing a cart up and down the supermarket aisles and filling it with our favorite manufactured foods made from high-carbohydrate whole grains, fruits, and starchy vegetables precooked and packaged in boxes, bags, and cans. Precooked frozen meals are a favorite of the working mother who rushes home, pops them in the oven or microwave, and 15 minutes later calls the family to the dinner table. This is the wrong way to shop and wrong food to eat. Very few of the items on the supermarket shelves are acceptable on this diet program.

Shop the Perimeter of the Supermarket

You must shop for fresh whole foods in the meat, dairy, and vegetable sections. Most supermarkets in the United States have these departments along the perimeters of the store and the manufactured high-carbohydrate foods in the center aisles. Avoid the bakery that may also be on the perimeter. The marketing strategy that supermarkets use is to make you walk through all the aisles where high-profit manufactured foods are shelved in order to get to the milk and bread. I do not mean to imply that milk and bread are acceptable on my diet program because they are not. Erase your brain of all former nutritional guidelines and start learning scientific nutritional truth.

Erase your brain of all former nutritional guidelines.

Hard cheeses are the only acceptable foods that come from a manufacturing plant. Meat, chicken, fish, and seafood are either fresh or fresh frozen. These foods are not to be precooked or processed.

372

You may eat low-glycemic non-starchy vegetables that are fresh or fresh frozen. The goal is to minimize the size of the vegetable serving because of the low calorie content. This is not a calorie-restricted diet program. You are not to stuff yourself full of low-glycemic vegetables in order to create a full feeling as is commonly recommended. A large serving of vegetables will leave you hungry and looking for a high-glycemic snack later. Eating a low-calorie meal only serves to make you hungry for carbohydrates.

Avoiding fat in the meal is wrong as well. Fat suppresses the appetite and satisfies for a longer period of time. You will avoid the desire to snack on high-glycemic foods if you eat a high-fat meal. Fat actually lowers insulin and glucose. Lean meat allows the body to make glucose from the amino acids. Diabetics must learn to balance the fat content to prevent hypoglycemia, and they should always be prepared to satisfy hunger with acceptable meat and fat to maintain glucose levels.

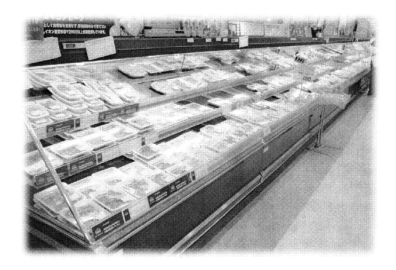

Supermarket Meat Display Case in Japan

Recipe No. 1

Two of My Favorite High-Protein, High-Fat, and Low-Carbohydrate Meals

This meal is a good way to use leftover meat such as beef, pork, lamb, chicken, or turkey. It is especially good for adding moisture and fat to dry, lean meat such as turkey breast.

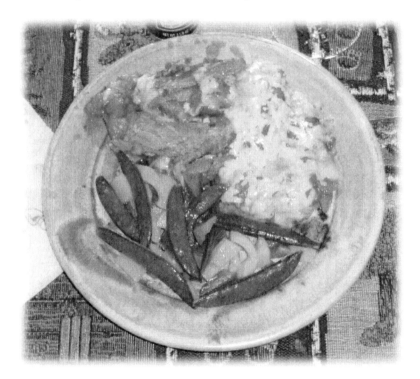

Ingredients:

Refined coconut oil with no flavor
Pre-cooked meat such as beef, pork, lamb, chicken, or turkey
Fresh green and/or yellow zucchini and snow peas
Eggs: one or two per serving
Coarsely-grated or sliced Swiss and cheddar cheese

Directions:

Dice the meat into 1/2" (12mm) cubes.

Slice the zucchini lengthwise and cut into 1/4" (6mm) half-round slices.

Sauté the meat, zucchini, and snow peas in coconut oil on low heat until the zucchini are soft but not mushy.

Break the eggs into a bowl and whisk until well blended.

Pour the eggs over the meat and zucchini and stir until the eggs are cooked.

Spread the cheese over the top of the meat, zucchini, and eggs, and cover with aluminum foil until cheese is melted.

Serve with water, tea, or coffee.

Restaurant Fancy Dinner Suggestion

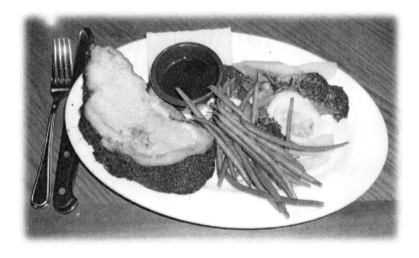

Roast Beef Prime Rib with Steamed Vegetables

Chapter 4

Recipe No. 2

Egg Cheese Burger with Sliced Tomato

This recipe is so quick and easy to prepare that even an ex-vegan could do it.

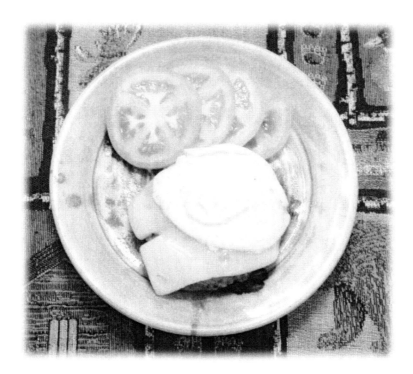

Ingredients:

1 ground meat patty (beef, pork, chicken, or turkey) per serving. Select high-fat beef for better taste; avoid added flavorings.

Eggs: one per serving
Sliced Swiss, cheddar, Monterrey Jack, or cheese of your choice
1 medium tomato
Condiments such as ketchup (low-sugar content) or canola mayonnaise

Directions:

Fry the meat patty in butter, coconut oil, lard, suet, or any other natural animal fat.

Fry the egg when the meat is almost done.

Place a slice of cheese on the patty, and place the fried egg on the top of the cheese.

Use condiments as desired.

Serve with sliced raw tomato.

Canola mayonnaise is excellent with the tomato.

Alternate Dinner Suggestion

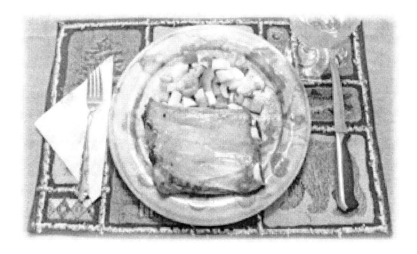

Grilled Beef Ribs with Sautéed Zucchini
Fatty side is up. Do not overcook. Eat all the fat.

Foods We Should Eat

- **Red Meat.** Eat red meat and natural fats, including saturated animal fats. A new study shows fresh red meat has no connection to colon cancer, but manufactured meat products increase colon cancer. A high-protein diet boosts healthy antioxidant levels, but a low-protein diet induces oxidative stress. Avoid labels listing "natural flavors." These additives could contain sugar and MSG, a nerve toxin that makes cancers incurable.

- **Meat, Fish, & Fowl.** Eat beef, lamb, pork, fish, seafood, fowl, and wild game of any kind. Do not cut off any of the fat—eat it all. Do not skin chicken, duck, or other fowl; eat all of the skin. Eat cold water fish such as salmon or fresh sardines (not canned), which are high in omega-3 essential fatty acids. Eat animal protein and animal fats at every meal.

- **Fried Pork Rinds.** Fried pork skins are deep fried in their own fat and sold as fried pork rinds. They would be considered an awesome snack food except for the fact that the raw skins are heavily salted to prevent the growth of bacteria during shipping, handling, and storage prior to cooking. The unhealthy salt is heavily concentrated in the cooked rinds. Some of the salt can be removed by dunking or rinsing in hot water and eating quickly before they get soggy, but a lot of unhealthy salt remains. Eat them in moderation, and completely avoid them if you have high blood pressure.

- **Saturated Fat.** Eat fat, including saturated fat. The North American Indians ate pemmican, a mixture of dried, crushed, and shredded meat mixed 50/50 with the animal fat to yield a food product that provided 75% of its calories from fat. Dried berries were sometimes added. This mixture would keep for many years. Eskimos lived all winter on nothing but caribou meat. They prepared a mixture using 80% fat and 20% caribou meat. Explorers Vilhjalmur Stefansson and Karsten Anderson found their health to be excellent. Dr. Blake F. Donaldson, MD.'s book, *Strong Medicine,* is about the Inuit-style meat-only Eskimo diet.

- **Eggs.** Eggs are highly recommended as the perfect food.

- **Cooking Oils.** Fry in coconut oil, butter, lard, suet, chicken fat, or any other animal fat, and use them generously in recipes. Do not cook with vegetable oils or olive oil.

- **Vegetables.** Eat well-done boiled or steamed asparagus, eggplant, green or yellow string beans, red tomatoes, spinach, celery, peppers, zucchini, or yellow squash. Green, red, gold, and yellow peppers are more easily digested if they are well cooked. Other low-carbohydrate vegetables are also acceptable. They are good when stir-fried in refined coconut oil. Make a nice lunch or dinner by adding cubed precooked or leftover meat to stir-fried vegetables. **Avoid large servings of vegetables. This diet is primarily meat, fish, fowl, seafood, eggs, and cheese with the natural fats.**

- **Avocados.** Eat avocados fresh or as a dip for vegetables. Avoid prepared dips with additives.

- **Cheese.** Hard cheeses are acceptable. Eat only hard cheeses which list no more than 1g of carbohydrates on the nutrition label. Low-salt Swiss cheese is a very good choice and can be eaten without limit. Cheeses with sodium content above 200mg per serving should be avoided, especially by those with hypertension (high blood pressure). Steven Jenkins' *Cheese Primer* is the best reference book for a good education about cheeses. Avoid low-fat, low-cholesterol cheese, but part-skim milk cheese is acceptable. Do not eat cream cheese, cottage cheese, soft cheese spreads, dry curd cottage cheese (DCCC), or Farmer's cheese. Some good cheeses are made from sheep's milk and goats' milk, but goats' milk cheese offers nothing special or better than cows' milk cheese. Blue-veined mold cheeses may promote candida more than other types and should be limited. Do not drink or cook with kefir milk, a fermented liquid product made with active yeasts and bacteria from kefir grain and goats' or sheep's milk. Do not eat kefir yogurt.

- **Omega-3 Fatty Acids.** Supplement with omega-3 essential fatty acids by taking Carlson's® Lemon Flavored Cod Liver Oil. Start with one tablespoon twice a day. Avoid flaxseed oil because it contains more inflammatory omega-6 fatty acids than essential omega-3 fatty acids. Flax is a poor source of omega-3 fatty acids. Your body must convert the shorter ALA fatty acid found in flaxseed oil into EPA and DHA fatty acids before you will receive major benefits, something most of us don't do well. Do not take krill oil as a substitute for cod liver oil. Krill oil is only 17 percent as effective in omega-3 fats at the recommended serving size and the same cost.

- **Borage Oil.** Supplement with omega-6 gamma-linolenic acid (GLA) by taking one borage oil capsule per day. The body cannot produce essential fatty acids—you must get them from the food you eat. Your body uses GLA and omega-3 fatty acids to make E1 series prostaglandins which help reduce inflammation, aid digestion, and help regulate metabolism. Avoid all other omega-6 vegetable oils as found in nuts, seeds, and grains.

- **Vitamins and Minerals.** Supplement with a complete vitamin, mineral, enzyme, probiotic, and amino acid program as described later in this chapter.

- **Reverse Osmosis Water.** Install a reverse osmosis water (R.O.) system with ultraviolet (UV) lamp for all drinking and cooking. The UV lamp kills all viruses and bacteria. Avoid domestic water, which contains chlorine and fluorine. Avoid mineral, natural, or spring water sold in stores as many contain undesirable minerals and contaminants. Some have been pulled from the shelves because of these contaminants.

- **Coffee, Tea, and Soft Drinks.** Regular coffee and black teas are acceptable. Two cups of regular black coffee a day are well tolerated by most people. Don't drink decaf coffee or decaf black tea because toxic chemicals are used to remove the caffeine. Peppermint tea is preferred. A small amount of fresh lemon or lime juice can be added to water or tea. Ginger root tea is great. Cut a piece of ginger root about the size of the small fingertip. Remove the skin. Chop and squeeze with a garlic press. Put the juice and pulp in a cup, French press, or tea ball and add boiling water. Steep for two minutes and strain out the pulp. Ginger has a spicy flavor and is very soothing to the stomach and digestive tract. Diet sodas containing aspartame and regular sodas are absolutely forbidden. Do not drink apple cider vinegar because the health claims are unfounded. The malic and acetic acids in apple cider vinegar can burn the throat and promote bacterial vaginosis (overgrowth of bacteria in the vagina).

- **Beware of Bacteria-Contaminated Coffee.** Many coffee shops and restaurants use a fresh-brewed coffee dispenser that contaminates the coffee with pathogenic bacteria. These bad bacteria upset healthy digestion without the consumer knowing the source of the food poisoning. The worst type of dispenser can be recognized as an insulated tank with a pump on the top. The internal parts of the pump are rubber or plastic diaphragms and tubes that cannot be cleaned. Some coffee shops and restaurants make no attempt to clean the pump mechanism. Rubber and plastic parts easily harbor bad bacteria that continue to multiply. The coffee in the pump also cools easily. The temperature of the coffee is not high enough to sterilize the parts. The best coffee dispenser is the type with a spherical clear glass pot that is very easy to clean and inspect. The coffee filter mechanism should be a stainless steel cone which is also easy to clean. Ask your coffee shop or restaurant about its coffee brewing and dispensing system. Inspect the clear glass serving pots for cleanliness. Don't drink coffee that is brewed and dispensed from a poorly-designed system.

- **Coconut.** Eat and cook with refined or virgin coconut oil, and eat unsweetened shredded coconut in limited amounts. Do not eat processed coconut flour because has fiber and carbohydrates.

- **Nuts and Seeds.** Limit most nuts and seeds because they contain high levels of omega-6 fatty acids. Hazelnuts (filberts), macadamia nuts, and pine nuts (pinion, pinon, pinyon or pignolia) are great snacks with the lowest amount of omega-6 fats. Cashews and walnuts are acceptable. Raw, blanched peanuts are actually a legume but are acceptable in limited amounts. Avoid nuts and seeds if weight loss is a concern because they will stop a good weight-loss program dead in its tracks.

- **Candida Restrictions.** Avoid yeast, vinegar, mushrooms, cheese, and fermented products, including Miso, for an anti-candida diet. These may be included in the diet for those without a candida or other yeast infection.

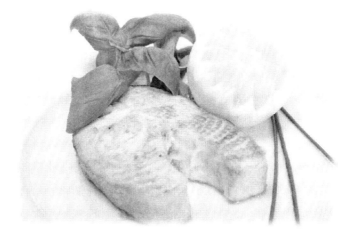

Healthy Salmon Steak

Don't be Afraid to Eat Meals that are 100% Meat and Fats

I lost weight and reversed my heart disease while gorging myself on a 100% meat lunches at a Chinese buffet restaurant. I avoided salt, coatings, monosodium glutamate (MSG), noodles, rice, pastries, and desserts. I also avoided carbohydrates as much as possible. My lunch consisted of three plates loaded with beef, steamed clams, shrimp, roast pork, pork ribs, chicken, frog legs, crab legs, bacon-wrapped imitation crab, imitation crab baked with melted cheese topping, and jasmine hot tea. I only ate a few pieces of bacon because of the high salt content. You can eat more salty foods if you do not have a salt sensitivity that raises blood pressure. I chose the fatty pork ribs in preference to the lean meat.

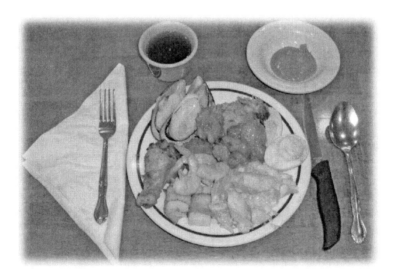

I weighed myself on the morning before the first lunch. Two days later, my weight was down three pounds (1.35 kg). Remember, this was after I ate three heaping plates of food in one meal. I ate the same lunch a week later. After two days, my weight was four pounds (1.8 kg) less than the first weigh-in.

Forbidden Foods

- **Carbohydrate Addiction.** As previously discussed, carbohydrates are very addictive; therefore, do not have them in your house and do not shop when you are hungry. Avoid the snack food aisle.

- **Detox Diet Plans.** Never participate in any of the popular detox diet programs. All of these programs recommend many foods that are very harmful to people with food-caused autoimmune diseases, cancer, heart disease, diabetes, and many others. These plans typically forbid eating the healthy foods listed here. Detox diet plans are always low-fat, which means they are high in harmful carbohydrates. The detox concept is a fraud and a scam. The body does not build up toxins except in cases of rare trace metals such as mercury or lead. The detox diet programs will not remove poisonous metals from the body. A standard scientific laboratory should be used to test for mercury or lead poisoning. Most alternative medicine tests for toxins and food allergies are scams as well. Detox diet plans also run the risk of causing leaky gut syndrome, the major cause of autoimmune diseases.

- **Sugar and Sweets.** Do not eat sugar in any form. Sugar raises the levels of free-radicals and blood insulin, which cause heart disease and diabetes. Do not eat corn syrup, fructose, honey, sucrose, maltodextrin, dextrose, molasses, cows' milk, rice milk, soy milk, grape juice, fruit juice, brown rice syrup, maple syrup, date sugar, cane sugar, corn sugar, beet sugar, succanat, or lactose. Do not eat candy, cookies, ice cream, cakes, dates, crackers, soft drinks, or yogurts, which are all high in carbohydrates. I have described diabetes, heart disease, and cancer as *Carbohydrate Addicts' Syndrome*.

- **Honey.** Do not eat honey. Honey is pure carbohydrate sugar consisting of fructose, glucose, sucrose, maltose, isomaltose, maltulose, turanose, kojibiose, erlose, theanderose, and panose. It is very confusing why people worship honey. They claim it is acceptable because ancient cavemen may have eaten it and somehow adapted to honey as a healthy food. That is an incorrect conclusion. Ancient Paleolithic men may have eaten it once in a lifetime but probably not. They didn't want to be stung by bees any more than we do, and they didn't have any protective netting.

- **Sugar Alcohols.** Many of the "sugar free" sweeteners are classified as *sugar alcohols*. Sugar alcohols affect the blood glucose levels less dramatically than regular table sugar, but they quickly add up to too many carbohydrates. They contain a little more than one half the amounts of carbohydrates as an equal amount of table sugar. Common sugar alcohols are mannitol, sorbitol, xylitol, maltitol, maltitol syrup, galactitol, erythritol, inositol, ribitol, dithioerythritol, dithiothreitol, and glycerol, as well as hydrogenated starch hydrolysates that are found naturally in fruit. These sugar alcohols generally have unpleasant side effects such as abdominal discomfort and bloating. They also have a laxative effect.

- **Processed Meats.** Do not eat processed meats, such as sausage, hot dogs, ham, deli meats, injected turkey, and injected chicken, due to the added chemicals, sugar, and salt content.

- **Starchy Vegetables, Lettuce, and Spinach.** Limit carbohydrates in all forms except low-starch vegetables. Avoid starchy vegetables that grow below the ground, such as potatoes, yams, turnips, beets, radishes, and carrots. Avoid pumpkin and winter squash. Never eat lettuce and raw spinach because of the risk of pathogenic bacteria contamination. Cooked spinach is okay. Salad bars are a high risk for food poisoning.

- **Fruits and Fruit Juices.** Do not eat fruits of any kind because of the sugar, and do not drink fruit juices. Fructose has been linked to insulin resistance, the primary cause of diabetes. Fruit promotes the growth of pathogenic intestinal bacteria, candida yeast, and fungi.

- **Margarine and Trans Fats.** Do not eat margarine, commercial mayonnaise, or any product that contains hydrogenated oils (trans fats). Mayonnaise made with canola oil is becoming popular and is acceptable in small quantities.

- **Omega-6 Fatty Acids.** Strictly avoid omega-6 polyunsaturated vegetable, seed, or grain oils made from corn, soybean, safflower, sunflower, cottonseed, almond, apricot, grapeseed, peanut, poppyseed, rice bran, sesame, teaseed, tomato seed, walnut, and wheat germ. Do not take omega-6 oils such as flaxseed or primrose oil. The omega-6 oils cancel the benefits of the good omega-3 fat. One beneficial omega-6 fatty acid is gamma-linolenic acid (GLA), which can be obtained by supplementation with borage oil. Solid scientific research shows omega-6 fatty acids are highly inflammatory and should never be eaten by anyone with bowel disease, heart disease, arthritis, or any other autoimmune disease. Healthy people should seriously limit these omega-6 fatty acids. Dr. Robert C. Atkins' *Age-Defying Diet Revolution* and Dr. Michael

384

Eades' *Protein Power Lifeplan* both have long sections describing the unhealthy effects of these oils.

- **Milk.** Do not drink cows' milk. Lactose in cows' milk is one of the most allergenic foods, and the symptoms are commonly described as *lactose intolerance*. Milk does not prevent osteoporosis. Do not drink goats' milk, rice milk, soy milk, lactaid milk, acidophilus milk, almond milk, or nut milks of any kind. Do not drink or cook with kefir milk, a fermented liquid product made with active yeasts and bacteria from grains and goats' or sheep's milk. Do not eat kefir yogurt. "Likewise, higher intakes of total dietary calcium or calcium from dairy foods were not associated with decreased risk of hip or forearm fracture." ("Milk, dietary calcium, and bone fractures in women: a 12-year prospective study". *American Journal of Public Health.* 1997 Jun;87(6):992-7.)

- **Heavy Whipping Cream.** Do not use cream or heavy whipping cream because it contains an unacceptable level of lactose called *buttermilk* after separation from the fats. Commercial whipping cream also has thickening additives such as carrageenan which may promote cancer and inflammation in the gastrointestinal tract.

- **Pre-Whipped Cream and Toppings.** Do not eat pre-whipped cream or low-fat, non-dairy whipped cream because these contain sugar or trans fats.

- **Yogurt.** The acidophilus in yogurt is simply killed by stomach acid and does not provide the desirable probiotics for the intestinal tract. The lactose in yogurt feeds candida yeast and pathogenic bacteria. All yogurts are bad food. Goats' milk yogurt is also bad food.

- **Soy Products.** Do not eat any soy products. Fermented foods are not acceptable for those with yeast overgrowth infections. Do not use soy protein powders, but whey protein powders are acceptable. Soy protein is missing several of the amino acids, one of which is classified as an essential. Do not eat soy protein chips or cereals. Tofu made from soybeans has been shown to shrink the brain and cause cognitive impairment (brain fog).

- **Wheat, Corn, and Other Grains.** Do not eat grain products made from wheat, corn, oats, rye, rice, barley, millet, kamut, or spelt. Corn is missing three of the essential amino acids. Grains are allergenic. Multiple sclerosis, lupus, rheumatoid arthritis, and asthma are rare in populations that do not consume grain products.

- **Packaged Foods and Snacks.** Do not eat breakfast cereals, pancakes, waffles, bread, biscuits, tortillas, taco shells, bagels, pasta, noodles, corn chips, popcorn, croutons, spreads, dressings, desserts, soups, soy snacks, rice snacks, candy, cakes, or pastries because they usually contain partially-hydrogenated vegetable oils, omega-6 fatty acids, MSG, chemical thickeners, colorings, and preservatives. They are all very high in carbohydrates.

- **Potatoes and Yams.** Do not eat any potatoes, sweet potatoes, yams, French fries, or potato chips. French fries are not only very high in unhealthy carbohydrates, but they're generally cooked in hydrogenated soybean oil or other rancid vegetable oils that are known to generate cancer-causing chemicals at high temperatures and are high in inflammatory omega-6 fatty acids. Always use coconut oil, butter, lard, suet, or other animal fats to fry other foods.

- **Bananas and Citrus.** Do not eat bananas, oranges, or grapefruits because they are very high in carbohydrates. One slice of lemon in tea or on food is permitted. Do not drink citrus juices.

- **Legumes.** Do not eat beans and legumes because of their high carbohydrate levels. Limit peanuts because they are a legume and contain an unhealthy fat.

- **Bad Cheeses.** Do not eat soft, dark orange cheeses that are made from partially-hydrogenated oils (trans fats). Avoid processed cheese foods that contain corn oil instead of butterfat. Do not eat cream cheese or cottage cheese since they contain lactose and other sugars. Contrary to popular belief, cottage cheese has been proven to cause bone loss and osteoporosis.

- **Smoking.** Stop smoking—but stop eating sugar first. Sugar will destroy your health faster than smoking.

- **Low-Fat Products.** Do not eat any product labeled "low-fat."

- **Hydrogenated Oils.** Do not eat anything containing hydrogenated oils (trans fats). Read every label.

- **Low-Cholesterol Products.** Do not eat any product labeled "low cholesterol."

- **Carbohydrates.** Avoid carbohydrates from all sources except low-starch vegetables.

- **Starch Blockers.** Do not take starch-blocking supplements or drugs. They promote fermentation of the starch by yeast in the colon. The undigested starch also provides a high-energy food source for pathogenic bacteria and toxin-producing fungi.

- **MSG.** Avoid monosodium glutamate (MSG) and the dozens of flavors and seasonings that have deceptively hidden the MSG glutamic acid ingredient.

- **Carrageenan.** Avoid carrageenan, a gum extracted from red seaweed and used as a fat substitute to thicken many food products. Unfortunately, carrageenan is used in many otherwise acceptable low-carbohydrate foods such as processed meats and heavy whipping cream. Carrageenan may promote malignancy and inflammation in the gastrointestinal tract and other cancers.

- **Fast-Food Restaurants.** Avoid fast-food hamburgers that are bulked-up with soy protein and/or cooked in trans fats or polyunsaturated fats. Burgers that are labeled as 100% beef and cooked by grilling or frying in their own fat are the best. Avoid French fries as well because the frying oils are either trans fats, polyunsaturated fats, or fat that has become rancid from overuse. Grilled chicken breast is an acceptable choice. Don't eat the bun. Don't eat any coated or deep-fried foods.

- **Restaurant Chicken Wings.** Restaurants ruin most of the good foods they touch. Chicken wings are a good example of awesome food that is destroyed by deep frying in trans fats or unhealthy omega-6 polyunsaturated fats, such as soybean, corn, safflower, or peanut oil. These fats easily become rancid, which makes them unhealthier. Baked chicken, fish, and red meat are okay if they are not heavily salted or treated with tenderizers such as MSG. You can ask the restaurant manager, but he may not tell you the truth.

Chapter 4

Cheating and Snacks on this Diet Program

Most people are tempted to cheat on this diet program. The first question they ask concerns **Forbidden Foods**. They want permission to eat them. Cheating a little will not derail my diet program if the carbohydrates do not raise insulin and you do not sink back into the old habit of gorging on extremely addictive carbohydrates. The following are some tasty suggestions to enjoy in limited amounts without disrupting the program.

- *Dove*® dark chocolate *Silky Smooth Promises*® made by Mars are only 43.4% sugars after digestion. Limit the quantity to one a day. They are not sugar sweet and add a nice flavor when eaten with black coffee or hot tea.

- Nuts in moderation, meaning two mouthfuls only.

- Strawberries, blackberries, and raspberries are relatively low in carbohydrates. A serving equal to five medium-size strawberries per day should not be a problem.

- Real extra creamy heavy whipped cream in a pressure can tastes great on the berries or on fried pork rinds. Pick a brand with the fewest additives and thickeners. The sugar content should not exceed 1 gm per 2 tablespoons. The goal is to pick a brand with the most fat from real heavy cream. Limit the amount.

- Taste the free sample of watermelon or cantaloupe that may be offered in the supermarket but don't buy one.

- One quarter of an apple once a day either raw or baked.

- Fat suppresses the appetite. For a high-fat, low-carb snack, place a pat of butter on each of four or five saltine crackers that have unsalted tops. Pick a brand of cracker without sugar and fewer additives. It's impossible to avoid the bad fats, but the amount is small. This treat also works wonders

388

as a midnight sleeping aid. Drink a little water with or after the cracker/butter snack and stay up for a few minutes to let it all settle. Go to sleep on the right side because it allows the stomach to drain into the small intestines more easily and completely.

- A rare treat of ice cream will not derail the program, but it should be limited in amount and frequency. Choose a high-fat, low-sugar ice cream instead of the low-fat varieties. Fat satisfies the appetite and slows digestion of the sugars.

Don't combine all of these permissible cheats within the same day because the total carbohydrate intake must be kept low. Avoid all candy, fruit, breads, desserts, and drinks that cause intestinal gas—a sure sign of bacterial fermentation.

Most people who are carbohydrate addicts have difficulty eating small portions or one bite of a favorite high-sugar treat. This leads to a complete pig-out. Carbohydrate addicts are hooked on a chemical blood glucose surge and the feeling of euphoria that becomes a psychological escape from reality. They should treat the problem the same as drug addiction and alcoholism— topics beyond the scope of this book.

People do not develop a compulsive addiction to food. They become addicted to carbohydrates and to the alcohol that is produced in the colon when the sugars are fermented. People do not become addicted to meat, protein, or fats. A protein or fat craving may occur on the standard low-fat, low-meat diet, but this is not an addiction. The body is simply screaming for healthy nourishment.

Chapter 4

Initial Low-Carb Symptoms Are More Severe in Diabetics

This diet produces a wide range of reactions among individuals. I can't tell you how you will respond because everyone does not respond in the same way. Diabetics have special considerations, but I have very good news for them also. My regimen is perfect for Type 1 or Type 2 diabetics, and this diet may allow them to taper off drugs with their doctors' permission. It reverses hypoglycemia and is 100% effective in preventing Type 2 diabetes mellitus in those who are not yet afflicted.

Going from a standard high-carb diet to the low-carb diet can initially cause several negative symptoms depending on other health problems. Healthy individuals have few negative reactions when they switch to my diet, but undiagnosed health problems may be exposed in those who are not as healthy as they thought. The following are some of the typical symptoms that some people experience:

- **Headache** – The low-carbohydrate diet can cause a slight headache in the forehead. I simply ignore it.

- **Ketosis** – Ketosis is a condition in which the liver produces a group of harmless elements called *ketone bodies*, which may create a strange taste in the mouth. This will only last for a few weeks at most. Claims that ketosis is unhealthy are scientifically false. Ketosis is not the same as ketoacidosis, a dangerous condition seen in diabetics.

- **Low-blood sugar symptoms** - A low-carbohydrate diet will reveal other health problems such as hypoglycemia or diabetes by exhibiting symptoms of low-blood sugar, e.g., headache, dizziness, blurred vision, difficulty concentrating, etc. Mix 1/2 teaspoon of glutamine in a glass of water or unsweetened

390

tomato juice to relieve the systems. Snack on fatty meat to prevent these symptoms. Don't go hungry. See your doctor if symptoms persist and are moderate to severe.

- **Constipation** - Constipation or a sluggish fullness can result because the digestive system is not accustomed to a healthy diet. The common opinion that it is necessary to have one or several bowel movements each day is a myth. Skipping one or even two days without a bowel movement is normal. Constipation can be prevented by taking the probiotics along with extra magnesium. Magnesium is a natural and safe laxative when taken in excess. People are commonly magnesium deficient, so this supplement is highly recommended. Take one KAL® Magnesium Glycinate 400 (200 mg) three times a day with meals.

- **Leg muscle weakness** - Leg muscle weakness appears in some people, particularly at the beginning of a hike or when climbing stairs. The best advice is to try to ignore it and keep going. The strength will return in a few minutes, and the legs will be stronger than ever as you continue on the hike.

- **Low energy level** - This diet can result in a lower energy level. Weakness is typical when people have been on a low-fat, high-carbohydrate diet and the body is not accustomed to burning fat for energy. Marathon runners experience this switchover that they call *hitting the wall.* Exercising after breakfast is the best way to kick-start the metabolism for the day. The low-carbohydrate diet lowers the body's metabolism, and a low metabolism is excellent for longevity. A high metabolism simply wears out cells faster, causes disease, and shortens life spans.

- **Weight loss** - This diet will help overweight people to lose weight. If weight loss is desired, the serving should be a piece of meat the size of the palm of your hand for each meal. Fatty cuts are okay but avoid excessive fats to reduce the calories. Chicken thighs are great but don't eat the skin. Don't buy the dry, lean cuts such as breast meat. Saturated fats are healthy and heal the body, but you must place a restriction on your caloric intake as well as your carbohydrates. Eat fats in moderation. Use very little butter on vegetates or none at all. Snack on low-carb vegetables only.

- **Weight gain** - If weight gain is desired, simply increase the fat by using butter generously on cooked vegetables from the acceptable list. Buy extra fatty meats and eat all the fat. Eat the skin on chicken and salmon. Eat a lot of hard cheeses and increase the amount of protein. Underweight people should never go hungry but should eat additional amounts of the acceptable foods to maintain weight or gain as desired. Underweight people easily gain weight on this diet.

- **Carbohydrate cravings** - Carbohydrates are highly addictive, but people don't believe this until they try going without them. This is the main reason people give up on the low-carb diet—especially those who are prone to addictive behaviors and have weak self control. They make up all kinds of excuses for quitting low-carb, but the truth is they can't overcome their addiction to carbohydrates. Addiction to high-sugar fruit is a serious problem among adults and children. A study of the shopping carts of adults and the eating habits of children easily proves this unhealthy addiction exists in all age groups. They would rather be sick than give up the addiction.

392

- **Nighttime Leg Cramps** - I have finally discovered the cause of nocturnal leg cramps in those on my high-fat, high-protein, low-carbohydrate, and low-fiber diet. The muscle cramps usually occur toward morning and appear just as one begins to awake, or perhaps it is the cramps that awaken them.

  My diet causes the body to discharge undesirable intercellular fluid, a great health benefit for those with hypertension and fluid retention. As the night progresses, the body becomes less hydrated, and it is this dehydration of the leg muscles that causes the cramps. A reduced level of potassium in the muscle cells contributes to the problem. The cure is simple. Keep a bottle of water near the bed and take two swallows of water each time you arise to use the bathroom. Add 1/8 teaspoon (305 mg) of potassium chloride in the form of Morton's Salt Substitute® to the water. I never get leg cramps when I follow this protocol. The extra water may increase the need to urinate, but I have not found this to be the case. Instead of urinating more frequently, the volume is simply increased. The extra water could also have other health benefits such as flushing the kidneys and removing more of the undesirable waste products from the blood.

  You may get a nocturnal leg cramp if you forget to hydrate during the night or if you think drinking water during the night is unnecessary. The cramps can be very painful. I have found that fighting against the tightening muscle is the best approach. Try to get out of bed as soon as possible and immediately stand up. This relieves the cramping faster than waiting a few seconds for it to dissipate. The wait time seems like forever.

Drug Therapy to Prevent and Reverse Cardiovascular Blood Clots

Cardiologists often prescribe Plavix® and aspirin to prevent platelets from sticking together to form life-threatening blood clots. These drugs are typically prescribed for patients who have a stent, have had heart artery bypass surgery, or have an irregular heart rhythm. The physician may also prescribe these drugs for people who have hypertension, coronary plaque, peripheral artery disease, arterial calcium deposits, or for those who have symptoms of oxygen deprivation to the brain. Coronary plaque is often the cause of hypertension. Plavix® plus aspirin greatly reduces the risk of a clot formation at the site of a plaque rupture and thereby reduces the risk for heart attack.

- **Plavix®** - Take one 75 mg tablet with dinner each day or as prescribed by your physician.

- **Aspirin** - Take one 81 mg over-the-counter tablet with breakfast each day or as prescribed by your physician.

Plavix® (75 mg) with dinner and aspirin (81 mg) with breakfast are taken to keep a ruptured plaque deposit from causing a blood clot and the resulting heart attack, stroke, or blockage in other arteries throughout the body. Your cardiologist will prescribe this treatment to prevent a blood clot from forming inside of a coronary artery stent. You may be busy in your daily routine and never know that a heart attack or stroke was prevented.

Plavix® (clopidogrel bisulfate) works to make blood flow more easily, and the effectiveness is not influenced by vitamin K in the diet or in supplements. Plavix® is generally the drug of choice for people with arterial plaque or those who have had stent placement or artery bypass surgery.

What is Plavix?
http://www.drugs.com/plavix.html

"Plavix (clopidogrel) keeps the platelets in your blood from coagulating (clotting) to prevent unwanted blood clots that can occur with certain heart or blood vessel conditions.

Plavix is used to prevent blood clots after a recent heart attack or stroke, and in people with certain disorders of the heart or blood vessels.

Plavix may also be used for other purposes not listed in this medication guide."

Aspirin has been used for many years as a blood thinner and anticoagulant. The effect is very positive and predictable, but it has side effects that can present serious complications. Aspirin has been known to trigger an asthma attack in sensitive individuals. Aspirin has long been known to cause stomach ulcers to bleed to the point of being life-threatening. Often the victim is unaware of the blood loss until he collapses from low blood pressure. Even so, a daily 81 mg aspirin tablet presents no side effects in most people and could save your life.

Aspirin can save your life if you are having a heart attack. If you think you could be having a heart attack, take two (2) full-strength 285 mg aspirin tablets immediately. Although they can perform like a miracle, you may have a false sense of security that the crisis is not serious. Don't ignore your symptoms. Always go the hospital emergency room if you suspect you have had a heart attack. Mild symptoms could make the decision to go to the emergency room difficult. It is better to have someone drive you to the hospital and wait in the visitors' area where help is seconds away rather than to wait at home. People often wait too long before going to the hospital. It could cost you your life.

A relative knew she was having a heart attack and went to the hospital emergency room. The doctor could not find anything wrong and suggested she return home, but she refused to leave and insisted on further tests. Sure enough, she did have a heart problem that required placing a stent in one of her heart arteries.

An aspirin a day could keep heart attacks away
Telegraph.co.uk - August 24, 2008
By Joanna Corrigan

"Men and women should take aspirin every day to help prevent heart attacks and strokes once they reach middle age, according to research.

Experts believe everyone over an age threshold - possibly as young as 50 - should be told to take the simple painkillers to ward off serious cardiac problems.

Aspirin lowers the chance of suffering a heart attack or stroke because it helps stop blood clots forming in the arteries of the heart or brain.

Under current guidelines, GPs only prescribe it to a patient who has already had a heart attack or stroke, or who is considered at high risk of another attack in the near future.

Previous studies have already suggested taking aspirin could cut the chance of having a heart attack or stroke by a third and the risk of a fatal attack by 15 per cent.

New joint research by Nottingham and Sheffield universities bolsters the view that blanket prescriptions could help millions of people later in life.

Analysis of 12,000 patients indicated men as young as 48 and women from the age of 57 could benefit from taking the drug every day.

Researchers, writing in the journal Heart, also claimed many of those who should be receiving aspirin under the current system were falling through the net.

The study suggests it would be easier to have a specific age threshold as a catch-all to ensure everyone is treated.

It found that by the time men are 47 and women 58, the risk of coronary heart disease was 10 per cent, which it deemed a proportion worth tackling.

Only if the patient could suffer dangerous side effects, for example if they had a stomach ulcer, diabetes or were at high risk of bleeding, should they be exempt, it concluded."

This treatment with Plavix® and aspirin is not without side effects. The combination reduces the clotting ability of the blood, and therefore cuts or injuries bleed more freely, and the body bruises much more easily. Your physician may recommend that you suspend Plavix® before elective surgery.

Coumadin® is another frequently prescribed blood thinner for patients who are at high risk for blood clotting or who have had a heart attack or stroke. Hemorrhage is the most serious risk associated with Coumadin® therapy. An acquaintance had been on Coumadin® for years after a stroke. While on a cruise, she fell and had uncontrollable internal bleeding. She nearly died before getting to a hospital. If you are taking blood-thinning drugs and have any fall, bad bump, or bruising, seek medical attention before severe symptoms begin.

What is Coumadin?
http://www.drugs.com/coumadin.html

"Coumadin (warfarin) is an anticoagulant (blood thinner). Coumadin reduces the formation of blood clots by blocking the formation of certain clotting factors.

Coumadin is used to prevent heart attacks, strokes, and blood clots in veins and arteries.

Coumadin may also be used for purposes other than those listed in this medication guide."

Coumadin® is often compared to rat poison for good reason. Both Coumadin® and some rat poisons inhibit vitamin K. Rat poison depletes vitamin K to the extent that the animal bleeds to death, while Coumadin® controls the vitamin K level to prevent blood clotting in individuals with conditions such as heart arrhythmias, heart valve prolapse, atrial fibrillation, and other complications that present a high risk for thrombosis (blood clots).

Vitamin K is a blood-clotting factor. Since vitamin K deficiency leads to bleeding, a deficiency while taking blood thinners is a serious concern. Drugs such as Coumadin® (warfarin sodium) inhibit vitamin K, and routine blood tests are required to ensure the correct dosage. Eating food high in vitamin K or taking a vitamin K supplement is not recommended with these drugs.

These blood thinners are not the initial causes of spontaneous bleeding, but rather they prolong bleeding as a result of injury or disease, e.g., ulcerative colitis and stomach ulcers. One should be very cautious about excessive blood thinning. Never eat garlic or take garlic supplements while on blood-thinning drugs. Garlic is a very potent blood thinner. Be extremely cautious also about taking any herbal remedies and supplements. A wide assortment of herbal products, including St. John's Wort, Coenzyme Q_{10}, vitamin K, bromelain, dan-shen, dong quai, garlic, and ginkgo biloba are known to interact with Coumadin® or otherwise affect coagulation.

Pradaxa® (dabigatran etexilate) is an alternate drug to Coumadin® that keeps the platelets in the blood from coagulating. The drug functions in a different manner and does not suppress vitamin K as is the case with Coumadin®. These two drugs are generally prescribed to prevent blood clots that result from atrial fibrillation.

Check the quotation below to see why taking the vitamin K supplement is important. Vitamin K is needed to prevent unhealthy bleeding. Vitamin K is necessary for the healthy healing of injuries, but it is not a blood thickener as many people claim. Taking vitamin K does not promote blood clots in healthy individuals and should not be a concern for those who are not taking blood-thinning drugs. Always talk to your doctor before taking vitamins, minerals, supplements, and herbal products in combination with prescription drugs.

Why Should We Take Supplemental Vitamin K?
http://www.nlm.nih.gov/medlineplus/druginfo/natural/983.html

"In the body, vitamin K plays a major role in blood clotting. So it is used to reverse the effects of "blood thinning" medications when too much is given; to prevent clotting problems in newborns who don't have enough vitamin K; and to treat bleeding caused by medications including salicylates, sulfonamides, quinine, quinidine, or antibiotics. Vitamin K is also given to treat and prevent vitamin K deficiency, a condition in which the body doesn't have enough vitamin K. It is also used to prevent and treat weak bones (osteoporosis) and relieve itching that often accompanies a liver disease called biliary cirrhosis.

People apply vitamin K to the skin to remove spider veins, bruises, scars, stretch marks, and burns. It is also used topically to treat rosacea, a skin condition that causes redness and pimples on the face. After surgery, vitamin K is used to speed up skin healing and reduce bruising and swelling."

Vitamin K has been shown to prevent and reverse calcification in the arteries. A deficiency can cause cardiovascular disease known as *hardening of the arteries*. This is bad news for people who are taking Coumadin® to treat other cardiovascular problems. Vitamin K is also needed for strong bones and reduces the incidence of prostate cancer.

Bruising and Bleeding Exacerbated by Blood Thinners

Blood thinners such as Coumadin®, Plavix®, aspirin, omega-3 fatty acids, garlic, and vitamin C can exacerbate bruising from small blood vessel ruptures below the skin and external bleeding from scrapes or cuts. Minor injuries can be treated at home, and emergency first aid can be performed on serious injuries prior to receiving professional treatment. The following procedures make the injury less serious and promote faster healing.

While taking blood thinners, bruises can appear spontaneously without realizing that any injury has occurred. A burning or stinging sensation is an indication that bleeding below the surface of the skin is occurring, and a dark blue bruise quickly appears. The bleeding may cause a pooling of blood and a lump called a *hematoma*. Take immediate action to keep the bruise or hematoma as small as possible.

A small bruise should be treated by applying medium pressure to the affected area with the fingers or thumb in an attempt to stop the subsurface bleeding. Hold pressure on the area for at least 10 or 15 minutes. Release the pressure slowly and do not rub or agitate the affected area. Keep the muscles in the area at rest. Observe the injury for at least 30 minutes to ensure the bleeding does not reoccur.

Deep bruises or bleeding that hurts but cannot be seen can occur as the result of a pulled muscle, tendon, or ligament. I found the best treatment to be an elastic athletic bandage wrapped lightly during the day but removed before bedtime. Healing could take ten days or more. You can expect the injury to become very painful during the night whenever you awake.

Bruising can result from a blood draw or an IV insertion if precautions are not taken. Always remind the nurse that you are on blood thinners. I had an IV removed by a nurse who placed gauze and thumb pressure over the site, but she made the mistake of releasing the pressure to take a little peek. Because she was in a hurry, a hematoma immediately formed that required extra treatment and took two weeks to heal. Since that incident, I ask the nurse to allow me to apply my own pressure. I request that a pressure wrap be used and leave it on for at least 20 minutes before slowly and cautiously removing it.

 A hematoma can suddenly appear when the injury causes a volume of bleeding larger than a small bruise. Medium pressure should immediately be applied to the area in an attempt to stop the bleeding. This measure will usually be successful but should be followed by applying a pressure wrap while continuing to hold pressure on the area. A hematoma on a finger can be treated by wrapping with a band aid, but avoid wrapping too tightly as this will cut off normal blood circulation. Arm or leg injuries will require an elastic wrap as commonly used for sports injuries. A padding of folded gauze should be applied directly on the injury prior to the elastic wrap. Care must be taken to get a proper tension on the wrap. Avoid a tight wrap that will strangle the limb and prevent normal blood flow. The elastic wrap has the added advantage of reducing the hematoma by allowing the blood to be absorbed. Do not leave the wrap on longer than 30 minutes and never go to sleep without first removing the wrap.

Surface cuts tend to bleed persistently and continue to weep when on blood thinners. Two methods can be used to stop the weeping.

- The first is to apply medium pressure with the fingers or thumb. Hold the pressure for 10 to 15 minutes and release slowly. Observe the injury for another 15 minutes to make certain weeping has not resumed, which is likely to occur.

- The second and more effective method is to apply the point of an aluminum sulfate (65%) stick, called a *styptic pencil*, directly on the area that is weeping. These old-fashioned medicinal pencils look like a piece of hard chalk and have been sold for years to stop bleeding caused by a cut from a shaving razor. Hold pressure by pressing the pencil on the injury for 5 to 10 minutes and release slowly. The injury will sting when the pencil is in the correct place. Release the pencil slowly and observe the injury for another 15 minutes to make certain weeping has not resumed. Reapply the pencil as many times as needed and increase the time if bleeding is persistent. The styptic pencil seems to discourage infections. Do not apply an antibiotic for at least 30 minutes after bleeding has stopped as this will cause the bleeding to resume. Keep the pencil dry. To clean prior to use and/or storage, scrape the point with a knife to remove some of the pencil.

Vitamin and Drug Therapy to Prevent and Reverse Cardiovascular Disease

Cholesterol can be dialed to perfect numbers using nicotinic acid (vitamin B3) and simvastatin, a popular cholesterol-lowering prescription drug. This relatively inexpensive but very effective therapy reduced my arterial plaque by 50% in only 25 months as determined by accurate procedures. In my case, the cardiologist performed an angiogram in September 2007 that showed two coronary plaque restrictions of 50% and 40%. Twenty-five months later, he performed another angiogram that showed the occlusions were reduced to 25% and 20%—a 50% reduction in the size of the plaque deposits.

Plaque removal is achieved by taking 2000 mg per day of real niacin (nicotinic acid) plus 10 mg of Zocor® (simvastatin). These doses are typical for a large male and should be half as much for a small female. Lifestyle and treatment must address all of the risk factors and promote the protective factors such as high HDLs. The high-fat, high-protein, low-carbohydrate diet I present reduces LDL cholesterol, insulin, glucose, triglycerides, fibrinogen, and Lp(a), and raises the good HDL cholesterol. All of these changes were necessary to reverse my heart disease. I believe they will also prevent Type 2 diabetes and cardiovascular plaque 100% of the time. The prevention of Alzheimer's disease and cancer may be an additional health benefit.

High doses of vitamin B3 reverse heart disease.

My vitamin and drug therapy has produced awesome cardiovascular improvements and has been enthusiastically approved by my cardiologist. The angiogram revealed that my heart disease has been reversed. I believe the combination of nicotinic acid and simvastatin has removed arterial plaque and calcium deposits throughout my body. This is not an unproven theory or conjecture as many books, news articles, medical clinics, government health organizations, and medical colleges present. This reversal is a cardiologist-verified reality. It has already occurred. However, this treatment does much more than reverse heart disease. I believe it has reversed and prevented vascular disease in other areas of my body.

Most books and articles simply parrot other publications without verifying that the references are not pure conjecture and unsubstantiated theories. I discarded all of this material and built my foundation and recommendations on the science of basic human anatomy and physiology. This is why the material I present is in stark contrast to most references.

Nicotinic Acid and Simvastatin Therapy

The niacin must be in the form of the nicotinic acid molecule. Other niacin formulas are worthless in treating cholesterol. Do not substitute other products.

Niacin must be the nicotinic acid molecule.

Over-the-counter nicotinic acid (niacin) plus 10 mg per day of simvastatin achieved a 93 point drop in LDL cholesterol from 168 to 75, or 55%. Nicotinic acid is also available as a very effective prescription drug with the trade name Niaspan® made by Abbott Laboratories®. Niaspan® achieved a better decrease in LDL cholesterol from 168 to 68, or 60%, a full 100-point drop. This result is astonishing.

Over-the-counter nicotinic acid plus 10 mg per day of simvastatin increased HDL cholesterol from 57 to 68, or 19%, a nice 11-point increase. Niaspan® was slightly less effective but still produced a good result, with HDL cholesterol increasing from 57 to 66, or 16%. Either source of niacin has excellent effectiveness. Niaspan® has the benefit of assuring a consistent pharmaceutical grade drug.

Niaspan, 500 mg Controlled-Release Nicotinic Acid
http://www.drugs.com/niaspan.html

What is Niaspan?

"Niaspan Controlled-Release works by reducing LDL ("bad") cholesterol and triglycerides and increasing HDL ("good") cholesterol. Niaspan contains niacin, also called nicotinic acid, a B vitamin (vitamin B3). It occurs naturally in plants and animals and is present in many multiple vitamin supplements.

Niaspan lowers cholesterol levels, reducing the risk for a second heart attack, slows or treats hardening of the arteries, and lowers very high serum triglyceride levels. It is used in combination with diet."

Niaspan side effects
http://www.drugs.com/niaspan.html

"Get emergency medical help if you have any of these signs of an allergic reaction: hives; difficulty breathing; swelling of your face, lips, tongue, or throat. Call your doctor at once if you have any of these serious side effects:

- feeling light-headed, fainting;
- fast, pounding, or uneven heart beats;
- feeling short of breath;
- swelling;
- jaundice (yellowing of your skin or eyes); or
- muscle pain, tenderness, or weakness with fever or flu symptoms and dark colored urine.

If you are diabetic, tell your doctor about any changes in your blood sugar levels.

Less serious side effects of Niaspan include:

- mild dizziness;
- warmth, redness, or tingly feeling under your skin;
- itching, dry skin;
- sweating or chills;
- nausea, diarrhea, belching, gas;
- muscle pain, leg cramps; or
- sleep problems (insomnia).

Side effects other than those listed here may also occur. Talk to your doctor about any side effect that seems unusual or that is especially bothersome."

How to Take Nicotinic Acid and Simvastatin

The time of day and method for taking the nicotinic acid and simvastatin are very important in order to improve effectiveness and minimize the side effects. Two thousand milligrams of nicotinic acid is a very large dose that must be started slowly and increased over time to minimize the flush (warmth, redness, or tingly feeling under your skin). It is very important to avoid fats 45 minutes before and several hours after the dosage. I found the following to be the best procedure based on dinner at 5:00 PM and the last fatty snack at 6:30 PM:

1. At 7:30 PM, take one 500 mg tablet of nicotinic acid and one 10 mg tablet of simvastatin. I have found that ½ of a medium-size tomato is a good snack to eat at the same time. Continue this each day for the first week. You most likely will experience a strong flush on day one. This is harmless.

2. After your body becomes accustomed to the nicotinic acid and the flush reaction subsides, increase the

nicotinic acid to two tablets with the 10 mg of simvastatin and tomato snack. Continue this regime for one more week before increasing the nicotinic acid.

3. Increase the nicotinic acid to three 500 mg tablets plus 10 mg of simvastatin. Always begin at about 7:30 PM. Space the tablets over a 30-minute period.

4. Increase the nicotinic acid to four 500 mg tablets plus 10 mg of simvastatin beginning at 7:30 PM, and space the tablets over a 45-minute period. A low-fat, low-carbohydrate vegetable snack is recommended.

Adverse Reactions to Nicotinic Acid Therapy

After nearly four years of nicotinic acid therapy, I experienced a rash on my thighs. I noticed an unusual niacin taste for several mornings before the rash appeared, and I believe this may have been related to the rash. Although the rash is not common, I discontinued the therapy for a few days and began to slowly increase the dosage.

Approximately eight months prior to the rash, I developed tenderness on the balls of both feet. Two podiatrists (foot doctors) were positive that the problem was not related to my cholesterol therapy, but my suspicion was confirmed when I discontinued the nicotinic acid for a few days and resumed at half the dosage, 1000 mg per day.

Shortly after struggling to solve my foot problems, I developed tenderness on the sides of my hips during sleep that could have been related to my blood thinning drugs, cholesterol control program, or both. My hips were also stiff and tender while walking. My thighs were weak, and I experienced tingling in the lower legs. The tingling, muscle weakness, pain, and tenderness may also be caused by damage to the sheath cells covering the nerves in the legs and feet. All of these problems began about four years after I started the program. I remembered that I had stopped taking Coenzyme Q_{10} a couple of years earlier because I thought it was unnecessary with the niacin therapy. That assumption was wrong. Niacin blocks Coenzyme Q_{10} just like statin drugs do. A major adjustment in my blood thinning, cholesterol, and nutritional supplement programs was needed to correct and restore the strength and health of my legs. I discontinued Plavix with my doctor's permission but continued to take 81 mg of aspirin per day. I stopped taking niacin for three weeks.

New Program to Restore Strength and Health to the Legs

After I realized the Coenzyme Q_{10} deficiency had caused problems with my feet and legs, I began to aggressively supplement my diet with ubiquinol, a reduced and more bioavailable form of Coenzyme Q_{10} that the cells need to produce energy. I started with a therapeutic dose of two 100 mg gel caps four times a day, two with each of three meals and two during a mid-morning or afternoon snack. The results were dramatic. My feet were the first to feel better and soon my legs began to improve. The recovery takes many weeks and possibly several months.

Keep in mind that this is a therapeutic dose of ubiquinol. The label on the bottle may only state one per day at the 200 mg dosage. My research indicates that higher doses have no adverse effects, but you must always proceed at your own risk when exceeding the supplier's recommendations. The ubiquinol must contain Kaneka QH® as the only qualified supplier because they hold the patent. Do not accept any product identified as *regular* or *quick absorbing* Coenzyme Q_{10}. It is not the same. I like the

NOW Foods® product because the gel caps are smaller. The primary or secondary oil in the products should be medium chain triglycerides (MCTs), not entirely vegetable oils. My preferred brands are:

Now Foods®, Ubiquinol Kaneka's QH® 100 mg Softgels

Jarrow Formulas®, Ubiquinol QH-Absorb® 100 mg Softgels

I began taking 500 mg of nicotinic acid again in the evening for two weeks before slowly increasing the dosage as determined by the condition of my legs and feet. My cardiologist suggested I build the niacin dosage up to 1500 mg per day rather than 2000 mg and combine it with 10 mg of simvastatin. These adjustments placed me back on a good program.

Stopping and Pausing Nicotinic Acid Therapy

Nicotinic acid therapy can be stopped abruptly at any time without any negative reactions, but starting the therapy again requires a gradual increase in the dosage as previously described.

I don't believe that pausing nicotinic acid therapy will cause the cardiovascular plaque to suddenly increase. Cholesterol is not the direct cause of arterial plaque, but cholesterol-lowering therapy is certainly necessary to remove existing deposits.

Important Niacin Update

I began a new niacin testing program a few months before this book was published. I take two 500 mg nicotinic acid tablets in the afternoon at about 3:00 PM and another tablet at 8:00 PM along with 10 mg of simvastatin. This approach kept total cholesterol at 153, LDL at 73, and HDL at 56.

Chapter 4

How Nicotinic Acid Therapy Works

The science to support nicotinic acid therapy for reducing LDL cholesterol and increasing HDL cholesterol is well known. The results are proven, backed by science as explained in the following report, and approved by the U.S. Food and Drug Administration (FDA). The effectiveness of nicotinic acid is not a wild sales pitch or questionable conjecture as are many cholesterol-lowering claims. This is the best therapy available.

How does nicotinic acid modify the lipid profile?
European Heart Journal, M. John Chapman
http://eurheartjsupp.oxfordjournals.org/content/8/suppl_F/F5
4.full

"Abstract

An atherogenic dyslipidaemic phenotype, characterized by low HDL-cholesterol levels, hypertriglyceridaemia and small, dense LDL, is commonly observed in patients with type 2 diabetes, the metabolic syndrome, or pre-existing cardiovascular disease and is inadequately addressed by current guidelines for the management of cardiovascular disease. Moreover, low HDL-cholesterol, in particular, is common among patients treated for dyslipidaemia and is little affected by statin treatment. Incomplete suppression of lipolysis by insulin in the fed state in insulin-resistant subjects leads to increased lipolysis in adipose tissue with elevated circulating free fatty acids (FFA). This metabolic abnormality leads directly to the development of the atherogenic dyslipidaemic phenotype. Nicotinic acid increases levels of HDL-cholesterol, probably largely through suppression of lipolysis in adipocytes secondary to activation of specific, G-protein-coupled nicotinic acid (HM74A) receptors. The reduction in FFA flux after nicotinic acid treatment also results in reduced levels of circulating triglycerides, mainly in the form of VLDL, and increased size and buoyancy of LDL.

> Treatment with nicotinic acid equally increases the size of HDL particles, which may promote increased reverse cholesterol transport from macrophages in the atherosclerotic plaque via the ABCG1 cholesterol transporter. The effects of nicotinic acid on the lipid profile are thus potentially anti-atherogenic and may address a major source of cardiovascular risk in insulin-resistant populations, such as those with the metabolic syndrome, type 2 diabetes and/or cardiovascular disease."

We can see from this description that nicotinic acid has the positive effect of moving the blood lipids and cholesterol in the right direction as has been shown by my own blood tests. Other positive effects of my drug and diet regime are:

- HDL cholesterol is increased.
- HDL particles have more of the safer, larger-size subfraction.
- LDL cholesterol is greatly reduced.
- LDL particles have more of the safer, larger-size subfraction.
- Triglycerides (free fatty acids blood lipids) are reduced.

Niacin must be the nicotinic acid molecule.

Several niacin compounds are sold and advertised to reduce cholesterol without causing a flush. They may not cause a flush, but I don't believe they are as effective as pure nicotinic acid. All niacin compounds that are not pure nicotinic acid should be avoided. I do not recommend the following:

- Inositol hexanicotinate (IHN)
- Niacin (no identification of the compound)
- 5-hydroxy-L-tryptophan (5-HTP)

411

Statin Cholesterol-Lowering Drugs Boost the Effectiveness of Niacin

My cholesterol therapy also included Zocor® (simvastatin), a statin cholesterol-lowering drug that provided a huge, very desirable increase in the HDL cholesterol while lowering LDL and total cholesterol levels. The combination of niacin and a statin drug appears to give a boost that neither could achieve independently. This great result occurred even though the daily 10 mg dose of simvastatin was small.

Niacin and simvastatin are a powerful combination for treating cholesterol.

The niacin alone actually lowered the HDL from 57 to 49, which was undesirable. Perhaps the 49 point reading was a laboratory error because it appears to be inconsistent with the three other measurements. However, it did lower LDL from 168 to 111, or 34% and total cholesterol from 241 to 173, or 28%, which are both significantly beneficial achievements. The HDL/CT ratio decreased from 0.28 to 0.24—the wrong direction. The HDL/LDL ratio decreased from 0.44 to 0.34, also in the wrong direction. Even though the HDL cholesterol measurement of 49 was suspect, a retest was not done. The action of niacin by itself is of no concern since the combination is the recommended therapy. My personal cholesterol program of 10 mg of simvastatin proves it was a very important factor in boosting the effectiveness of the 2000 mg of nicotinic acid.

Zocor® (simvastatin) is the only statin cholesterol-lowering drug that I can recommend. The following is a description of the product provided by the manufacturer:

"What are statins and how do they work?"

"Statins (or HMG-CoA reductase inhibitors) are a class of drugs that reduce cholesterol in individuals who have dyslipidemia (abnormal fats in the blood) and thus are at risk for cardiovascular disease. Dyslipidemia may involve an elevation of total cholesterol, a reduction of low density lipoprotein (LDL) cholesterol and/or triglycerides, or a reduction of high density lipoprotein (HDL) cholesterol in blood. Statins work by blocking the enzyme in the liver that is responsible for making cholesterol. This enzyme is called hydroxy-methylglutaryl-coenzyme A reductase (HMG-CoA reductase)."

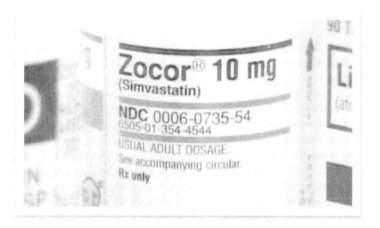

Laboratory tests prove my diet and drug cholesterol therapy gives awesome results.

Chapter 4

Why My Nicotinic Acid and Simvastatin Therapy Reversed My Heart Disease and the NIH Niaspan® Study Failed

The United States National Institutes of Health (NIH) conducted a study according to the guidelines established by Abbott Laboratories®, manufacturer of Niaspan® and Zocor®, two drugs approved by the U.S. Food and Drug Administration for reducing LDL and total cholesterol and increasing HDL cholesterol. The NIH study failed as I would have predicted, because the participants were required to eat a low-fat diet.

> **NIH stops clinical trial on combination cholesterol treatment**
> NIH News – National Institutes of Health
> May 26, 2011
> http://www.nih.gov/news/health/may2011/nhlbi-26.htm
>
> "Lack of efficacy in reducing cardiovascular events prompts decision.
>
> The NHLBI funded the AIM-HIGH study with additional support from Abbott Laboratories, a pharmaceutical company based in Abbott Park, Ill. Abbott also provided Niaspan and Merck Pharmaceuticals, based in Whitehouse Station, N.J., provided Zocor. All drugs used in the study were approved for marketing in the United States and Canada and have been on the market for many years.
>
> The National Heart, Lung, and Blood Institute (NHLBI) of the National Institutes of Health has stopped a clinical trial studying a blood lipid treatment 18 months earlier than planned. The trial found that adding high dose, extended-release niacin to statin treatment in people with heart and vascular disease, did not reduce the risk of cardiovascular events, including heart attacks and stroke.

Participants were selected for AIM-HIGH because they were at risk for cardiovascular events despite well-controlled low-density lipoprotein (LDL or bad cholesterol). Their increased risk was due to a history of cardiovascular disease and a combination of low high-density lipoprotein (HDL or good cholesterol) and high triglycerides, another form of fat in the blood. Low HDL and elevated triglycerides are associated with an increased risk of cardiovascular events. While lowering LDL decreases the risk of cardiovascular events, it has not been shown that raising HDL similarly reduces the risk of cardiovascular events.

During the study's 32 months of follow-up, participants who took high dose, extended-release niacin and statin treatment had increased HDL cholesterol and lowered triglyceride levels compared to participants who took a statin alone. However, the combination treatment did not reduce fatal or non-fatal heart attacks, strokes, hospitalizations for acute coronary syndrome, or revascularization procedures to improve blood flow in the arteries of the heart and brain.

"Seeking new and improved ways to manage cholesterol levels is vital in the battle against cardiovascular disease," said Susan B. Shurin, M.D., acting director of the NHLBI. "This study sought to confirm earlier and smaller studies. Although we did not see the expected clinical benefit, we have answered an important scientific question about treatment for cardiovascular disease. We thank the research volunteers whose participation is key in advancing our knowledge in this critical public health area, and the dedicated investigators who conducted the study."

The AIM-HIGH trial, which stands for Atherothrombosis Intervention in Metabolic Syndrome with Low HDL/High Triglycerides: Impact on Global Health, enrolled 3,414 participants in the United States and Canada with a history of cardiovascular disease who were taking a statin drug to keep their LDL cholesterol low. Study participants also had low HDL cholesterol and high triglycerides, which meant that they were at significant risk of experiencing future cardiovascular events. Niacin, also known as Vitamin B3, has long been known to raise HDL and lower triglycerides. Eligible participants were randomly assigned to either high dose, extended-release niacin (Niaspan) in gradually increasing doses up to 2,000 mg per day (1,718 people) or a placebo treatment (1,696 people). All participants were prescribed simvastatin (Zocor), and 515 participants were given a second LDL cholesterol-lowering drug, ezetimibe (Zetia), in order to maintain LDL cholesterol levels at the target range between 40-80 mg/dL."

The above NIH study was stopped because the experimental group (1,718 people taking Niaspan®) were having adverse reactions or worse results compared to the control group (1,696 people taking a placebo). Both groups were taking Zocor®. We can see that the participants were selected because they had high triglycerides—an instant and accurate indication that the participants had been on a low-fat, high-carbohydrate diet. We know the diet was left unchanged because Abbott Laboratories® specifies a low-fat diet on the instruction sheets for both drugs, and the study had to be conducted according to the manufacturer's instructions. It's standard practice to stop a study when the experimental group has adverse results because studies should not be performed in a manner that is harmful to the participants. The experimental group must always have a better intermediate and final result than the control group in order for the study to be completed.

Two studies were conducted with people on a low-fat diet who took a statin drug or the Niaspan® and Zocor® combination. They did not have a reduced incidence of coronary artery disease or a reversal of heart disease. My regimen reversed my heart disease because my diet was 70% fat.

I reversed my heart disease with a diet of 70% fat. The low-fat diet recommended by the NIH failed.

I believe the low-fat diet recommended by the National Institutes of Health and Abbott Laboratories® failed to reduce the progression of coronary artery disease for the following scientific reasons:

- Insulin remained high because a diet high in carbohydrates increases insulin, and insulin is one of the primary direct causes of coronary artery disease.

- Glucose remained high because the excessive amount of carbohydrates increases glycation, which is one of the primary causes of coronary artery disease.

- Triglycerides remained high because fruits in the participants' diet contained fructose that was converted by the liver directly into triglycerides. The excess glucose was also synthesized into triglycerides. High triglycerides are a primary risk factor for coronary artery disease.

- HDL cholesterol may have increased because of the drugs but was not high enough because the low-fat diet suppresses HDL cholesterol. Low HDL cholesterol is a primary risk factor for coronary artery disease.

- LDL cholesterol did not increase, but the dangerous LDL_b small, dense subfraction most likely became prominent.

Carbohydrates digest into sugars that in turn cause insulin to soar. Insulin is the most powerful hormone in the body and will overpower any statin or nicotinic acid cholesterol-lowering therapy. Insulin packs the small, dense LDL_b subfraction of cholesterol into the arteries throughout the body, causing the formation of arterial plaque. You can gorge yourself with cholesterol-lowering drugs and still develop coronary artery disease when insulin is high. This is the reason that 65% of diabetics die from heart disease. I do not believe I could have reduced my coronary plaque by eating the high-carbohydrate diet recommended by the American Heart Association®, American Medical Association®, Harvard Medical School®, Mayo Clinic®, and the U.S. National Institutes of Health®.

List of Laboratory Tests You Can Obtain Yourself

It is easy to obtain a vast array of laboratory tests without going to a physician. The following method may be the most cost effective if you don't have health insurance. You can purchase and pay for many discounted laboratory tests from HealthCheckUSA® through the Internet without a physician's prescription, or you can visit your physician first for his advice and a prescription. Explain that you wish to obtain the tests yourself and will have a copy sent to his office.

HealthCheckUSA®
Blood and Urine Tests You Can Order Yourself Online
http://www.healthcheckusa.com/

Laboratory Corporation of America® (LabCorp)
https://www.labcorp.com/wps/portal/

You can place the order on the Internet, pay with a credit card, print your order, and take it to the nearest LabCorp® testing facility. This procedure is less expensive than simply walking in without a prepaid order.

Two good packages of tests, Men's Profile and Women's Profile, can be performed at any local LabCorp® facility. Cholesterol and other tests require a fasting period of up to twelve hours. Call in advance to see what is required for your particular test. An appointment is generally not necessary. Simply find the nearest office and walk in with your order.

A professional interpretation of the test results is needed. LabCorp® offers the service of a licensed physician who will review your test results and provide recommendations, or you can take your results to your personal physician for review and consultation.

Everyone would benefit from learning about how each of the many blood and urine tests are used to measure health status. Doctors seem to be more relaxed when they talk to a patient who understands both the reasons for the tests and the results. The patient will also have a better understanding of the doctor's comments. Many Internet websites contain information about the tests.

Blood Tests and Interpreting Blood Test Results
http://www.flash-med.com/Lab1.asp

Blood Test Normal Values and Ranges
http://www.flash-med.com/LabNormal.asp

How to Interpret Your Blood Test Results
Amarillo Medical Specialists, LLP
http://www.amarillomed.com/howto

Premium Blood Testing for Cardio Health Analysis

The premium blood testing available from Berkeley HeartLab®, Inc. must be obtained from your cardiologist. Unfortunately, some cardiologists may not be aware of the importance of these tests or be able to interpret all of the nuances. Berkeley HeartLab® performs many advanced tests that are not available from your physician's local laboratory.

Reversing heart disease requires a very low level of LDL cholesterol as well as the lower-risk subfraction sizes. The HDL cholesterol level must be high and consist of the most beneficial subfraction sizes. Insulin, glucose, and triglycerides must be consistently low throughout the day—not just after a 12-hour fast when blood is drawn. The Berkeley HeartLab® measurements provide the information necessary to determine if the diet, supplement, and drug regimen is optimal.

My personal blood test results were excellent, proving that my diet, drug, and supplement regimen was scientifically correct. These excellent results were obtained on a diet composed of 70% fat, 30% of which was saturated animal fats. My blood tests prove the low-fat diet theory recommended by major medical and health organizations is false.

The following brief descriptions of the major test groups are quoted from the Berkeley HeartLab® literature:

- **LDL-S$_3$GGE***
  LDL-S$_3$GGE is a Berkeley HeartLab proprietary test that measures LDL particle size as a distribution of seven subclasses. Measurements of LDL determined as part of the conventional lipid panel may be normal while LDL-S$_3$GGE subclass analysis may indicate increased cardiovascular disease (CVD) risk.

- **HDL-S$_{10}$GGE***
  HDL-S$_{10}$GGE is a Berkeley HeartLab proprietary test that measures HDL particle size as a distribution of five subclasses. Standard HDL measurements may be normal while HDL-S$_{10}$GGE subclass analyses may indicate increased CVD risk.

- **ApoB** (ApoB-Ultra*)
  ApoB is the scientifically accepted measurement for LDL particle number. Monitoring statin therapy requires an accurate and reliable measurement of apoB.

- **Lp(a)**
  Lp(a) is an inherited abnormal protein attached to LDL. Lp(a) increases coagulation and triples CVD risk.

- **Homocysteine**
  Homocysteine is a metabolic by-product of methionine metabolism. Progressively elevated blood levels of homocysteine are a documented risk marker for cardiovascular events.

- **ApoE***
  Apolipoprotein E (apoE) is an inherited trait. ApoE genotype predicts lipid abnormalities and responsiveness to different dietary fat intake.

- ***CYP2C19* Genotype Test***
  The FDA has placed a warning on the label of Plavix[®] (clopidogrel) indicating that patients who are CYP2C19 poor metabolizers may not receive the full benefits of the drug.[Δ] Poor metabolizers treated with Plavix at recommended doses have exhibited higher cardiovascular event rates following an acute coronary syndrome (ACS) or percutaneous coronary intervention (PCI) than patients with normal CYP2C19 function.

- ***LPA*-AspirinCheck™ Genotype Test***
  Recently published studies indicate that a variant of the *LPA* gene predicts increased CVD risk and event reduction from aspirin therapy[†]. The polymorphism associated with risk of

CVD consists of an isoleucine residue (Ile4399) that can be replaced with a methionine residue (4399Met).

- **_KIF6_-StatinCheck™ Genotype Test***
  Recent research indicates that _KIF6_ predicts risk of coronary heart disease (CHD) and event reduction during statin therapy[‡]. In large, peer-reviewed publications, statin therapy has been shown to significantly reduce the increased risk of CHD events in carriers of the _KIF6_ gene variant.

- **9p21-EarlyMICheck™ Genotype Test***
  Recent research indicates that a polymorphism on chromosome 9 predicts increased risk for early onset myocardial infarction (early MI), abdominal aortic aneurysm (AAA), and MI/coronary heart disease (CHD)[#]. Identification of 9p21 carriers may allow health care providers to take steps to characterize and reduce risk factors that may contribute to the development or progression of disease.

- **Lp-PLA$_2$**
  Lp-PLA$_2$ is a marker for vascular-specific inflammation and also plays a causal role in the vascular inflammatory process, leading to the formation of vulnerable, rupture-prone plaque. Elevated levels have been shown to be powerful predictors of ischemic stroke and heart attack risk.

- **hsCRP**
  hsCRP is one of a number of acute phase reactant proteins that increases in response to inflammatory stimuli. In large epidemiologic studies, elevated levels of CRP have been shown to be a strong indicator of CVD.

- **Fibrinogen**
  Fibrinogen is a plasma glycoprotein that can be transformed by thrombin into a fibrin clot in response to injury. The combination of elevated fibrinogen with other CVD risk factors can substantially increase disease potential.

- **Insulin**
  Insulin is associated with the characterization of the Atherogenic Lipid Profile and Metabolic Syndrome. Abnormal

fasting insulin, especially when combined with other risk factors, identifies patients at significantly higher risk for CVD.

- **NT-proBNP**
  NT-proBNP is a progressive CVD risk marker with powerful independent prognostic value for detection of clinical and subclinical cardiac dysfunction. Elevated levels indicate the presence of ongoing myocardial stress and potentially an underlying cardiac disorder.

- **Q-LDL**
  Atherogenic Subclass Quantitation — Q-LDL provides a measurement of atherogenic particles based upon results from apoB and LDL-S$_3$GGE. Q-LDL is a useful monitoring metric for following response to lipid therapies particularly when pursuing aggressive LDL lowering goals.

- **Additional Tests**
  Berkeley HeartLab provides: Apolipoprotein A1, Total Cholesterol, Creatine Kinase, Glucose, HDL-Cholesterol, Hemoglobin A1c, LDL-Cholesterol, Hepatic Functional Panel[±], Renal Functional Panel[±], Triglycerides, Thyroid Stimulating Hormone (TSH), and Uric Acid.

Berkeley HeartLab, Inc.
http://www.bhlinc.com/
Berkeley HeartLab Headquarters
468 Littlefield Avenue
South San Francisco, CA 94080
Phone: 650-651-3100
Fax: 650-697-8741

Laboratory
960 Atlantic Ave., Suite 100
Alameda, CA 94501-1086
Phone: 510-747-1740

My Personal Cholesterol Test Results

Blood Test Cholesterol Readings (mg/dl)	Baseline Without Cholesterol Treatment Nov. 19, 2007	After 5 Months on Carlson's® Niacin- Time 2000 mg Therapy May 20, 2008	After 2 Months on Niaspan® Extended- Release 2000 mg Plus Simvastatin 10mg Therapy July 31, 2008	After 6 Months on Carlson's® Niacin- Time 2000 mg Plus Simvastatin 10mg Therapy January 19, 2009 Test by Berkeley HeartLab, Inc.®
Remember, these awesome cholesterol results were achieved in a diet of 70% fat.				
Total Cholesterol	241	173	153	157
HDL Cholesterol	57	49	66	68
LDL Cholesterol	168	111	68	75

Berkeley HeartLab, Inc.
Test Descriptions
http://www.bhlinc.com/clin_test.php

VLDL Cholesterol	16	13	19	14
Triglycerides	81	65	93	71
CT / HDL	4.23	3.53	2.3	2.3
LDL / HDL	2.95	2.27	1.0	1.1
TG / HDL	1.42	1.33	1.41	1.0
Overall Rating CHD Risk where: Men CT/HDL 5.0 = 1.0 Risk	Acceptable ratio but with high LDL <0.9 Risk	Very Good <0.7 Risk	Awesome <0.5 Risk	Awesome <0.5 Risk

Important Measurements and Cholesterol Subfractions

Lp(a) (mg/dl) < 30			5.0	14
IDL < 20			9.0	
Remnant Lipo. IDL + VLDL3 < 30			21	
HDL-2 Most Protective > 10			22	28
HDL-3 Less Protective >30			42	49
VLDL-3 Small Remnant < 10			12 (high)	
LDL1 Pattern A			7.9	27

425

LDL2 Pattern A			17.5	21
LDL3 Pattern B			28.0	10.4
LDL4 Pattern B			5.2	0.5
LDL Density Pattern where: A = Good Large, Buoyant A/B = Intermediate Size and Density B = Bad Small, Dense BB	Unknown	Unknown	Pattern "A" Excellent Lowest Risk LDL	"A" Excellent Lowest Risk LDL Carlson's® OTC niacin was actually better with more low risk "A" LDL than prescription Niaspan®
Lpo B (mg/dl) <60				64
Lpo E Genotype				Genetic Type 3/3
KIF6 Genotype 719				Genetic Type Trp/Trp
Homocysteine <15 ATP III Goal <10				13.1

Lp-PLA2 (ng/dl) <419 ATP III Goal <200				249
CRP (hs)(mg/l) <5.0 ATP III Goal <1.0				0.8
Fibrinogen (mg/dl) <436 Goal <350				407
Insulin (microU/mg) <25 Goal <10				20
NT-proBNP (pg/ml) <125				41

Note:

Carlson's® Niacin-Time nicotinic acid (time release) has been unavailable at times for some unknown reason; however, there are many equivalent products available. I have tested the following replacements and found them to be equally effective:

True Niacin, Time-Release, 500 mg
Meridian Naturals®

SLO-NIACIN®, Polygel Controlled-Release, 500 mg
Upsher-Smith Laboratories, Inc. ®

Nicotinic Acid and Simvastatin Side Effects

The first tablet of nicotinic acid will likely cause a side effect called a *flush*, which may last up to one hour. It feels like sunburn and may appear on the face, neck, or elsewhere; but the flush is considered to be harmless according to many references. It's very important to start with the smallest dose of 500 mg or less and gradually increase the dose as the body adjusts and the flush diminishes. It's also important not to eat any food containing fat within 45 minutes before taking the niacin and several hours afterward. I prefer to take the niacin between 7:30 and 8:15 PM, one tablet at a time equally spaced. Take the 10 mg simvastatin with the first niacin tablet.

Women can increase the dose in steps to a maximum of two or three tablets per day depending on weight with an adjustment period of one to two weeks between steps. Men should increase the dose in steps as the flush diminishes to reach the maximum three or four tablets depending upon weight. Follow the same instructions for the over-the-counter nicotinic acid as for Niaspan® Extended-Release, the prescription drug variety of time-release niacin.

Niacin flush is a harmless side effect.

The flush caused by the nicotinic acid is shocking to some people who do not want any side effects whatsoever, and this may cause them to discontinue the treatment. This decision is unfortunate because taking a statin drug alone has never been shown to reverse heart disease or diminish the size of arterial plaque. In addition, cardiologists normally require their patients to have periodic blood tests to measure liver and kidney functions when statin drugs are taken at the high levels recommended by the manufacturers. The patients may not feel any side effects, but the blood tests show that the liver and kidneys are under stress.

Nicotinic acid can cause muscle weakness as is common with higher doses of statin drugs. The weakness is generally felt in the legs, but a hidden side effect could be heart muscle weakness— not a pleasant thought. I have explained this in detail in this chapter.

Nicotinic acid may also leave a strange taste in the mouth for several hours. This can be removed by brushing the teeth or rinsing with a little lemon water. This side effect is very minor.

Nicotinic acid does have a positive side effect in addition to reversing heart disease. It tends to shrink the sinuses and relieve chronic congestion. Unfortunately, the benefit only lasts a few hours and the congestion returns. It would be great if this side effect lasted all day, but it doesn't.

Kidney and Liver Function Tests

I recommend that you have periodic blood tests to measure liver and kidney functions while taking the niacin and simvastatin combination. After several months on a high dose of a statin drug alone, test results may be out of range. My cholesterol-lowering treatment gives better results. The 2000 mg of nicotinic acid plus the small 10 mg dose of simvastatin did not cause any adverse blood test results. My results were all perfectly normal and near mid-range on every test.

I had perfect kidney and liver function test results.

Many heart patients who are placed on a statin drug alone are often very disappointed with their cholesterol test report, and they are even more disappointed because liver and kidney tests show these organs are under stress. The patients on statin cholesterol-lowering drugs alone are often faced with this problem. If they reduce the dose to improve their liver and kidney functions, their cholesterol numbers become worse.

Genetic Factors Determine Effectiveness of Nicotinic Acid

Because of genetic differences, not everyone responds to nicotinic acid therapy in the same way. I was very fortunate to have the genotype that responds well to the niacin and simvastatin combination. My genetic factors were tested by Berkeley HeartLab, Inc. as explained below.

> **Berkeley HeartLab, Inc.**
> Test Descriptions
> http://www.bhlinc.com/clin_test.php
>
> **KIF6-StatinCheck™ Genotype Test**
>
> "KIF6 genotyping provides significant information beyond traditional risk factors to help with the identification of patients at risk for CHD events and the personalization of their treatment. Kinesin-like protein 6 (KIF6) is a protein involved in intracellular transport. A single nucleotide polymorphism (SNP) of KIF6 (719 Arg) has been shown to predict increased coronary heart disease (CHD) risk and event reduction during statin therapy*. The genotypes of KIF6 carriers include either one or two 719Arg alleles (e.g., Arg/Trp or Arg/Arg), and the KIF6 noncarrier genotype lacks the 719Arg allele (e.g., Trp/Trp).
>
> About 60% of the studied populations** were carriers of the KIF6 genetic variant (719Arg) that was found to substantially increase their risk for coronary heart disease (CHD) events.

**Studied populations predominantly consisted of Caucasians 45 years of age and older. Studies in other ethnic groups are ongoing."

I tested as a KIF6 719Arg allele Trp/Trp type. Therefore, I do not have the higher risk for coronary heart disease according to genetic types.

ApoE (LpoE on my report)

Apolipoprotein E is present on chylomicrons, VLDLs, and HDLs and functions as a ligand for lipoprotein receptors. The apoE gene has three common alleles (E2, E3, E4) that code for three isoforms of the apoE protein (E2, E3, E4). The alleles are inherited in a co-dominant manner resulting in six genotypes (e2/e2, e2/e3, e2/e4, e3/e3, e3/e4, e4/e4).

Clinical Implications:

Individuals who are e2/e2 are prone to develop Type III hyperlipidemia. The E4 allele is associated with increased plasma cholesterol levels and subsequent increased risk for coronary heart disease. ApoE genotype can play a significant role in predicting patient responsiveness to cardiac-related environmental factors, statin therapy, and dietary therapy.

Treatment considerations:

Compared to "standard" treatment recommendations for the "normal" apo E3 patients, and considering associated cardiovascular disease risk marker abnormalities, personalized recommendations for lifestyle changes and pharmacotherapy may be modified with apo E2 and apo E4 genotype patients.

* Apo E2:

- Respond particularly well to statins.
- Moderate alcohol intake may have positive effects.
- Low fat diet may increase small dense LDL.
- Moderate (35%) fat dietary restriction recommended.

* Apo E3:

- Normal treatment guideline recommendations.
- Preventive (25%) fat or moderate (35%) fat dietary restriction determined by overall lipid profile.

* Apo E4:

- Limited responsiveness to statins.
- Alcohol intake may have negative effects.
- Very low (20%) fat dietary restriction recommended.

My apolipoprotein type is LpoE 3/3 (ApoE E3/E3), and therefore standard treatment is recommended. People who are E2/E2 are prone to Type III hyperlipidemia (high cholesterol), and E4/E4 types are at increased risk for high cholesterol levels and subsequent coronary disease.

Based on my LpoE 3/3 (ApoE 3/3) test result, dietary fat should be restricted to no more than 25% to 35% according to Berkeley HeartLab, Inc., but I reversed my heart disease and reduced my coronary artery plaque by 50% in 25 months on a diet composed of 70% fat. Obviously, more research is needed on the high-fat, high-protein, and low-carbohydrate diet. It appears to have been given no consideration and was rejected without testing because nearly everyone has been brainwashed to believe dietary fat causes heart disease. The researchers have apparently concentrated their investigations on various levels of dietary fat below 35% instead of using dietary carbohydrates as the variable. This is the reason that reversing heart disease in the general population is nearly impossible. As stated in previous chapters, bacterial and viral infections, blood levels of insulin, glucose, and triglycerides are the primary causes for coronary artery disease. The low-fat diet normally recommended as heart healthy actually increases insulin, glucose, and triglycerides. All of these were extremely low on my diet of 70% fat. The diet recommended by most cardiologists, professional nutritionists, medical schools, government health authorities, and professional medical associations is backward.

Professional organizations have heart disease risk factors backward.

ApoB (ApoB-Ultra)(LpoB on my report)

"Apolipoprotein B is the predominant apolipoprotein attached to LDL. It is part of every non-HDL lipoprotein (VLDL, IDL, LDL). ApoB is the scientifically accepted gold standard measurement for LDL particle number. An accurate and reliable measurement of apoB is of great benefit in monitoring efficacy of statin therapy. In fact, the ADA and the ACC released a consensus statement in 2008 that recommends guiding therapy for cardiometabolic risk patients with apoB measurements.

ApoB Ultra: When a patient has elevated triglycerides, apoB measurements may be skewed to the high side because of the presence of apoB-containing chylomicrons and VLDLs. Only Berkeley HeartLab performs an ultracentrifugation procedure that removes the influence of chylomicrons and VLDLs and reports this highly accurate measurement as apoB Ultra.

Clinical Implications:

Elevated apoB (>120 mg/dL) may signify two to three-fold increased cardiovascular disease risk even when LDL-cholesterol is within normal range. Several decades of scientific literature support the measurement of apoB as the most accurate indication of the amount of atherogenic particles. ApoB is therefore an excellent metric for monitoring response to statin therapy.

Treatment considerations:

* Common first-line pharmacological considerations:

- Statins

* Additional pharmacological considerations:

- Cholesterol absorption inhibitors.
- Nicotinic acid.
- Bile acid sequestrants.
- Fibrates.

* Lifestyle changes:

- Fat-restricted, cardioprotective diet.
- Weight loss.
- Regular exercise.

Combination therapy including statins and nicotinic acid and/or fibrates can be effective in patients with excess apoB and small dense LDL disorder."

I tested LpoE = 64 (ApoE = 64) versus a range less than 60, so I was slightly over the desirable limit but much below the elevated limit of 120. I did not have small, dense LDL disorder, as my LDL subfractions were greater in the large, less-dense "A" subfraction. In other words, my total regimen consisting of a high-fat diet, nicotinic acid, moderate statin, and moderate exercise was very effective as evidenced by this measurement. All the blood tests show that my regimen should have been effective for reversing and preventing heart disease, and indeed it was. Like they say, "The proof is in the pudding." But don't eat the pudding on my diet program.

My wife, Marti, did not have the same result with nicotinic acid, but she didn't need the therapy. Her HDL cholesterol level is consistently over 100 and has tested as high as 125, prompting her doctor to say, "You have enough HDL for the entire family." She also tends to bleed and bruise easily, which indicates that her blood is naturally thinner than mine. Her triglycerides have tested as low as 45, and her glucose always tests below 100 because she is on the same diet as I am. Her insulin level was also low, giving her a very low risk for heart disease without any cholesterol modification therapy. She is not salt sensitive. Her blood pressure is consistently as low as 90/60, and her veins show she has no vasoconstriction—all heart-favorable conditions.

Cholesterol Control Program Summary

Other books and references about reversing heart disease typically give emotional pleas to refrain from eating animal fats and eggs, but they give very little in the way of scientific facts to support their false claim that the fats and cholesterol in these foods clog arteries. Free cardio health literature available in the cardiac units of most hospitals and prestigious medical clinics will condemn saturated animal fats and advise people to eat lots of fruits and vegetables. Medical Internet websites, medical associations, and government health departments all support this, but my experience has shown it to be wrong. We continue to see an epidemic of cardiovascular diseases and the progression of these diseases in patients who are under the care of highly-credentialed physicians practicing in the world's most respected treatment centers.

My cholesterol modification therapy is based on pure science and is verified by the most sophisticated proprietary testing methods available from Berkeley HeartLab, Inc®. They have done an outstanding job of testing and analyzing body chemistry and genetics related to heart disease, and I highly recommend them. However, Berkeley HeartLab, Inc. has fallen for the false anti-fat propaganda, and they promote a diet with less than 30% fats on a calorie basis. Do not follow their dietary advice as presented above.

A low-fat diet is a high-carbohydrate diet. There are no other options. There are only three dietary macronutrients: fats, proteins, and carbohydrates. Calories must come from carbohydrates when the fats and protein are limited. My diet composed of 70% fats has reversed my heart disease because it is based on the scientific fact that carbohydrates cause heart disease.

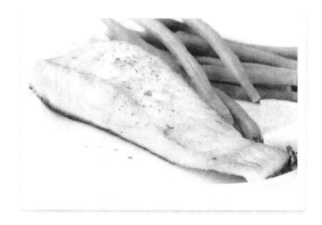

Salmon Steak with Green Beans

Supplement Nutritional Therapy

Dr. Atkins' Vita-Nutrient Solution: Nature's Answer To Drugs is the best book for determining the correct vitamin and mineral dosages, therapeutic effects, and normal recommendations. Dr. Atkins discusses the vital functions of vitamins and nutritional supplements, and the book provides a list of diseases and ailments that the supplements can help to cure or alleviate.

Many people question my diet regimen, and their questions are generally expressed as follows: "If I follow your diet program, will I be getting all of my necessary vitamins and minerals?" "Do I have to take all of the vitamins, minerals, and other supplements that you recommend?" "Why do you take supplemental vitamins if your diet program is so good?" These are very good questions because they reveal the nature and extent of the false nutritional information that has pervaded our society. They never question whether the high-carbohydrate diet recommended by the *USDA Food Guide Pyramid* is deficient in essential amino acids and essential fatty acids. I explain that my diet regimen will supply all of the essential vitamins, minerals, amino acids, fatty acids, and other nutrients. The supplemental vitamins, minerals, and other nutrients I recommend are intended to provide the body with an overwhelming supply rather than simply meeting some theoretical minimum daily requirement. The intent is to provide the body with maximum nutrition in order to reverse diseases and overcome damaged body functions caused by the previous high-carbohydrate diet. Yes, diets high in whole grains, fruits, and vegetables will severely damage your body. The current epidemics of cancer, heart disease, and diabetes are evidence beyond doubt. The North American Plains Indians of centuries past carefully observed the connection between optimal health and their diet, but our current professional nutritionists ignore the obvious connection.

Many people think the Atkins' low-carbohydrate diet lacks essential nutrients because it doesn't match the *USDA Food Guide Pyramid*. They base nutritional requirements on the *Nutrition Facts* label required on all processed foods in the United States for nutritional Daily Values (DV) and the U.S. Food & Drug Administration (USFDA) *Recommended Daily Allowance (RDA)*. This is unfortunate because the *USDA Food Guide Pyramid* was developed by vegetarians with an agenda. Nathan Pritikin and Senator George McGovern appear to have been the perpetrators who formulated the first *USDA Food Guide Pyramid*. They ignored opposing scientific data and many highly qualified objectors. It was a scam from the beginning—a make-believe nutritional plan to limit the consumption of animal products, particularly saturated fats.

The *USFDA Nutrition Facts* are based on the *USDA Food Guide Pyramid* rather than on scientific facts. This is easy to prove. Simply go to a food count book and analyze a 2000-calorie diet according to the pyramid. The results will show that the diet perfectly meets every nutritional requirement. It is not scientific. The *USFDA Recommended Daily Allowance* was simply adopted because it was based on the *USDA Food Guide Pyramid*. There is no hard science behind the establishment of the USFDA daily nutritional requirements. The USFDA recommended daily allowance for carbohydrates is 300 grams or 60% of calories, but the scientific requirement is zero. There are no essential scientific reasons why carbohydrates are required. Optimal health is achieved by limiting carbohydrates to a minimum, not by making them 60% of the diet. Carbohydrates cause diabetes, heart disease, cancer, and intestinal diseases.

Reverse and Prevent Heart Disease

Supplements are listed in order of priority.
The most important are at the top.

Vitamin, Mineral, or Supplement (R) = Refrigerate	Capsule or Tablet Size 1000 mcg = 1 mg	Breakfast	Lunch	Dinner
The following seven supplements are required for cardiovascular therapy.				
Nicotinic Acid Time-Release for Cholesterol Treatment	500 mg			2 to 4 Tablets 7:30 to 8:15 PM
Aspirin	81 mg	1		
Ubiquinol Kaneka QH®	100 mg	1	1	1
L-Taurine	850 mg	1	1	1
P5P, Pyridoxal-5-Phosphate	275 mg	1		1
Astaxanthin	4 mg	1		1
L-Proline	500 mg		1	

Multivitamin Multimineral Centrum Silver®	---	1		
Carlson's® Lemon Cod Liver Oil (R)	Tablespoon	1		1
Borage Oil with 300mg GLA (R)	1300 mg	1		
Bacillus Coagulans probiotic by Thorne Research® (R)	100 mg	1		
Multidophilus Lactic Flora by Solaray® Buy Locally (R)	100 mg	1		
NOW® Colloidal Minerals (R)	Cap Full	1		
KAL® Magnesium Glycinate 400	200 mg	1	1	1
Betaine Hydrochloric Acid (HCL) with Pepsin	650 mg	1	1	1

Reverse and Prevent Heart Disease

Lutein and Zeazanthin	20 mg/1 mg		1	
Mega 10X Digestive Pancreatin Enzymes (R)	Capsule	1	1	1
L-Lysine	500 mg	1		1
Other supplements and recommendations.				
Boron Complex	3 mg			1
Zinc, Chelated	30 mg		1 Every other day	
Copper, Sebacate 22mg	3 mg		1 Every other day	
Manganese	10 mg			1
Potassium	99 mg	1	1	1
Chromium	500 mcg			1
Vitamin A	10,000 IU	1		
Vitamin B-50	30 mg		1	
Vitamin C	500 mg		1	
Vitamin D$_3$	5,000 IU	1		
Vitamin E, Mixed Tocopherols (R)	200 IU	None		

Vitamins K1 and K2 Complex	9 mg/1 mg	Every other day		
Folic Acid	1000 mcg		1	
NutriCology® Germanium	150 mg			1
Biotin	5 mg	1		
Iodine as Norwegian Kelp	225 mcg	1		1
Vanadium, Chelated	2 mg			1
Selenium	200 mcg	Twice a week only		
Phosphatidyl serine Complex	1000 mg (2)		1	
L-Glutamine Powder (R)	½ Teaspoon	As desired		
Ultimate Lo Carb Whey Powder Biochem (R)	Heaping tablespoon	As desired		
Branched Chain Amino Acids	Heaping teaspoon	As desired		

Why Take Supplemental Vitamins and Minerals?

I receive many emails with the following question. "If your diet program is as healthy as you say, why do you recommend taking so many vitamins, minerals, and supplements?" The answer is easy. I take supplements for one reason, and that is to overwhelm the body with optimal nutrition. My recommend foods—fresh meat, wild game, fish, fowl, seafood, shellfish, vegetables, eggs, and cheese—are nutritionally dense, unlike the manufactured foods in boxes and bags. None of these foods except cheese is processed in a manufacturing plant. Therefore, the essential nutrients have not been stripped away as occurs with heavily processed foods. The natural vitamins, minerals, essential amino acids, and essential fatty acids are very abundant in these fresh foods. We know that minerals are not available in the food if the soil where the animal grazed or the vegetables grew lacks these minerals. The North American continent is extremely deficient in chromium; therefore, the foods grown here contain very little. The same applies to all essential nutrients.

> **Supplements are intended to overwhelm the body with optimal nutrition.**

Manufactured foods and domestic drinking water contain excessive amounts of some minerals and totally lack others. Tap water varies throughout the country, and some of the minerals in tap water should be completely avoided. Therefore, I strongly recommend installing a reverse osmosis (RO) water system. The system should have an ultra violet (UV) lamp that disinfects the water by killing pathogenic bacteria, viruses, yeast, fungi, protozoa, and parasites. Tap water is not sterile—RO water is.

443

Because the RO unit strips good and bad minerals, chemicals, heavy metals, fluorine, chlorine, radioactive isotopes, hormones, and drugs from the water, my supplement program replaces minerals in the proper amount for optimal health. The heart is very sensitive to minerals and metals in the diet, and tap water is simply not acceptable for drinking in quantity. Certainly, we drink whatever is provided in restaurants, but even though many restaurants have water purification systems, the purity is not guaranteed unless they are RO systems.

Bottled water made by the same RO process is available in supermarkets and vending machines. Some of the primary minerals are usually added for flavor enhancement and health, but many essential trace minerals are not added. Though this water appears to be healthy, it may not be any better than tap water because many vital trace minerals are missing.

Bottled water is deficient in trace minerals.

Toothpaste containing fluoride is recommended. It's better to receive the lower dose of fluoride in the toothpaste than to ingest fluoride that most U.S. communities add to tap water.

Highly Recommended Supplements for Heart Health

Omega-3 Fatty Acids obtained from Carlson's® Lemon Flavored Cod Liver Oil are an absolute must for preventing and treating heart disease. Do not substitute any other brand. Don't be concerned about the taste. Cod liver oil that has a strong fishy taste and odor is actually rancid and should be avoided. Don't buy cod liver oil in capsules because encapsulation is used to disguise the bad taste and odor of a rancid product. This is the best quality available and is shipped directly from Norway to worldwide retailers. I take two tablespoons per day, one with breakfast and one with dinner. This quantity exceeds the recommendation on the bottle but is perfectly acceptable according to several physicians whom I highly respect.

I was very disappointed to find my recent blood test showed vitamin D to be below the recommended range. This was a total shock because cod liver oil contains more than the minimum daily value, and I was taking six times the regular dose. I believe the deodorizing process must be removing the vitamin D. Always have your vitamin D measured on a routine blood test.

Taurine is involved in the stabilization of heart rhythm. Loss of intracellular taurine in the heart leads to arrhythmias. Taurine is used in hospitals to treat congestive heart failure (CHF). Take one 850 mg tablet three times a day for a large male or two times a day for a female. Read more about the advantages of taurine in Chapter 2.

Taurine and omega-3 fatty acids are heart foods.

Astaxanthin is one of the most powerful antioxidant and anti-inflammatory supplemental nutrients. It reduces pain in the joints, tendons, and muscles caused by overuse, stress, or injury

445

and is said to be effective for arthritis and tennis elbow. Astaxanthin helps to prevent skin aging and has been shown to help the skin resist damage and autoimmune reactions caused by sun exposure. I hiked for two hours in the snow, high in Rocky Mountains on a sunny winter day, and my face didn't even turn red. Normally I would have been sunburned. Astaxanthin is an awesome supplement.

Astaxanthin may prevent cardiovascular plaque.

All of these benefits make astaxanthin a prime heart supplement, especially as a protector and healing agent for the tender heart valves and linings of the arteries and veins. Other major organs, such as lungs, liver, kidneys, intestines, eyes, and brain, could also benefit from its powerful antioxidant and anti-inflammatory properties.

Astaxanthin is a free radical scavenger that inhibits lipid peroxidation and thereby protects cell membranes from damage. Astaxanthin may reduce arterial plaque formation by reducing oxidative damage of LDL-cholesterol. It is a much more effective antioxidant than other carotenoids and antioxidants such as beta-carotene and vitamin E. It does not convert to vitamin A like other beta-carotenoids, so toxicity is not a concern. I take two 4 mg capsules of astaxanthin daily.

After I started taking astaxanthin, I stopped taking less effective antioxidants such as alpha lipoic acid. You will not be eating fruit on my regime, but don't be concerned about a lack of antioxidants. Astaxanthin provides a mega dose of antioxidants compared to that found in fruits. I have included this special section about astaxanthin because it is very important.

Serrapeptase (serratiopeptidase) has been getting considerable attention and interest as an enzyme supplement that may help to remove cardiovascular plaque, cysts, prevent blood clots, reduce varicose veins, liquefy mucus, clear capillaries of the brain, and remove dead, fibrous protein tissues throughout the body. Serratiopeptidase is a proteolytic (protein destroying) enzyme found to be produced by bacteria in the digestive system of the silkworm. The silkworm uses the enzyme to dissolve the protein fibers of the cocoon to release the butterfly. It has the unique ability to dissolve dead protein while ignoring live, healthy protein tissues. The butterfly inside the cocoon is not harmed even though the protein fibers of the cocoon are dissolved. The hope is that serrapeptase would dissolve the dead protein in and around plaque deposits in arteries to hasten the reversal of coronary and carotid artery disease. It is readily absorbed in the intestines and has been found in the blood after being taken orally but is not readily discharged in the urine.

Serrapeptase may help to remove artery plaque.

Arteries in the heart and neck are prone to the development of arthrosclerosis which the artery becomes narrowed and hardened due to the deposit of cholesterol (atherosclerosis), fats, fibrous protein tissue, and calcification (arteriosclerosis). Physicians are reluctant to apply stents in the carotid artery or to perform surgery because of the high risk that the procedure will release debris into the smaller cerebral vessels and cause a stroke. The future may see serrapeptase injections as a procedure that removes or reduces the plaque deposit without this risk. Trials have been fairly encouraging and effective, but the procedure would be expensive because it must be repeated several times over many months. Oral serrapeptase has interesting prospects where the plaque is near a junction, corner, or small arterial branch. Stenting is not possible in these areas, and the high risks associated with bypass surgery can thus be eliminated.

Oral serrapeptase supplementation is recommended as a preventative measure to hopefully reduce the formation of new artherosclerotic plaque and clear small arterioles and capillaries in the brain, heart, kidneys, liver, lungs, and elsewhere. Serrapeptase has been shown to clear airways and blood vessels of the lungs when the patient was given two 20,000 SPU (serratiopeptidase units) capsules four times a day away from food and the amount reduced as the patient improved. Some patients with arterial blockage have been treated with three 120,000 SPU capsules per day in divided doses on an empty stomach for seven days. The results showed a substantial reduction in symptoms. The dosage was then reduced to one capsule per day.

Serrapeptase has been used successfully to treat fibrocystic breast disease and sinusitis. It has also been shown to be a good anti-inflammatory agent for relieving pain. The health improvements appear to be numerous without harmful side effects. The hope that serrapeptase would prevent or improve Alzheimer's disease is exciting because some theories suggest that the disease is caused by a rogue protein deposit in the arterioles and capillaries of the brain. Serrapeptase may remove these deposits.

Keep in mind that I reduced my coronary plaque without taking serrapeptase, so the addition of serrapeptase to my regime could be another major improvement. I generally take one 120,000 SPU capsule per day on an empty stomach.

Common Vitamins, Minerals, and Supplements That Are Not Recommended on This Therapy Program

Some of the vitamins, minerals, and supplements that many people hope will prevent heart disease or lower cholesterol are not recommended for the following reasons:

- Red yeast rice is an herbal product that has been shown to increase blood pressure without delivering on the promise to significantly reduce cholesterol.

- Selenium can have negative side effects and should be limited to 200 mcg every other day.

- Calcium in excess presents a cardiovascular risk. It can contribute to heart rhythm irregularities and possibly cause plaque and calcification in the arteries. The daily multi-vitamin and mineral tablet contains more than enough calcium. In addition, cheese is a very good source and this diet is rich in hard cheeses.

- Vitamin C and vitamin E tend to cause an undesirable increase in blood thinning when on Plavix® and aspirin therapy. Take vitamin C if you discontinue Plavix®.

Avoid Whole Food Vitamins

Never eat vitamin products that are classified as *whole food* vitamins. The final product is concentrated fiber, cellulose, starches, and sugars that are made by dehydrating fruits, vegetables, and grain grasses. Humans should not eat grass, and we should avoid fiber, cellulose, starches, and sugars. The vitamins and minerals are not concentrated enough for a therapeutic dose, but the concentrated carbohydrates promote heart disease, diabetes, and cancer. Do not take whole food vitamin supplements.

Beware of Fraudulent Vitamin, Mineral, and Supplement Claims

The vitamins, minerals, and supplements on the list that I have prepared have been thoroughly researched, tested, and shown to provide significant health benefits without harmful side effects. The list is long, so I did not want to waste my money or yours on supplements offering negligible benefits. There is an abundance of fraudulent claims about vitamins, minerals, and supplements, and some have the potential to be very detrimental to your health. For this reason many countries have placed or are considering placing tighter controls on nutritional supplements.

Beware of companies that sell unusual chemical products that they claim will miraculously heal every imaginable ailment. Purchase my recommended supplements from manufacturers that are dependable and provide factual information rather than from high-pressure, high-hype suppliers who make outrageous claims.

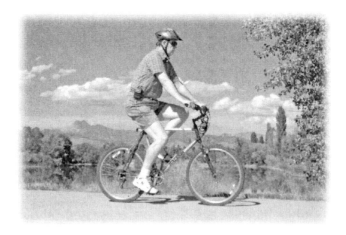

Kent on St. Vrain River Bike Path
Longmont, Colorado, October 1, 2011

Reversing Heart Disease and Preventing Diabetes

Chapter 5

Lower High Blood Pressure

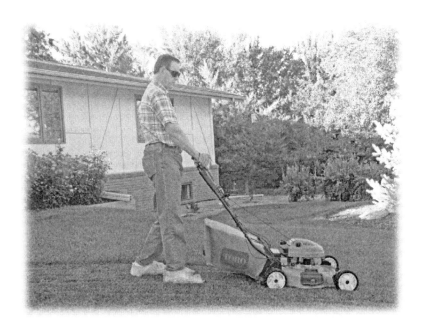

Move It! Move It!

Chapter 5

I had normal blood pressure until 1983 when I was 44 years old and it suddenly rose to 150/100. During the next 24 years, it fluctuated but generally averaged 150/90. The high pressure was very persistent, and because the side effects from drugs were annoying, if not unacceptable, it remained untreated until my heart attack in September 2007 at the age of 68.

High blood pressure (hypertension) is a cardiovascular condition in which the blood pressure in the arterial system is elevated. Hypotension is the reverse in which the arterial blood pressure is considered to be lower than normal. Medical references and medical professionals almost universally proclaim that hypertension increases the risk for cardiovascular and heart disease. Persistent hypertension places a prolonged load on the heart without giving the heart muscles the opportunity to recover, rest, and heal. This leads to an enlarged heart, congestive heart failure, and abnormal heart rhythms.

Hypertension can be the result of coronary disease, not the cause. Cardiovascular diseases usually result in abnormal blood pressure and irregular pulse rate, and these diseases are the major causes of hypertension. For example, any restriction in a major heart artery reduces the blood and oxygen flow to the heart muscle. The body reacts harshly by trying to restore the blood flow to the afflicted part of this vital organ. The hormonal systems and the heart itself react to the restriction by taking the following actions:

- The heart attempts to restore blood and oxygen flow to the heart muscle by increasing the force of the contractions. The heart muscle literally contracts faster and harder.

- The hormonal system reduces blood flow to the peripherals in order to deliberately increase the blood

452

pressure. The high blood pressure is necessary in order to provide adequate flow through the restricted heart artery. The body accomplishes this adjustment by producing vasoconstricting hormones to constrict the arteries, arterioles, and capillaries of the peripherals. Vasoconstriction can be observed in the veins in the back of the hands that appear flat rather than bulging with blood flow. The hands and feet are cold to the touch because of the reduced flow. Doctors attempt to use vasodilators to treat hypertension, but these drugs fight against the real problem and don't provide a lasting resolution.

- The resulting hypertension increases the blood and oxygen flow to the heart muscle, thereby overcoming the effects of the artery restriction.

Placing a stent at the location of a plaque deposit anywhere in the body can immediately cure hypertension that was caused by the restriction. Stents placed in the arteries of the heart, neck, kidneys, and legs are very effective.

Hypertension that persists over a long period of time can weaken and enlarge the aorta and cause an aneurysm. When left untreated the aneurysm can suddenly rupture and result in sudden death. Persistent high blood pressure is also the leading cause of chronic kidney failure and contributes to the frequency and severity of hemorrhagic strokes.

Hypertension also increases the risk for ischemic stroke. The following definition of cerebrovascular disease explains why people are at risk for both types of strokes.

Cerebrovascular disease
http://en.wikipedia.org/wiki/Cerebrovascular_disease

"Cerebrovascular disease is a group of brain dysfunctions related to disease of the blood vessels supplying the brain. Hypertension is the most important cause; it damages the blood vessel lining, endothelium, exposing the underlying collagen where platelets aggregate to initiate a repairing process which is not always complete and perfect. Sustained hypertension permanently changes the architecture of the blood vessels making them narrow, stiff, deformed, uneven and more vulnerable to fluctuations in blood pressure.

A fall in blood pressure during sleep can then lead to a marked reduction in blood flow in the narrowed blood vessels causing ischemic stroke in the morning. Conversely, a sudden rise in blood pressure due to excitation during the daytime can cause tearing of the blood vessels resulting in intracranial hemorrhage. Cerebrovascular disease primarily affects people who are elderly or have a history of diabetes, smoking, or ischemic heart disease. The results of cerebrovascular disease can include a stroke, or occasionally a hemorrhagic stroke. Ischemia or other blood vessel dysfunctions can affect the person during a cerebrovascular accident."

The endocrine glands (pituitary, pancreas, ovaries, testes, thyroid, and adrenal) directly regulate heart rate and blood plasma volume that in turn affect blood pressure. The actual cause of hypertension may be difficult to diagnose and treat effectively because the pathways to hypertension are numerous and complex.

Disease or abnormality can cause hypertension by triggering the affected organ to excrete hormones that cascade throughout the body. The brain, heart, and kidneys have also been shown to affect blood pressure. The kidneys produce a hormone called *renin* that has a direct effect on blood pressure, and renin overproduction may be one of the most common reasons for hypertension. Cushing's syndrome is a disease of the adrenal glands caused by high levels of cortisol. Stress increases adrenaline that in turn increases blood pressure to prepare the body for heightened physical activity often called the *fight or flight* response. Hyperthyroidism (high thyroid hormone) and hypothyroidism (low thyroid hormone) can also affect blood pressure.

Hormones regulate blood pressure.

Approximately 5% of pregnant women develop high blood pressure, one of the symptoms of a condition called *preeclampsia*, which is most likely the result of problems in the placenta. Excessive protein in the urine is another symptom of preeclampsia. The high blood pressure can't be treated effectively but normally disappears when the baby is born. The hypertension is very dangerous as it can damage the endothelial lining of the blood vessels in the brain, lungs, kidneys, and liver and lead to the failure of multiple organs, convulsions, coma, and death. Women with preeclampsia often have a premature delivery, and the preeclampsia can affect the baby and cause it to be underweight and be born prematurely.

The aorta is the primary discharge artery of the heart that arches up and over the right pulmonary artery. The upper part of the arch has branches that lead to the upper body. Hypertension can be caused by a congenital defect called *coarctation of the aorta,* a sharp restriction that occurs as the aorta turns down toward the lower body. This condition can be life-threatening when the restriction is severe.

Vitamins and minerals such as vitamin D or potassium can directly affect blood pressure when they are deficient. Herbal products, prescription drugs, illegal drugs, alcohol, and common over-the-counter supplements can cause hypertension. The list is almost endless. The side effects seem to be hypertension rather than hypotension; otherwise, the products or chemicals would quickly become popular hypertensive treatments. Red yeast rice is an herbal product recommended to lower cholesterol. It does little to lower cholesterol but it does raise blood pressure. Melatonin is effective for improving sleep but also raises blood pressure.

Some herbal products can cause hypertension.

This book attacks hypertension with dietary restrictions; vitamin and mineral supplements; prescription drugs; surgically opening restricted heart arteries with stents; and removing arterial plaque from the heart, kidneys, legs, neck, brain, and other organs.

Those with hypertension should seriously consider a medical examination to determine the precise condition of the heart arteries. A treadmill stress test is not the best method if you feel you could have a heart problem because of the serious risk of heart attack or death during or soon after the test. It is ironic that a treadmill test presents no risk to a healthy person who doesn't need the test, but it can be extremely risky to a person with undiagnosed heart disease as explained in Chapter 1.

Normal blood pressure certainly reduces the incidences of stroke, congestive heart failure, myocardial infarction, and sudden death. However, investigators were surprised to learn that the all-cause mortality was not affected by actively treating hypertension when the diastolic blood pressure was less than 95 mmHg. Those who took blood pressure medications died at the same all-cause rate as those in the control group who received no treatment.

The Systolic Hypertension in Europe (Syst-Eur) Trial
http://www.hypertensiononline.org/slides2/slide01.cfm?q=systolic+blood+pressure&dpg=4

"The Systolic Hypertension in Europe (Syst-Eur) Trial enrolled 4,695 patients >60 years old, with hypertension, for a median follow-up of 24 months (range 1-97 months). All patients were initially started on masked placebo. After three run-in visits one month apart, average sitting systolic blood pressure was between 160 and 219 mmHg, with diastolic blood pressure <95 mmHg. During randomization, participants were assigned to nitrendipine 10-40 mg daily (n=2,398), plus enalapril 5-20 mg daily and hydrochlorothiazide 12.5-25 mg daily if needed, or to matching placebo (n=2,297). The primary endpoint was a composite of fatal and non-fatal stroke. Other endpoints included congestive heart failure (CHF), myocardial infarction (MI), sudden death, and all cardiac endpoints (a composite of CHF, MI and sudden death).

Sitting systolic and diastolic blood pressures fell by 23 mmHg and 7 mmHg, respectively, in the active-treatment group (n=2,398), and by 13 mmHg and 2 mmHg, respectively, in the placebo group (n=2,297). The rate for the primary endpoint, a composite of fatal and non-fatal stroke, was reduced by 42% with active treatment (P=0.003). Non-fatal stroke decreased by 44% (P=0.007). All cardiac endpoints decreased by 26% (P=0.03), while all-cause mortality was not affected by active treatment (-14%, P=0.22)."

Testimony Regarding Use of Diet Therapy for Lowering Blood Pressure

Dear Mr. Rieske,

I don't know if you remember me, but I wrote to you some months ago to thank you for the advice you gave to young women to refrain from aborting or relinquishing their children for adoption. I now would like to thank you again - this time for your dietary advice.

A few months prior to stumbling upon your website, Biblelife.org, I had told my doctor I did not wish to take medication for high blood pressure. I told her I wished to change my diet and lose weight to see if that would get it under control. The next morning, I began the DASH diet, which is the typical low fat, high grain diet. I restricted my kcal to about 1600 daily. I was losing weight, but I was hungry all the time and did not know if I could sustain this way of eating for the long haul. I was determined, though, because I didn't want to go back to the doctor empty handed and feel that pills were my only recourse.

After I'd been on this regimen for two months, I found your website and began reading. I then noticed your section about diet. I read the section and the next day I began to follow the Atkins' Induction Plan. I had lost 15 pounds at that point on the DASH plan. Since starting on the low-

carbohydrate, high-fat plan, I have lost another 20 pounds, and my blood pressure is now 117/77!

Since starting the Atkins' plan, I have done a great deal of reading and research into the politically-based history of the low-fat diet in our culture. It is shameful. I now share with people the benefits I have received eating fat and restricting carbohydrates. Not only is my blood pressure normal and my weight much better, but I no longer suffer from the acid reflux that plagued me daily for over two decades. I had resigned myself to a life of acid reducing medications and over the counter tablets to control this problem. I haven't had to use any of these for months now. The acid reflux is cured!

Here is how I now typically eat. I eat no grains, legumes, or starchy vegetables. I eat eggs, meat, fish, and fowl; including the fat and the skin. I eat butter, coconut oil, and olive oil on my foods. I eat non-starchy vegetables. I also eat almonds and walnuts. I eat small amounts of cheese and very occasionally, I will eat some berries. I do not eat other fruits, though.

I absolutely believe that God led me to your website. He knew that I was ready to make a commitment to better health this time, and it took me to where I needed to go to find the information that would help me. I have no doubt this is true. I had heard of Atkins and low-carb diets for several years but was convinced that they were unhealthy. I

459

believed dietary fat and cholesterol would harm me. I believed I had to eat grains to be healthy. I even believed that vegetarianism was probably the healthiest diet, and I had stopped eating meat on many days! I was adamantly against these low-carb diets. I had read information stating they were healthy, but I didn't believe a word of them. But, something changed in me when I read your website. Something told me I could trust what you were saying. I believe that "something" was God.

So, thank you very much for putting this information out there. I don't know if you hear from many people, but I want you to know that your website has helped to change my life for the better. I go back to it from time to time to read about other topics.

Sincerely,

Laurie

Blood Pressure Control without Drugs

Emotions and mood swings, such as excitement, anxiety, and depression, can have very negative effects, including high blood pressure, high pulse rate, poor digestion, constipation, or diarrhea. Controlling these emotions can assist in controlling hypertension and improving overall health.

Many medical references state that "normal" blood pressure for an adult is 120/80 mmHg. Others state that normal blood pressure is 130/85. Very few references state that high pressure is normal for older adults, but blood pressure below 150/90 was formerly considered to be normal. Authorities from the U.S. government's National Institutes of Health have dropped the normal blood pressure limit to 120/70 mmHg because strokes and heart attacks continued to occur in those within previously higher limits. Of course strokes and heart attacks continue for people at the lower limit, but they ignore that fact. They have published guidelines titled, *"Dietary Approaches to Stop Hypertension" (DASH)*. The DASH Diet has been summarized as follows:

> "The DASH Diet is a well-balanced way of eating that provides lots of choice and is easy to learn. It centers on real foods, not chemicals, food labels, or supplements. It is rich in fruits, vegetables, and low-fat dairy foods and reduced in red meat, fats, and sweets. This healthy way of eating has been thoroughly tested in several large studies sponsored by the National Institutes of Health and has been scientifically proven to help people lose weight, lower their blood pressure and cholesterol, and even improve how they feel!"

Don't eat the DASH Diet. Those on this plan have not reduced hypertension as promised. It's nothing more than another way to promote the *USDA Food Guide Pyramid* that gave us the cardiovascular and hypertension crises in the first place. The DASH Diet promotes carbohydrates in the form of glucose and fructose, both of which cause insulin spikes, weight gain, and cardiovascular diseases.

The DASH Diet will not resolve your hypertension.

Many studies draw the conclusion that the slightest increase in blood pressure above normal can increase the incidence of stroke or heart attack. These conclusions are highly suspect because the studies are not able to separate blood pressure from among the many variables. People who have a stroke or a heart attack typically have contributing factors, such as coronary artery disease, vitamin and mineral deficiencies, hormone abnormalities, fatty acid deficiencies, or amino acid deficiencies.

For example, vegetarians are at risk for hemorrhagic stroke caused by a ruptured blood vessel or capillary in the brain. Their low-fat, low-protein, and low-cholesterol diet commonly results in weak arteries that make them prone to strokes even though blood pressure is normal. The strength and health of the blood vessels are vitally important for stroke prevention. The low-carbohydrate diet with high levels of protein and natural animal fats provides the nutrition necessary to build strong, healthy blood vessels.

Pharmaceutical companies are emphasizing blood pressure in order to get more people to take their drugs. Many of the claims about blood pressure are simply scare tactics used by companies with an agenda. The medical profession places a high emphasis on prescription drugs for treating high blood pressure. At most they may suggest lowering salt intake, reducing weight, and increasing exercise. These steps do help but are still inadequate in most cases. The following steps are more extensive and successful at reducing high blood pressure.

Correcting Mineral Deficiencies and Imbalances

The following is a multi-step approach to treating hypertension. All of the steps should be employed since the cause for high blood pressure is often illusive and may have been incorrectly diagnosed.

Step No. 1

Correcting mineral deficiencies and imbalances is the most important step toward reducing high blood pressure. The first step is a close review and adjustment of sodium, potassium, calcium, magnesium, and all trace minerals.

Water

Do not drink tap water. Nearly all tap water has a serious mineral imbalance. Supermarket water labeled *natural spring water* or *distilled water* is not acceptable. Only buy water that has been processed by the reverse osmosis (RO) process, or install your own RO with UV lamp water system. Use RO water for drinking and cooking. Take it to the job and on vacation. My recommended supplements provide minerals in the proper proportions.

Do not drink large amounts of water. The supplements I recommended require a generous amount of water just to get them all down. Drink when you're thirsty, and keep in mind that drinking an excessive amount of water actually flushes vital minerals from the body. On several occasions, water-drinking contests have resulted in deaths. Several professional athletes have died as a result of mineral depletion from sweating and drinking excessive amounts of water. Since the recent death of a marathon competitor, many professional trainers advise giving special mineral water to professional athletes. This is good advice for the average person as well.

Important Supplements to Take and Avoid

A deficiency of any mineral can be unhealthy, and an excess of most minerals can be unhealthy. Therefore, the goal is to take a precise amount of minerals and other supplements and avoid excesses. The following supplements should be taken or avoided in an attempt to control hypertension.

Colloidal Minerals

Supplement the diet with colloidal minerals that contain all of the major minerals as well as the trace minerals. The importance of vitamins to good health is widely known, but many people do not know that trace minerals are also essential. Without minerals to act as catalysts, many vitamins cannot perform their necessary functions. Colloidal minerals are in a form that your body can readily absorb. The common metallic forms of minerals resist interaction with water and are not always easily absorbed by the body.

Take one 1 fl. oz. (2 tablespoons) of colloidal minerals per day in a glass of RO water or low-sodium tomato juice. The caps on the containers of many colloidal minerals can be used as measuring devices as described on the labels. I suggest taking colloidal minerals with breakfast.

Selenium

Take selenium with caution. Selenium can have toxic symptoms when taken in excess. Your doctor may advise against selenium if you are taking certain drugs. Selenium deficiency causes many heart problems, including irregular heartbeat, heart palpitations, cardiomyopathy (deterioration of the heart muscles), sudden heart attack, and death. Other deadly diseases include liver failure, cancer, and pancreatitis.

Taurine

Take taurine or taurine amino acid. The highest concentration of taurine is in the heart where it is involved in the stabilization of heart rhythm. Loss of intracellular taurine in the heart leads to arrhythmia. Taurine is used to treat congestive heart failure (CHF). Take one 850 mg tablet 3 times per day for a large man and 2 times per day for smaller individuals.

Vitamin P5P

Vitamin P5P (pyridoxal-5-phosphate, the active form of vitamin B6) is needed to promote taurine use in cell metabolism. Take one or two 50 mg capsules per day. Conventional vitamin B6 is not an acceptable substitute. Both can be taken at the same time, but vitamin P5P is needed for taurine metabolism.

Copper

Take a copper supplement. Copper is vital for healthy arteries. Copper deficiency is widespread and leads to many serious diseases, including cerebral aneurysms (rupture causes a stroke), abdominal aorta aneurysms (rupture causes instant death from internal bleeding), nerve damage, birth defects, cerebral palsy, and mental deterioration. Do not take high doses of zinc because it depletes copper. I suggest taking copper and zinc together with lunch. Supplement with 3 mg of copper four times per week.

Chapter 5

Zinc

Take a zinc supplement with copper, but avoid taking other minerals at the same meal. Zinc prevents many minerals from being absorbed by the digestive tract. I suggest taking zinc with lunch and the minerals below with dinner or as listed in the supplement table in Chapter 4. Supplement with zinc and copper four times per week (every other day) in the range of 30 mg zinc and 3 mg copper in a 10/1 ratio. Excessive amounts of zinc have been found to be detrimental to the cardiovascular system.

Manganese

Take a manganese supplement. It's important in enzyme systems, blood sugar control, energy metabolism, and thyroid function. Manganese is required for the body to make the powerful antioxidant enzyme superoxide dismutase (SOD) that reduces cell damage from free radicals as well as inflammation. Because high doses of some minerals can deplete manganese, I recommend supplementing the diet with 10 mg every day.

Magnesium

Perhaps magnesium should be classified as the most important supplement for reducing hypertension, heart palpitations, and arrhythmia. A magnesium deficiency is common in nearly everyone and is related to arthritis, osteoporosis, migraine headaches, and asthma. Since it is difficult to raise the amount of magnesium in the cells, several weeks or months may be required to build it up in the body. However, heart palpitations may stop within a few weeks, and the heart rate should be very steady and equally spaced. Magnesium is a natural and safe laxative when taken in excess. A large male should take one 200 mg tablet of KAL Magnesium Glycinate 400® three times per day with a meal. Smaller individuals should take only two. Take less if it causes loose bowels, or take more if constipation is a problem.

KAL Magnesium Glycinate 400® is the highly-absorbed form of magnesium chelated with amino acids. It can be taken at twice the dosage as other brands without causing intestinal distress. Do not substitute another brand. Magnesium is essential for a healthy heart and cardiovascular system, and the current deficiency in the general population is going largely unrecognized even thought it contributes to a decline in health. Calcium gets all the attention and displaces magnesium in the minds of the health-conscious public in the same way that it displaces magnesium in the cells. Magnesium deficiency contributes greatly to the current decrease in bone, skeletal, and cardiovascular health. Magnesium is very important for building strong bones, but the dairy industry has convinced people that broken hip joints are caused by a calcium deficiency. Actually, hip joints break because of a protein deficiency. My diet program corrects all of these problems and builds super-strong bones. Take magnesium and give up calcium.

Magnesium is essential for strong bones and a healthy heart and cardiovascular system.

Diuretic prescription drugs for hypertension also deplete the body of electrolytes, particularly potassium and magnesium, which most likely are already deficient. If you take diuretics, be prepared to reduce the dosage according to your doctor's instructions because blood pressure could drop when taking these minerals. Correcting the electrolyte balance reduces the need for diuretics.

WARNING: Magnesium can be toxic for those who have either renal (kidney/liver) problems or atrioventricular blocks.

Chapter 5

Sodium

Sodium should be avoided. Excess sodium depletes both potassium and calcium. Fifteen percent of the general population responds negatively to common table salt (sodium chloride). Many diet and medical books claim the outcry against salt is unwarranted, but the authors must not be salt sensitive. If they were, they would know that salt causes water retention and hypertension in sensitive individuals.

A high-potassium, low-sodium diet protects the body against cancer and cardiovascular disease. Consuming salty foods or drinks can cause arrhythmia and a blood pressure surge in minutes. Getting too much sodium chloride coupled with diminished potassium is a common cause of high blood pressure. Strictly reduce the intake of all sodium compounds. Most people become addicted to salt and can't control their addiction even though they've been told of the harmful effects. People who lack self-control usually fail to control their blood pressure, weight, and health. Salt becomes toxic to them because they do not excrete it as is required to maintain health, and the body becomes heavily laden with excess sodium. The symptoms include water retention in tissues and cells that increases during the day. Blood pressure increases accordingly and is typically higher in the evening. During the night, the body begins to dump the water and sodium in the urine. A very low-sodium diet begins to show some benefits after about one month, and these benefits continue to increase for many months. Purging the excess sodium from the cells could take as long as one year.

Potassium

Take potassium because it is an extremely important electrolyte that functions to maintain water balance, water distribution, and acid/base balance. Potassium is needed for the proper function of muscles, nerve cells, heart electrolytes, kidneys, and the adrenal glands. Everyone should increase the consumption of potassium chloride, which is readily available as Morton's Salt Substitute®. Never take other brands that contain monopotassium glutamate or any glutamate compound such as MSG.

The sodium chloride salt added to food in manufacturing and preparation causes an imbalance in the sodium/potassium ratio. Vegetables, fruits, and unprocessed meats and fish are high in potassium and low in sodium. However, restricting fruits is strongly recommended because they contain a high level of fructose that is associated with hypertension. Processed foods can have a 10 to 1 ratio of sodium to potassium, while natural foods have a ratio of only 1 to 10. Use a potassium chloride salt substitute instead of table salt.

The sodium-potassium pump is the body process that maintains a proper balance between sodium and potassium. Cell membranes allow sodium to enter when the sodium ion potential is high and the potassium ion potential is low. Sodium moves inside the cell where it attracts water and makes the cell hydrate and swell. Eating less salt reduces the sodium ion potential that allows potassium to enter the cell and force the sodium and water out as the potassium enters. This is the diuretic effect that reduces water retention and lowers blood pressure.

If you have high blood pressure and/or an irregular pulse, take ¼ teaspoon of potassium chloride (610mg) in a cup of water. Recheck your blood pressure and pulse after 60 minutes. If both have improved, supplement daily. Do not supplement with potassium if you are taking a potassium-sparing diuretic.

Chapter 5

Calcium

Calcium is rarely mentioned as a cause of hypertension. The reason for this is intuitively obvious. Calcium is the *holy mineral that prevents osteoporosis*. Health and nutrition experts have a serious conflict of interest. Physicians and health authorities continue to advise women to gorge themselves on calcium as a means of preventing bone loss and osteoporosis, but they cannot bring themselves to expose the fact that calcium also raises blood pressure and causes heart disease. Women are constantly being told to eat lots low-fat yogurt, low-fat cottage cheese, low-fat milk, and fruit and to avoid meat in order to protect their bones. This advice has failed to prevent osteoporosis. In fact, these recommendations have caused the current osteoporosis epidemic.

Calcium has a serious negative ramification in that it depletes magnesium from the body, and 75% of the people in the United States eat a diet that is deficient in magnesium. My low-carbohydrate diet allows a generous quantity of hard cheeses that are high in calcium. The daily multivitamin tablet also has calcium; therefore, do not supplement with calcium tablets if cheese is consumed. My cardiologist agrees completely with my calcium restriction. The following study explains why calcium causes hypertension.

> **Acute hypercalcemic hypertension in man: Role of hemodynamics, catecholamines, and rennin**
> *Kidney International* (1981) 20, 92–96
> http://www.nature.com/ki/journal/v20/n1/abs/ki1981109a.html
>
> "Acute hypercalcemic hypertension in man: Role of hemodynamics, catecholamines, and renin. The effect of acute hypercalcemia on blood pressure, blood volume, hemodynamic parameters, plasma norepinephrine,

epinephrine, dopamine, renin, and aldosterone concentrations was investigated. After 1 hour of equilibration, 10 patients received an infusion of calcium gluconate in 5% dextrose (calcium 15 mg/kg of body wt in 3 hours). The calcium infusion increased the mean serum calcium from 8.7 to 13.0 mg/dl, the systolic blood pressure from 144 10 to 184 (SEM) 12 mm Hg (P < 0.001), the diastolic pressure from 78 4 to 93 5 mm Hg (P < 0.01). The plasma volume was decreased by 9% (P < 0.001), whereas the hematocrit was increased (P < 0.05). Heart rate and cardiac output remained unchanged. Total peripheral resistance was increased from 1643 223 to 2256 387 dynesec/cm5 (P < 0.05). The plasma epinephrine concentration rose from 4.5 0.7 to 6.9 1.2 ng/dl (P < 0.01). The plasma norepinephrine concentration was unchanged after 2 hours and increased only slightly after 3 hours of calcium infusion. Plasma renin, aldosterone, and dopamine concentrations were not significantly changed. These findings demonstrate that acute hypercalcemic hypertension is mediated by an increase in peripheral vascular resistance. Hypercalcemic hypertension may be induced by a direct effect of calcium on blood vessels; calcium-mediated increase in adrenal epinephrine release may play a mild contributory role, and plasma volume contraction, an inhibitory role."

Calcium is an essential mineral needed to build and maintain bones and teeth as well as provide efficient muscle contraction and blood clotting. Calcium chloride is added as a firming agent in many canned vegetables, including tomatoes, carrots, mixed vegetables, potatoes, and zucchini. For this reason, canned vegetables should be limited. Eat fresh vegetables instead. Calcium chloride can raise systolic blood pressure by 20mm Hg and diastolic blood pressure by 15mm Hg within one to two hours and can completely overpower blood pressure medication.

Calcium in the cells of the heart increases the force of the contractions, constricts blood vessels, and raises blood pressure. As a result, blood supply and oxygen to the heart muscles are decreased. Calcium channel blockers are a group of drugs prescribed for hypertension. They reverse the negative effects of calcium by preventing it from moving into the cells of the heart and blood vessels. They relax blood vessels and increase the supply of blood and oxygen to the heart, thereby reducing its workload.

Excessive calcium is hypertensive.

Many medical references and professionals claim that calcium can lower blood pressure. This is highly questionable since doctors commonly prescribe calcium channel blockers to treat hypertension. Doctors also administer IV calcium chloride as an emergency treatment for patients with dangerously low blood pressure.

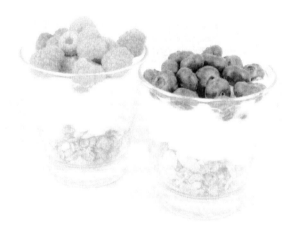

Yogurt, Fruit, and Cereal are "Forbidden Foods"

Step No. 2

Adopt the Low-Carbohydrate Lifestyle

Adopt the low-carbohydrate lifestyle as outlined in Chapter 4. This alone can reduce elevated blood pressure because it acts as a powerful diuretic that eliminates excess water from the body. Dietary carbohydrates are stored as glycogen, and one gram of glycogen holds three grams of water. The low-carbohydrate diet forces the body to use stored glycogen and in doing so, the stored water is excreted. Therefore, the low-carbohydrate diet acts as an effective natural diuretic to reduce blood pressure.

The low-carbohydrate diet is a powerful diuretic.

However, it is only effective when the amount of carbohydrates in the diet is below 20 grams per day, and the diuretic effect may be completely lost at 40 grams per day. Eating carbohydrates after eliminating the stored water will result in immediate water retention and a corresponding increase in blood pressure.

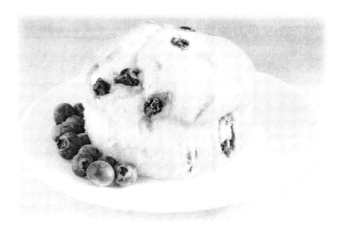

Blueberry Muffins are "Forbidden Foods"

Chapter 5

Step No. 3

Avoid Harmful Food Additives

A panic disorder or anxiety attacks can send blood pressure and pulse rate soaring for no apparent reason. This is caused by hormones that trigger a fight or flight response. These panic or anxiety attacks can be greatly reduced by taking commonly available supplements without the need for costly prescription drugs that may have dangerous side effects. Emotions and mood swings, such as excitement, anxiety, and depression, can have very negative effects on the body, including high blood pressure, high heart pulse rate, poor digestion, constipation, or diarrhea.

Don't consume any diet soft drinks that contain aspartame, and don't eat any foods sweetened with aspartame. Aspartame is commonly used to sweeten diet sodas and foods and can cause vasoconstriction and hypertensive reactions that completely overpower everything in this program. Aspartame can also overpower prescription blood pressure-lowering medications. It is imperative that all aspartame be eliminated from the diet.

> **Aspartame converts to powerful excitatory neurotransmitters that raise blood pressure.**

One diet soda per day will nullify all of the anti-hypertension treatments presented here. The body converts aspartame to the amino acid phenylalanine that is the precursor of tyrosine, which in turn is the precursor of dopamine and the excitatory neurotransmitters epinephrine and norepinephrine (also called *adrenalin* and *noradrenalin*). These neurotransmitters are powerful vasoconstrictors that constrict the blood vessels and raise blood pressure dramatically.

474

Aspartame hypes the hormonal system and causes hunger, anxiety, and insomnia. Do not take phenylalanine or tyrosine supplements except as normally present in low-carbohydrate whey protein powder. Phenylalanine and tyrosine are both helpful in treating depression, but both should be avoided by people with hypertension.

Phenylalanine can be a dangerous amino acid and can cause the following problems in sensitive individuals or complications in certain situations:

- Hypertension

- Prostate - Exasperates urination difficulties caused by benign prostatic hyperplasia (BPH or enlarged prostate)

- Pregnancy - Can harm the baby

- Cancer - Can stimulate pigmented melanoma, the deadliest form of skin cancer

- Phenylketonuria (PKU) - Harmful to those with improper phenylalanine metabolism

- Anxiety - Can exasperate panic disorders and anxiety attacks

- Insomnia

These comments are not simply prejudicial. Most of the negative claims against aspartame are false. For example, most critics claim that aspartame turns to formaldehyde in the blood. This is scientifically false. Ten percent of the aspartame can be converted to methanol in the small intestines. It could possibly be converted to formaldehyde, but this does not occur because formaldehyde is not found in the blood of people who consume aspartame sweetened diet drinks or foods. However, it is a scientific fact that aspartame is broken down into phenylalanine during digestion. Diet drinks containing aspartame give this warning on the can or bottle for those people with PKU who cannot metabolize phenylalanine.

Acceptable drinks are unsweetened tomato juice, tea, water, and coffee. Coffee has the short-term effect of increasing blood pressure but is not nearly the problem that is commonly claimed. The rash of caffeine criticism is mostly false except for the tendency to cause breast tenderness in women and high blood pressure in some people. The most common short-term effect of caffeine is an elevated pulse rate. Don't drink decaf coffee or decaf black tea because toxic chemicals are used to remove the caffeine. Peppermint tea is preferred. A small amount of fresh lemon or lime juice can be added to water or tea. Ginger has a spicy flavor and is very soothing to the stomach and digestive tract. Ginger root tea is great.

- From fresh ginger root, cut a piece about the size of the small fingertip.

- Remove the skin.

- Finely chop and place pieces in a garlic press.

- Press the juice into a cup or French press.

- Add the pulp from the garlic press and fill the cup with boiling water.

- Steep the tea for two minutes.

- Strain out the pulp and enjoy.

Beware of coffee, tea, and energy drinks that are spiked with herbal products known to send the heart rate skyrocketing and the blood pressure soaring. Don't drink any fruit juice or regular soft drinks because they contain high levels of fructose and sugar. Don't drink cows' milk, goats' milk, rice milk, soy milk, or any energy drinks because they contain sugar, fructose, lactose, and other carbohydrates. Limit alcoholic beverages. Don't drink anything containing more than two calories per 16 oz. (0.47 liters).

Hypertensive Foods, Drugs, and Herbal Products to Avoid

The following additional foods, drugs, supplements, and herbal products have been found to increase blood pressure. These should be avoided.

- Alcohol in excess

- Birth control pills

- Ephedra (ma huang)

- Licorice

- Lobelia or other sources of lobeline

- Yohimbe

- Tobacco

Beware of coffee and tea spiked with uppers.

Step No. 4

Improve Breathing and Stop Bad Breathing Habits

Breathing exercises reduce high blood pressure, and improper breathing can cause a dramatic rise in blood pressure. Don't skip this last step as it may be the most important one for you. In a recent test, a blood pressure reading of 154/100 dropped to 129/79 in only 15 minutes simply by practicing the proper breathing technique. This technique can replace old breathing habits that cause elevated blood pressure. Mechanical Engineering principles are related to proper breathing.

Mechanical Engineering Principle

The lungs function much like the common internal combustion piston engine in a car, truck, motorcycle, or bus. The engine draws in air and fuel, burns the fuel to produce a power stroke, and discharges the products of combustion. Pistons move up and down in the engine block, and each stroke displaces a volume that is the area of the piston times the stroke. The total displacement (Vdisp) is commonly expressed in cubic inches (ci) or cubic centimeters (cc) to identify the size of the engine.

The space above the piston is the combustion chamber volume (Vcc) and is generally a part of the head that is bolted to the block. The total volume ratio (Vt) is according to the formula:

$$Vt = Vdisp / (Vcc + Vdisp)$$

The compression ratio (CR) for an engine is generally in the range of 8–10 for gasoline engines and 15–17 for diesel engines. The compression ratio (CR) is according to the formula:

$$CR = (Vcc + Vdisp) / Vcc$$

Smaller combustion chambers produce a higher compression ratio, and the power and efficiency are both improved with high compression ratios on both a theoretical and practical basis. Race engines have higher compression ratios but require more expensive fuel. Diesel engines have very high compression ratios and are much more efficient as a result.

Human Lungs and Breathing Principle

The human body draws in oxygenated air in the same way as an engine. The lungs absorb the oxygen into the blood for delivery to the cells where combustion takes place to give the muscles energy and to create heat that keeps us warm. Carbon dioxide is the product of combustion within the cells that is carried in the blood, transferred to the lungs, and discharged in the air we exhale.

Proper breathing can lower your blood pressure.

We can't exhale all the air because the lungs have small residual spaces that don't empty. The windpipe is a semi-rigid tube that doesn't collapse, and the windpipe volume can't be expelled. This remaining volume is very similar to the combustion chamber in an engine.

The volume of air taken into the lungs when we breathe is similar to the displacement in an engine, but the body is different because the volume is variable. The residual volume is also variable. We can stop exhaling with our lungs half empty and begin inhaling again. This recycle of carbon dioxide-laden air back into the lungs is a big problem. Shallow breathing leaves a large amount of air in the lungs that is low in oxygen and high in carbon dioxide. The transfer of oxygen to the blood and the carbon dioxide from the blood to the air is sharply reduced.

Shallow breathing creates the same effect as being at a high altitude. Many physicians advise patients not to go to high altitudes, but they may fail to advise the patient to breathe deeply.

Shallow breathing raises blood pressure.

Breathing is partly voluntary and partly involuntary. We can control our breathing rate by taking deep or shallow breaths, and we can breathe rapidly or slowly. Involuntary breathing takes over when we are asleep, deprived of oxygen (hypoventilation), or have excessive oxygen (hyperventilation). Most of the times we simply ignore our breathing and let the involuntary system take over. We tend to get lazy and establish a pattern that becomes a habit. Some people develop a very bad breathing pattern that leads to higher blood pressure, but this can be easily corrected.

The position of our body also changes our breathing. We compress the abdomen by sitting and leaning forward, which pushes the diaphragm up into the chest. The amount of air that can be inhaled is thereby reduced. This improper position is common with desk work or factory assembly line operations. You must not stay in a position that prevents a full intake of air with each breath. Body fat can contribute to breathing problems, especially when tummy fat restricts the amount of air we can draw into our lungs while bending forward. You may notice that you can't draw in a breath of air while bending forward and putting on your shoes. We then straighten up and begin gasping for air. This is a common problem with people who are obese.

The lungs of younger individuals easily assimilate oxygen from the air they breathe and efficiently discharge carbon dioxide when they exhale. This efficiency or ability to assimilate oxygen is greatly reduced as we age because of the many years spent inhaling air pollution, dust, chemicals, and cigarette smoke. Older people do not hyperventilate very easily as do younger people and children. As we age, breathing becomes less efficient to the point where additional oxygen must be administered to people with damaged lungs in order to keep the blood oxygen level within an acceptable range. This inefficiency greatly contributes to high blood pressure in older individuals and those who have smoked or have damaged lungs.

The Heart Increases Blood Pressure to Compensate for Improper Breathing

The heart and blood pressure operate involuntarily. We can't simply decide to change our heart rate and thereby decrease our blood pressure. The body automatically controls the heart to supply oxygenated blood to the body. The heart rate and blood pressure will change depending on the body's demand and the ability of the lungs to provide oxygen and remove carbon dioxide.

Shallow breathing deprives the body of oxygen, and the heart must automatically compensate by pumping more blood. This produces higher blood pressure and a faster pulse rate. Reducing activity also tends to reduce blood pressure and pulse rate as occurs during sleep.

Biofeedback and relaxation techniques reduce overall activity, change hormone levels, and lower blood pressure. However, these do not provide long-lasting blood pressure control during everyday activity because we forget to do them. You most likely will not do biofeedback or relaxation techniques while mowing the lawn or struggling to solve a computer problem.

Chapter 5

Blood Pressure Control Method

Breathing is work, and we tend to get lazy. The following steps will restore deep breathing, increase the number of breaths per minute, and help to lower blood pressure.

Step No. 4a - Breathe in deeply, sharply, and quickly using the chest and the diaphragm. Allow the tummy to expand as the diaphragm presses downward into the abdominal cavity. You may find it difficult to expand the chest, but this will allow more air to be inhaled. This technique reduces the pressure within the chest cavity to less than the atmospheric air pressure. The difference in pressure drops the blood pressure accordingly. You will immediately notice that you rarely inhale air to the full capacity of lungs. Taking a full breath of air is the second key part of this breathing technique. You must inhale a good supply of oxygen with each breath. A tight belt, clothing, body fat, or poor sitting position will prevent deep breathing.

Step No. 4b - Relax and exhale slowly. Exhaling should take twice as much time as inhaling. Simply relax and let the air flow out. Do not force the air out because compressing the chest to expel the air increases the blood pressure accordingly. Breathe out to empty the lungs of as much air as possible. You will notice that you rarely exhale all of your air, but this is a vital part of this breathing technique. You must dispel as much of the old air and carbon dioxide as possible. Practice inhaling and exhaling as completely as possible.

Step No. 4c - The breathing rate must be adjusted voluntarily. A more rapid rate than necessary will cause hyperventilation as a result of excess oxygen in the blood. A slow rate will deprive the body of oxygen and send the heart into action to increase the pulse rate and blood pressure. The tendency is to take a few shallow breaths per minute that fail to adequately oxidize the blood. The heart compensates for the low oxygen level by increasing the blood pressure and pulse rate.

Step No. 4d - Breathing exercises must be done several times a day to break the old patterns. You will be distracted by your everyday events and forget about breathing. I forget when I'm concentrating on my computer. You may hold your breath without being aware of it or slump back into your old involuntary breathing pattern. Concentrate on the proper breathing technique at least once every hour. Inhale deeply and exhale fully to reestablish a proper breathing pattern.

Step No. 4e - Your breathing pattern should automatically change over time as you become accustomed to breathing properly. Watch out for relapses. Go back to the beginning with hourly exercises to get back into the proper pattern that will become a new habit.

Obstacles to Proper Breathing

Breathing is ideally done through the nose. However, few people enjoy the pleasant feeling of being able to take an easy, deep breath through the nose because of chronic sinus problems or a deviated septum. Any restriction can greatly reduce the amount of air flow and make it harder to breathe. This is particularly true during sleep when many people are forced to breathe through the mouth. Breathing restrictions can be caused by:

- A broken nose that healed wrong and restricted the passage

- A deviated, bowed, or crooked nasal septum between the two passages

- A latent, mild nasal infection that may be undiagnosed

- Sinus infection or allergy that creates a restriction due to puffiness

- Candida yeast infection in the nasal passages that creates swelling of the tissues

- An adverse sinus reaction to low humidity

Nasal and Sinus Treatments Can Improve Breathing

Chronic sinus and nasal congestion can be a bacterial infection that should be treated with antibiotics, but this is generally a misdiagnosis. Doctors will prescribe an antibiotic that fails to bring relief, but they rarely test for a yeast infection or prescribe any treatment for yeast in the nasal passages. The symptoms may be caused by a yeast or fungal infection that causes itching and excess mucus. The fungi are attracted to and thrive in the moist environment. Treatment is easy because fungi are quickly killed by sodium bicarbonate (common baking soda), and a home remedy may be more effective than commercial products. Simply purchase a 1 oz. (30 cc) plastic nasal rinse or squirt bottle. Mix 1/4 teaspoon (1.25 cc) of sodium bicarbonate with reverse osmosis water in the bottle. Squirt or drip the mixture generously into each nasal passage. The treatment should be done twice a day for five days. The sodium bicarbonate may sting slightly at the back of the nasal passage, but it should quickly go away. Reduce the concentration if the stinging is uncomfortable. This is a mild and very effective treatment.

Nasal problems can raise blood pressure.

Breathe·ease XL® is an alternative for treating nasal and sinus congestion. This excellent product is formulated and sold by Dr. Murray Grossman, M.D., an otolaryngologist (ear, nose, and throat medical specialist), and is readily available on the Internet.

Eliminating yeast in the sinuses and nasal passages can cause bacteria to flourish and vice-versa. Therefore, a good antibiotic should be used in addition to the anti-fungal treatment. Mupirocin® nasal is used to prevent severe staph and other infections in the nose. It eliminates surface and hair-borne bacteria but may not be effective for deep sinus infections. Use an oral antibiotic such as Keflex® for sinus infections.

Snoring can be caused by restricted air flow in the throat. This condition is often seen in overweight people because fat within the tissues of the throat restricts the flow. The only practical way to eliminate such a restriction is to reduce body fat to the ideal range. The tongue can also relax into the back of the mouth and restrict the air passage by the rearward movement of the lower jaw. A device is available that fits in the mouth to prevent this.

Restrictions in the nasal passage can increase blood pressure when we exhale. The chest and diaphragm compress the lungs to exhale, and any resistance creates an increased pressure in the lungs and throughout the chest cavity. This extra resistance also pressurizes the outside of the heart. The extra pressure is added to the pressure developed by the heart muscle and propagates throughout the entire cardiovascular system.

Nasal and Sinus Treatment with Pharmaceuticals

Normal sinuses are air-filled spaces and are free of infection. They have openings that allow cilia to move mucus and bacteria out of the sinuses. Nasal and sinus treatments using prescription drugs can remove these chronic bacterial or fungal infections but are not always totally effective. Bacteria and yeast live on the surfaces of the nasal passages, sinuses, and hairs inside the nose;

and drugs taken into the bloodstream simply do not reach these external surfaces. When a fungal or yeast infection is suspected anywhere in the body, mouth, or nasal passages, I recommend taking a prescription antifungal drug such as Diflucan® (generic: fluconazole) or Sporanox® (generic: itraconazole); but do not take either with statin drugs or niacin. Take Keflex® (generic: cephalexin) for bacterial infections as directed by your physician.

The antibiotic I prefer for home use is ZYMAR® (gatifloxacin ophthalmic solution 0.3%) by Allergan that is generally prescribed as an antibiotic eye drop. It is available internationally from Magic Pharma at www.magicpharma.com. Use saline nasal spray from a pressurized dispenser several times a day to keep the nose moist and discourage bacterial and fungal growth. I prefer using lysine amino acid powder mixed with MCT oil as a treatment for suspected virus infections.

I saw a local otolaryngologist with symptoms of a nasal infection, but he only suggested surgery for a deviated septum. He made no attempt to check for any bacterial or yeast infection. I rejected the surgery and resolved my problem with the above treatments.

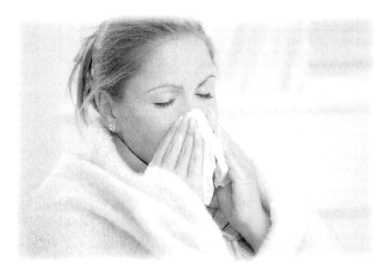

Step No. 5

This step is about exercise, but you must exercise correctly. Chapter 6 will explain how exercise can kill you.

Exercise is very important for overall health and vigor, and the lack of exercise will result in a tired feeling and reduced energy. The best time to exercise is after breakfast while the cortisol level is still high, but I prefer mid afternoon in colder weather. Exercising during the late afternoon or evening is less desirable because it stimulates the body too late in the day and may disturb sleep. A brisk 30-minute walk four times a week with some uphill effort is adequate. The exercise should include a 15-minute period of high output and heavy breathing. Those close to ideal weight should increase the activity, but those who are overweight require less because the extra weight provides a higher level of exertion.

Moderate exercise can reduce blood pressure.

Aerobic exercise is very helpful for lowering blood pressure and should be in accordance with your physician's limitations. It can be overdone and should not produce any negative side effects. The proper aerobic exercise can drop blood pressure from 155/95 to 125/78 within 20 minutes after completion.

Constriction of the arteries and arterioles is a major cause of high blood pressure. This condition can be seen by observing the veins in the back of the hand while relaxing. Veins that can easily be seen and make the skin rise indicate a high flow rate. Flat veins in the back of the hand indicate vasoconstriction and a low flow rate. High blood pressure is associated with flat veins and a low flow rate.

During a short period of aggressive aerobic exercise (15–25 minutes), the body releases vasodilating hormones in order to increase blood flow to the muscles. This action often lowers the blood pressure after the exercise is completed and you have had a cool down period. Bicycling, hill climbing, swimming, aggressive walking on an inclined treadmill, using an elliptical trainer, and pedaling a stationary bicycle are wonderful exercises. Whatever the exercise, it should be done three to seven times per week. I prefer to ride my bike aggressively for 15 minutes every day and will occasionally engage in longer and harder exercise like mountain climbing.

You should understand that the scientific techniques presented here are expected to lower your blood pressure and may require a change in your prescription medication because blood pressure could drop to an undesirably low level. You should discuss this with your doctor and be prepared to taper off your medications with his approval. The reverse is also true. You cannot go back to your old lifestyle after discontinuing your medications because your blood pressure will quickly go up again. You should be prepared to increase your medication if you discontinue these techniques.

False Advice about Hypertension

Many medical organizations, medical clinics, physicians, nutritional organizations, and professional nutritionists present long lists of recommendations that they claim will reduce hypertension. However, most of these recommendations do not work as has been proven by the high levels of hypertension in all English-speaking countries.

Don't be tricked by false advice about blood pressure.

The following are some of these false recommendations to disregard:

- **Red Meat and Eggs** - Many doctors and nutritionists claim we should avoid eating red meat and egg yolks because they contain arachidonic fatty acid (AA) that raises the blood pressure by causing vasoconstriction. This theory is false. Most people with hypertension already eat very little red meat and eggs, but they still have high blood pressure. Red meat and eggs do not cause high blood pressure in any way. The diet program presented here encourages eating high levels of red meat and eggs.

- **Saturated Fats** - Many medical organizations, physicians, and nutritionists claim saturated fats cause hypertension. This claim is false.

- **Vegetarian Diet** - Many medical organizations, physicians, and nutritionists claim the vegetarian diet prevents or cures hypertension. These claims are false. Many vegetarians develop high blood pressure.

- **Dietary Approaches to Stop Hypertension (DASH) Diet -** The DASH Diet emphasizes eating fruits, vegetables, whole grains, and low-fat dairy foods while avoiding red meat, saturated animal fats, and eggs. People with hypertension can quickly and easily test this diet for themselves to prove it does not reduce hypertension, and they will find the DASH Diet is simply another vegetarian ploy to stop people from eating animal products.

- **Manage Stress** - The claim is often made that managing stress can control hypertension. This can be true when a short-term, high-stress situation raises the levels of cortisol and adrenaline, but many people find that relaxing does not help their chronic hypertension because it is not caused by stress.

- **Sleep, Baths, and Snacks** - The recommendation that a warm bath and a snack before bedtime will give a more restful sleep that will reduce hypertension is false. Many people with hypertension also have sleep apnea, but a warm bath and a snack will not provide any cure for sleep apnea. In fact, the warm bath and snack will most likely raise blood pressure. If you have hypertension, simply test this false theory for yourself.

- **Soy Products** - A claim has been made that adding soy to cookies reduces blood pressure because of the higher protein content. The minor four point drop observed in the study (if true) was most likely caused by the reduction in sugar and grains. If eating protein were the answer for reducing hypertension, the study should have recommended a high-protein red meat diet.

- **Excessive Exercise** – Moderate exercise can certainly help lower blood pressure in some cases, but excessive exercise is not the panacea for achieving normal blood pressure when the cause is hormonal, disease, or a restriction in the coronary arteries. This is why exercise has such varied results.

- **Potatoes, Fruits, Cereals, and Chocolate** – Many foods are erroneously touted to reduce blood pressure. You can tests these food yourself to disprove the claims. Potatoes, chocolate, whole grain cereals, Ezekiel bread, bagels, dietary fiber, rice, tofu, bananas, nuts, seeds, legumes, vegetables, vegetable juices, beet juice, exotic fruits, berries, pomegranate juice, orange juice, and other fruits and fruit juices will not reduce your blood pressure.

Step No. 6

Prescription Drugs for Treating Hypertension

The following drugs may exhibit fewer and less severe side effects than many of those used for treating hypertension. Tekturna® is a direct renin blocker that relaxes blood vessels, thereby lowering blood pressure and allowing the heart to pump more easily. It can be taken anytime with or without food but should not be taken with fat as this reduces the absorption and effectiveness. The bioavailability is low (not easily absorbed) and requires 7 to 8 days to reach a steady-state level.

> **Some drugs for treating hypertension are safe, effective, and present very few side effects.**

Tekturna® (generic: aliskiren hemifumarate) is a renin blocker manufactured by Novartis® and sold internationally under the brand name Rasilex®.

> "Renin is secreted by the kidney in response to decreases in blood volume and renal perfusion. Renin cleaves angiotensinogen to form the inactive decapeptide angiotensin I (Ang I). Ang I is converted to the active octapeptide angiotensin II (Ang II) by angiotensin-converting enzyme (ACE) and non-ACE pathways. Ang II is a powerful vasoconstrictor and leads to the release of catecholamines from the adrenal medulla and prejunctional nerve endings. It also promotes aldosterone secretion and sodium reabsorption. Together, these effects increase blood pressure. Ang II also inhibits renin release, thus providing a negative feedback to the system. This cycle, from renin through angiotensin to aldosterone and its associated negative feedback loop, is known as the renin-angiotensin-aldosterone system (RAAS). Aliskiren is a direct renin

inhibitor, decreasing plasma renin activity (PRA) and inhibiting the conversion of angiotensinogen to Ang I. Whether aliskiren affects other RAAS components, e.g., ACE or non-ACE pathways, is not known."

Avapro® and Benicar® are angiotensin II receptor antagonists (blockers). Avapro® and Benicar® work by blocking certain hormones to prevent blood vessels from narrowing and reduce sodium and fluid retention, although they are not considered to be diuretics. These two drugs generally have less severe side effects than many other drugs. Blood pressure medications are known to inhibit libido, but Avapro® and Benicar® do not appear to have this negative side effect. Take either drug with or without a meal. I prefer Benicar®.

"Benicar® (generic: olmesartan medoxomil) is an angiotensin II type 1 (AT$_1$) receptor antagonist. Olmesartan is used for management of hypertension (alone or in combination with other classes of antihypertensive agents); may be used in fixed combination with amlodipine or hydrochlorothiazide when such combined therapy is indicated. Angiotensin II receptor antagonists are one of several preferred initial therapies in hypertensive patients with chronic kidney disease, diabetes mellitus, or heart failure. Angiotensin II receptor antagonists can be used as monotherapy for initial management of uncomplicated hypertension; however, thiazide diuretics are preferred by JNC 7 (The seventh report of the Joint National Committee on Prevention, Detection, Evaluation, and Treatment of High Blood Pressure.)"

Metoprolol is a beta blocker for treating hypertension and tachycardia, a faster-than-normal resting heart rate. It is very effective, fast acting, and has been shown in studies to lower the risk of death from a heart attack. Take 50 mg of Metoprolol XL instead of Tekturna® by cutting a 100 mg tablet in half. Increase to two 50 mg divided doses for persistent hypertension.

My Personal Blood Pressure Control Results

My symptoms suggest that my kidneys produce excessive renin, which causes a small amount of vasoconstriction and fluid retention. Since this is occurring more in the evening and during the night, I have been taking 150 mg of Tekturna® in the afternoon. I have also taken 150 mg of Avapro® with breakfast but recently switched to 20 mg of Benicar®. Both are receptor blockers for the angiotensin II hormone that causes vasoconstriction, and I have not experienced side effects from any of these drugs. My pulse rate remains low and steady even after drinking coffee. The results are excellent as shown in the table below. All hypertensive drugs were discontinued in February 2013 because they were no longer necessary.

I hike aggressively in the Rocky Mountains at 9,000 feet (3,000 m) elevation or ride my bike aggressively and never feel my heart beating. I performed a test on 3/18/2011 by taking my blood pressure before and after my 15-minute bike ride. You can see that my blood pressure after the ride had quickly dropped to 149/76 in the short time it took me to put my bike in the garage and come in the house.

My Personal Blood Pressure Data				
Date	Time	Systolic Diastolic	Pulse	Activity
9/18/2010	9:10 AM	125 / 74	63	Resting
10/20/2010	8:12 PM	126 / 68	67	Resting
1/10/2011	2:30 PM	134 / 74	58	Resting
3/18/2011	2:00 PM	119 / 74	67	Resting
3/18/2011	2:18 PM	149 / 76	84	After Bike Ride
3/18/2011	2:20 PM	136 / 72	84	Quick Retest

My Switch to Eplerenone

My blood pressure was very satisfactory as long as I avoided salty foods and took supplemental potassium. I am one of the fifteen percent of salt-sensitive people, so I began taking eplerenone.

Inspra® and Eptus® (generic: eplerenone) are very effective drugs that block the negative effects of too much aldosterone hormone in the body. Aldosterone is a steroid hormone of the mineralocorticoid family that is produced in the zona glomerulosa (outer section) of the adrenal cortex in the adrenal gland. Aldosterone receptors are located in the kidneys, heart, brain, and other areas of the body where important mechanisms are activated by the hormone.

Aldosterone has a major effect of increasing blood pressure by signaling the kidneys to increase the retention of sodium ions (NA^+) and reduce potassium ions (K^+) in the blood. Aldosterone also signals the intestines, bladder, and sweat and salivary glands to reabsorb sodium into the blood. The extra sodium circulating through the blood causes an increase in water retention inside and outside of cells and an increase in blood volume, while the potassium is excreted by the kidneys in the urine. An excessive level of aldosterone becomes pathogenic (disease causing) and leads to kidney and cardiovascular diseases.

People who are sensitive to the amount of salt in the diet as indicated by an increase in blood pressure have an excessive excretion of aldosterone by the adrenal gland. The symptoms make aldosterone testing unnecessary and include:

- Hypertension (high blood pressure)
- Swelling and tingling of the feet and ankles

- High serum level of sodium at or near the top of the normal range
- Low serum level of potassium at or near the bottom of the normal range

Physicians often miss the importance of the sodium and potassium readings in the patients' blood tests when they are within the normal ranges. The physicians may correctly recommend a lower sodium diet, but they may react very negatively to the thought of supplementing the diet with potassium since an excessive amount can cause a dangerous irregular heart rhythm.

Diuretic drugs have been used for decades to control fluid retention and hypertension, but the negative side effects are very undesirable. Eplerenone is a fairly new drug that the US Food and Drug Administration approved in 2002. It is classified as an aldosterone receptor antagonist, meaning that it blocks the aldosterone receptor sites and thereby prevents the high level of aldosterone from having negative effects on the body. It doesn't reduce aldosterone but shields the body from the negative effects. Eplerenone reduces the amount of sodium in the blood and controls high blood pressure directly rather than by treating symptoms. Even so, dietary salt should be limited and dietary potassium should be minimized.

The recommended dose of eplerenone is 50 mg per day with or without food, which results in a gradual increase of eplerenone in the blood over a period of several days. The effect is a steady control of blood pressure throughout the day and a proper balance of sodium and potassium. Care should be taken to check the level of potassium in the blood, especially if an irregular heart rhythm is observed.

Future Blood Pressure Testing and Control Methods

The body has a complicated blood pressure control system that communicates by excreting numerous hormones to activate and control organs in a number of different ways. This complicated system is under intense study, and much has been learned. We know that it is better to treat hypertension by controlling hormones than by trying to modify the symptoms. As described above, drugs to control renin and angiotensin II hormones are very effective and have few side effects.

Hopefully, more progress will be made in the future to control hypertension by treating the organs that are generating the hormonal signals. Future discoveries may make it possible to dial blood pressure to a desired number with hormonal drug therapy, but that day had not arrived.

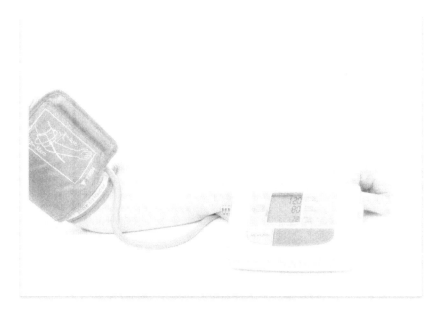

Automatic Digital Blood Pressure Monitor

Reversing Heart Disease and Preventing Diabetes

Chapter 6

Diet Therapy for Heart Valves, Palpitations, Arrhythmias, and Other Abnormal Heart Rhythms

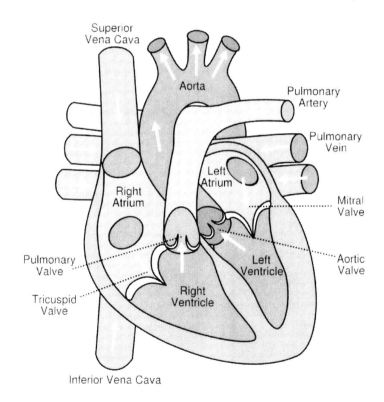

T his chapter will address diet therapy as a means of healing leaky heart valves and restoring normal heart rhythm. We are led to believe that these abnormalities can only be corrected with harsh prescription drugs, high-risk surgical procedures, or by following the diet recommendations of the *USDA Food Guide Pyramid*. Drugs can achieve some degree of improvement in preventing palpitations, arrhythmias, and other abnormal heart rhythms, and your physician's advice should be carefully considered as these conditions are often life-threatening.

A younger person may panic when he feels his heart skip a beat for the first time or when he feels an irregular rhythm. The heartbeat usually returns to normal before he has a chance to see a doctor, and he soon realizes that his health did not appear to suffer in any way. So he forgets about the episode until it happens again. Each time a person experiences an episode of irregular heart rhythm with no other ill effect, he becomes more accustomed to it and less concerned. This is dangerous because arrhythmias can result in blood pooling within the heart and the formation of a clot that can move to the lungs, brain, or extremities. A blood clot in the brain causes a stroke that often leads to brain damage and death.

Palpitations are rapid, irregular, or strong heartbeats that can be felt. They could be caused by a number of factors, including anemia (deficiency of red blood cells) or a thyroid hormone irregularity. Palpitations are common and usually present no immediate health risk.

Arrhythmias are a more serious condition in which the irregular heart rhythm is caused by abnormal electrical activity or nerve impulses in the heart. This abnormal activity is more serious because it can result in a cardiac arrest and sudden death called *sudden arrhythmic death syndrome.* See your cardiologist for any irregular heartbeat in order to resolve the underlying cause.

Heal Abnormal Heart Rhythms

Minerals are masters of the nerve impulses that control the heart muscles. The first approach to preventing palpitations, arrhythmias, and other abnormal heart rhythms is to correct electrolyte and mineral imbalances. The primary minerals, sodium, potassium, calcium, and magnesium, must be in balance. Most diets contain excess sodium and calcium but are deficient in potassium and magnesium. Trace minerals usually not found in a multivitamin tablet can be vital as well. We do not know as much about trace minerals as we should, so the best procedure is to supplement the diet as a precautionary measure.

The six steps in this chapter will correct common deficiencies in essential amino acids, essential fatty acids, vitamins, and minerals. I call this program the *Rieske Super Cardiovascular Tune-up (RSCT).* Other wonderful benefits occur because diet therapy provides optimal nutrition to the heart muscles, nerves, arteries, veins, and heart valves.

Giving your heart a tune-up may eliminate palpitations or arrhythmias.

Doctors often attempt to correct an irregular heart rhythm with electrical shock by installing a device called a *pacemaker.* The physician runs one or more electrodes through the veins to reach the heart, where the electrical leads pass through a valve and are attached to the muscle within the ventricle. This treatment is not without major risks, and the corrective effect may only be temporary. Aside from the fact that it may not work, damage can occur to the blood vessel walls including a possible rupture.

499

Plaque or other material can be dislodged from the blood vessel wall, travel to distant sites in the body, and form clots or blockages that can cause a stroke. The electrical shock also carries the risk of stopping the heart or causing the irregular heartbeat to become even worse. The wire or electrode can damage the heart valve over time or cause it to leak.

Healing Leaky Heart Valves

The dietary regimen for regenerating leaky heart valves is the same as for regenerating cervical discs, joint tissues, and other delicate membranes. We must overwhelm the body with essential nutrition far beyond the "minimum requirements." An abundance of essential amino acids, fatty acids, vitamins, and minerals is necessary for healthy heart valves. We know that it is possible to regenerate heart valves because people can have a heart murmur for years that will resolve without any medical intervention.

> Caution: Leaky heart valves can be life-threatening. Consult your physician before you proceed with any diet therapy suggested in this book.

The professional medical establishment makes little or no effort to repair heart valves by nutritional measures, and the idea is largely dismissed. The primary option is to replace the valve with a mechanical valve, cadaver valve (harvested from a dead body), or one from an animal—generally a pig. A few brave cardiologists have been able to regenerate heart valves by nutrition and supplements, but the majority offer diet therapy programs that prove to be ineffective. Research studies are rare because diet therapy as a cure for a leaky or regurgitating heart valve is simply not on the radar screen of the government health departments, medical schools, or medical heart associations.

Heart valve damage can be caused by bacterial infections such as rheumatic fever, essential amino acid deficiencies, or essential fatty acid deficiencies. Yes, not eating enough protein and fat from meat and fish can cause heart valve damage. Likewise, eating a diet that abounds in essential nutrients can help the heart valves to heal in the same manner that other tissues of the body heal and regenerate themselves.

We are constantly being brainwashed about the benefits of antioxidants and vitamin C while we are told to gorge ourselves on fruits and vegetables. Vitamin C is certainly an essential nutrient for humans, and antioxidants help to rid the body of undesirable, detrimental molecules and compounds. Vitamin C deficiency causes a disease called *scurvy*, and free radicals that damage cells can be eliminated by antioxidants. However, little is said about the illnesses caused by deficiencies of essential amino acids that are the building blocks of life. Professional nutritionists and health gurus brainwash the public to believe that they need very little protein but fail to list the diseases and health problems that occur as a result of protein deficiency. It has become the secret nutritional catastrophe that no one wants to talk about. Everyone wants to ignore it because meat is comprised of protein, and most fruits and vegetables have little or no protein.

Protein deficiency is estimated to cause 10 million deaths annually worldwide, but very few references give the actual diseases resulting from protein deficiency other than kwashiorkor malnutrition, learning disability, and mental retardation. Kwashiorkor produces edema (swelling from water retention as seen in third-world children), ulcers on the skin, and fatty liver disease. Protein deficiency in combination with an excess of fructose is a deadly combination for fatty liver hepatitis and death.

Protein deficiency has become a nutritional secret.

The health disorders caused by protein deficiency are treated like a leper who is shunned. Don't believe the modern nutritional claims that we don't need much protein. The following are just a few of the problems caused by protein deficiency.

- Endothelial cells that form a single layer (tunica intima) lining of the arteries are weakened by protein deficiency. The result is an increase in hemorrhagic strokes and plaque deposits.

- Weak collagen in the bones results in easy breakage, e.g., hip fractures in the elderly who are often protein deficient.

- Weak lining of the intestines resulting in leakage of partially-digested matter into the bloodstream sets off an immune response and causes autoimmune diseases as discussed in my previous book, *Absolute Truth Exposed – Volume 1*.

- Protein deficiency causes a weak immune system because all immune cells are made from amino acids derived from dietary protein.

- Bodily organs become weak, sickly and subject to disease.

- The entire body becomes weak, fragile, subject to infection, and at risk for hundreds of diseases. Children suffering from protein deficiency exhibit a condition called *failure to thrive*. They are small, weak, and sickly.

Heart valves are made from protein amino acids found in meat, fish, fowl, and seafood. Amino acids, essential fatty acids, vitamins, and minerals found in meat, fish, fowl, and seafood are all we need to build and regenerate heart valves.

Heart valves need essential amino acids and essential fatty acids for healing.

A leaky heart valve can create havoc in the cardiovascular system. The symptoms are irregular heart rhythm, abnormal blood pressure, blood clots, stroke, and cardiac arrest. In other words, it can easily kill you. The functions of heart valves have been described in detail in Chapter 1.

Essential Fatty Acids Help Heal Heart Valves

The three most nutritionally-important omega-3 fatty acids are alpha-linolenic fatty acid (ALA), eicosapentaenoic acid (EPA), and docosahexaenoic fatty acid (DHA). These are classified as *essential* because the body cannot make them from other fats, and deficiencies lead to many diseases. Flax seed oil contains alpha-linolenic fatty acid (ALA) but does not contain EPA or DHA fatty acids, which can become deficient. Some people lack the ability to convert ALA into EPA or DHA, and therefore flax seed oil is not a good source for the essential omega-3 fatty acids. Cod liver oil is the best choice because all three of these essential fatty acids are directly available to the body; they do not require conversion. Cod liver oil naturally contains vitamins A and D that are essential for healthy heart valves, bone formation, and cancer prevention, but it does not contain the unhealthy omega-6 vegetable fatty acids found in flax seed oil. Do not eat flax seed oil or ground flax seed.

Healthy Fatty Acid Foods		
Animal Fats	Arachidonic Acid	Saturated Fats
Fish Oils	EPA Omega-3	DHA Omega-3
Butter	Coconut Oil	Mono Fats
Palm Oils	Hard Cheeses	Eggs

Linoleic fatty acid (LA) and arachidonic fatty acid (ARA) are the two essential omega-6 linoleic fatty acids. In reality, only ARA is essential, but LA has also been listed because the body can make ARA from LA by a process known as *biosynthesis*. One or the other is needed—or both. They are essential fats that play a fundamental role in several physiological functions. Since a deficiency leads to many diseases, we must be sure our diet contains sufficient amounts of either linoleic acid or arachidonic acid. The body easily converts linoleic fatty acid—found mainly in grain, nut, and seed oils—into arachidonic fatty acid, but the process can create an unhealthy oversupply of ARA. Vegetarians get an unhealthy, pro-inflammatory, oversupply of ARA because linoleic acid is found in all vegetable oils Meat contains healthy, limited amounts of ARA.

The best resource for accurate scientific information concerning nutrition and fats is the book, *Know Your Fats: The Complete Primer for Understanding the Nutrition of Fats, Oils, and Cholesterol*, by Mary G. Enig, Ph.D.

Unhealthy Fatty Acid Foods		
Grain Oils	Seed Oils	Most Nut Oils
Vegetable Oils	Omega-6 Fats	Cottonseed Oil
Trans Fatty Acids	Soybean Oil	Corn Oil

In the following table, we can see the benefits of eating meat compared to the undesirable nutrition in grains, fruits, vegetables, and legumes.

Best Sources for Essential Nutrition		
Dietary Nutrient	**Meat, Fish, Fowl, and Seafood**	**Grains, Vegetables, Fruits, and Legumes**
Essential Amino Acids	Complete	Limited Requires Mixing Grains and Legumes to Achieve
Essential EPA and DHA Fatty Acids	Complete	Limited Requires Special Efforts to Achieve
Vitamins	Complete	No B12 Low Iron Low A, D, and K
Minerals	Complete	Grains Have High Phytic Acid That Causes Chromium, Vanadium, Lithium, and Zinc Deficiencies
Essential Arachidonic Fatty Acid	Correct Amount	Excessive Amount
Mycotoxins, Molds, Fungi, and Yeasts	None	Toxic Amounts

Chapter 6

The diet, vitamin, mineral, and supplement regimen presented in Chapters 4 and 5 must be followed to the letter in order to overwhelm the heart valves with optimal nutrition. Below is a testimony from a gentleman who used this diet therapy to treat his heart valve that was damaged as a result of rheumatic fever.

Aortic Valve Regurgitation Was Reduced

"Dear Sir,

More than 2 years ago, I emailed you and described my problem with aortic valve regurgition.

In the first Echocardiogram report dated 2/3/05, it is stated that:

> *"The color flow doppler study reveals moderate to severe aortic regurgition and least moderate mitral regurgition, with very early dilatation of the left ventricle and left atrium."*

In the Conclusion of Cardiac Catheterization, which was performed on 4/15/05, it is said that:

> *1- Moderate to severe (3+) aortic regurgition.*
> *2- Mild (1+) mitral regurgition.*
> *3- Normal coronary arteries.*
> *4- Rheumatic heart disease.*

After that I started to use cod liver oil and borage oil as described in your website. One year later, I had another Echo done on 04/05/06. The summary of the Echo is:

"A 2D echo with M-Mode and color Doppler was performed. The left ventricle systolic is normal. There is no evidence of left ventricle hypertophy. There is turbulent flow in the LOVT. The aortic valve is not visualized, cannot r/o a bicuspid valve. The aortic valve is not well visualized. There is turbulent flow in the LOVT, cannot rule out a bicuspid valve. There is mild aortic insufficiency."

I had another Echo done on 10/17/06 because I wanted to verify the last report of Echo. It is said in the report that:

"The impression was Mild Aortic Regurgitation.
Normal left ventricular function."

I had another Echo done about 3 months ago. I do not have the report, but I remember clearly the result is the same:

"Mild Aortic Regurgitation"

The Cardiogram I did last month is normal. I went to a new cardiologist with all my paper with old and new result (the first cardiologist believes only his Catheterization on 4/15/05). The new doctor noticed the difference between the old Echo and the new *ones, and he suggested me to make new Echo and Nuclear Stress test on 10/04/07. By the way, I have taken Benicar 20mg for more than 2 years.*

Your help has been greatly appreciated."

The above gentleman has had significant improvements in the functioning of his heart valves by taking the recommend fatty acid supplements. This awesome achievement was obtained even though he may have been lax in adhering to all of my recommendations in the following six steps. The tone of his letter clearly shows a relaxed attitude without any hint that he needs heart valve surgery.

Fruits will never heal leaky heart valves.

Fruits do nothing scientifically to heal heart valves because they are practically devoid of amino acids and fatty acids. In fact, fruits are harmful because the high concentrations of fructose and glucose stimulate the pancreas to produce insulin that in turn can promote adrenaline and cortisol production and create a catabolic state. This is a cascading effect as the catabolic state promotes destruction of the tissues, not healing and repair. Fruits, whole grains, vegetables, and legumes will never heal leaky heart valves because they do not have the abundance of amino acids and essential fatty acids as found in animal food sources. The following steps will overwhelm your body with powerful healing nutrition that enables the body to regenerate and heal delicate protein structures of the heart valves.

The following is a general outline of the nutritional steps that may regenerate and heal leaky heart valves and restore normal heart rhythm.

Step No. 1

Omega-3 and Omega-6 Fatty Acid Supplementation

Supplementation with the correct ratio of essential fatty acids has been shown to heal the delicate tissues of heart valves. The same has been shown to heal hard, cracked, and bleeding skin on the hands. These essential fatty acids will heal many other tissues and are very effective in healing the delicate lining of the intestinal tract.

- **Omega-3 Fatty Acids** - Take one tablespoon of Carlson's Lemon Flavored Cod Liver Oil twice a day with a meal. This brand is of the highest quality and has a very mild taste. **The importance of taking cod liver oil (EPA and DHA fatty acids) and borage oil (GLA fatty acid described below) cannot be over stated. This combination is absolutely required.**

- **Borage Oil** - Supplement the diet with omega-6 gamma-linolenic acid (GLA) by taking one borage oil capsule per day. The body cannot produce essential fatty acids; you must get them from the food you eat. Your body uses GLA and omega-3 fatty acids to make E1 series prostaglandins that help to reduce inflammation, aid digestion, and regulate your metabolism. Avoid all other omega-6 vegetable oils as found in nuts, seeds, and grains.

Fish oil is not considered to be as effective as cod liver oil. Krill oil does not have enough omega-3 fatty acids. Cod liver oil has a higher concentration of EPA and DHA essential fatty acids. Flaxseed oil is not acceptable because it contains a high concentration of other undesirable omega-6 fatty acids and a low-level of GLA fatty acid. Primrose oil is not considered to be as effective as borage oil. Borage oil has a higher concentration of GLA fatty acid.

Step No. 2

High-Fat, High-Protein, and Low-Carbohydrate Diet

It is very important to eat a low-carbohydrate diet because it will automatically make big changes in the hormones (e.g., reduce blood insulin levels) and provide an abundant supply of amino acids. This diet is presented in Chapter 4.

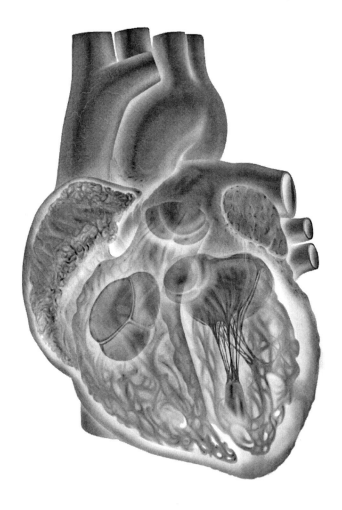

Cross Section of Ventricles and Valves

Step No. 3

Vitamins, Minerals, and Supplements

The goal is to overwhelm the body with vitamins, minerals, and supplements in order to create optimal health because a deficiency in just one element will prevent healing. Research has shown that 85% of patients with mitral valve prolapse have latent tetany due to chronic magnesium deficiency. Tetany is a condition marked by muscles spasms and is associated with deficient parathyroid secretions caused by low levels of calcium and magnesium and an excess of phosphates.

Supplemental potassium can correct an irregular heart rhythm. Take one 99 mg potassium chelate capsule. Recheck your pulse after 10 minutes, and if it improves, continue to take one capsule daily. Do not supplement with potassium if you are taking a potassium-sparing diuretic.

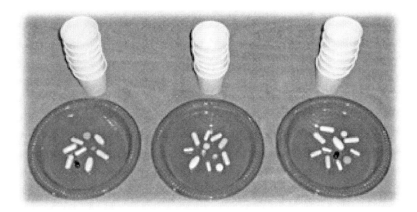

- **Vitamins and supplements are distributed weekly into 21 small paper cups for breakfast, lunch, and dinner.**
- **The supplements are displayed on the saucer to indicate the quantity taken with each meal.**

Chapter 6

Step No. 4

Human Growth Hormone Boost Using Amino Acid Therapy

Bodybuilders eat a high-protein diet and supplement with additional protein powder in order to build body mass, muscles, ligaments, tendons, and bones. Millions of bodybuilders have proved this over several decades of testing and refinement. The science behind the high-protein diet confirms the results found in actual practice.

Bodybuilders eat a high-protein diet.

Meat provides the full complement of all essential and nonessential amino acids needed to heal the cardiovascular system without adding undesirable carbohydrates. Vegetarian foods, such as whole grains, soy, and legumes, do not fulfill these requirements and are unacceptable substitutes.

Bodybuilders typically eat a lot of meat as a high-quality protein source. They also supplement with protein powder mixed into drinks and shakes. Whey protein powder contains all the essential and nonessential amino acids necessary to build a healthy body. The following product is made from cow's milk whey protein, and all of the lactose (milk sugar) has been stripped during manufacture. It is predigested using special healthy bacteria to break down the protein molecules into the individual amino acids and branched-chain amino acids. The amino acids can pass through the intestinal-blood barrier to quickly become available for healing the body and building bone collagen, tissues, ligaments, tendons, and muscles. Extra glutamine is also recommended.

Protein and Glutamine Drink - Prepare a drink made with whey amino acid protein powder that is enriched with extra glutamine amino acid. BioChem® Low Carb® whey protein powder is an excellent choice. It consists of a full complement of amino acid isolates that heal the body and require no digestion. Prepare the drink by blending 8–16 oz of reverse osmosis with UV lamp water or unsweetened, low-sodium tomato juice with 1 heaping teaspoon (12 gm) of whey protein powder plus 1 rounded teaspoon (8 gm) of glutamine amino acid powder. Stir vigorously with the teaspoon. The whey protein must be specified as "isolates from cross flow microfiltration and ion-exchange, ultrafiltered concentrate, low molecular weight, and partially hydrolyzed whey protein peptides rich in branched-chain amino acids and glutamine peptides." The low-carbohydrate type at 1 gm per scoop or less is best, but it should not be more than 4–5 gm of carbohydrates per scoop. Do not substitute protein from soy, egg, casein, or any other source. Sugar or any other sweetener is unacceptable. Use the natural flavor without additives. This amino acid drink can be enjoyed anytime with or without a meal. **Keep in the refrigerator after opening. Old product should be discarded because it can support bacteria and become contaminated. Whey protein powder can cause some gas and an unusually full feeling.**

This combination of amino acids has been shown to provide the following healing properties:

- Provides pain killing effects by healing the nervous system

- Absorbed without requiring digestion

- Stimulates insulin-like growth factor 1 (IGF-1) that functions similarly to insulin and enhances protein synthesis and healing

- Fight infections by stimulating the immune system

- Provides growth of protein collagen and strengthens bones

- Provides all of the amino acids required to heal and grow ligaments, tendons, joints, muscles, intestinal tract, heart muscle, heart valves, arteries, veins, and organs

- Prevents hypoglycemia (low blood sugar) symptoms

Human Growth Hormone (HGH) Frauds and Scams

Some products are sold with claims that they boost human growth hormone, but most of these claims are bogus. Human growth hormone is a large molecule and cannot be taken orally because it can't pass through the intestinal-blood barrier. The body simply digests the hormone by breaking it down into the individual amino acids from which it is made. Supplemental products containing HGH (human growth hormone) are a fraud. They don't work. Synthetic hormone injections were thought to be a great anti-aging discovery and did perform well, but it was soon discovered that the hormone caused many types of cancers. Do not take HGH supplements or HGH injections.

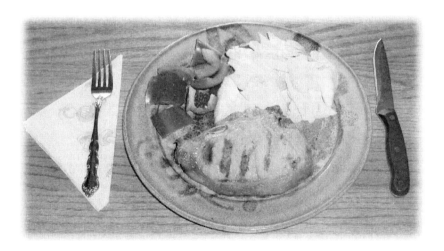

Grilled Pork Chop with Red Pepper and Cabbage
Typical High-Protein, Low-Carbohydrate Meal

Step No. 5

Do-It-Yourself Stem Cell Therapy

Yes, you can do your own stem cell therapy. It may not be effective, but I believe the possible benefits far outweigh the cost and risks that are considered to be very low or none at all. I have taken the following stem cell product along with this six-step program for a neck problem that has been complete healed.

Doctors and the U.S. Food and Drug Administration (USDA) are very much against these types of do-it-yourself treatments just like they are against all do-it-yourself alternative medicine. The USDA resisted approving the recommended product for use as a therapeutic drug. However, it worked to our advantage because we can now buy it without a prescription, and the research company that developed this stem cell product simply started selling it as a nutritional supplement. You can order it on the Internet without a prescription. It's safe and very easy to take orally. It's packed in dry ice to keep it frozen and shipped via one-day express in a special insulated box.

Most stem cell claims are false promises that will never be fulfilled. Stem cells will not cause a new heart to grow. Stem cells will not overpower the unhealthy effects of catabolic hormones, protein deficiencies, fat deficiencies, and the high-carbohydrate diet; but the stem cells recommended here may help heal damaged tissues and promote growth.

There are many myths, lies, and scams surrounding the topic of stem cells, and some universities and organizations have faked research results in their scramble for a share of the hundreds of millions of dollars from the governments of the United States and other countries worldwide. However, research has developed some stem cells that do encourage your existing cells to heal, regenerate, multiply, and propagate. Bovine embryonic mesenchymal cells (or mesenchyme) can be taken to help heal damaged heart valves. The following product is recommended even though the effectiveness is unknown. The theory is to provide overwhelming nutrition. Studies are not available to prove or disprove the effectiveness of bovine embryonic mesenchymal cells. Leaky heart valves are life-threatening, and every attempt should be made to regenerate them.

Mesenchyme: Little Known Rejuvenating Healer
by James Wilson, ND PhD DC and Carolyn McLuskie

Rejuvenate: Make young or as if young again.
(Concise Oxford Dictionary)

"A unique and unusual substance called mesenchyme has arrived on the American market with little notice or fanfare. However, you will be hearing a lot about it in the years to come. Mesenchyme will revolutionize the way we handle health problems because of its astonishing and well-documented ability to repair and rejuvenate damaged cells and tissues.

Mesenchyme is undifferentiated embryonic connective tissue, the true mother lode of cell growth and cell regeneration. Mesenchymal cells develop during the early embryonic stages of mammalian gestation and are the source material from which most of the mammalian body's organs and tissues are made - everything from bones, muscles, and connective tissue to the central nervous system. What is extraordinary about mesenchyme in that when it is ingested it migrates to the area of greatest injury in the body. Once there, it aligns itself with the damaged cells and/or tissues, becomes identical to them, and then starts replicating.

Regenerates Damaged Cells

The result is regeneration or replacement of the damaged cells. The implications for speedy and full recovery from everything from broken bones to herniated discs are enormous. We now have the potential to create healing where there was previously no hope of recovery. Later in this article, you will read how one of the authors restored severely herniated discs that should have required surgical. fusion, as well as greatly accelerated recovery from a ruptured Achilles tendon.

Interestingly, the mechanism for organ formation from mesenchymal cells is still present in some adult animal species. For example, it is the presence of mesenchymal cells that allows a salamander to regenerate its tail if cut off. In the human adult, the only mechanism where these cells normally function is in the healing of wounds.

The mesenchyme available on the US market is made from bovine embryonic mesenchymal cells. The cells are harvested from pregnant cattle destined for slaughter and subsequent human consumption. Only healthy fetuses from healthy cattle are used. Because mesenchyme is, by definition, undifferentiated fetal cellular material, it has not yet developed immune markers. It is therefore accepted by the human host without provoking an attack by the immune system and can freely work its magic on any number of physical injuries and traumas.

Mesenchyme has the ability to migrate to any tissue in need of repair and, once at the site, to take on the characteristics of the healthy cell it associates with. When mesenchyme is next to cartilage, it becomes cartilage and replaces or repairs damaged cartilage. This is true for organ tissues too; for example, when it is next to kidney, mesenchyme becomes kidney. If one has damaged cells from a broken bone, mesenchyme associates itself with the wounded tissue, assumes the specific characteristics of that type of bone, and begins to repair the damaged tissue and create new bone cells. It sounds incredible, but much research has verified this unique action. Thus, mesenchyme has great potential in regenerating diseased or injured tissues of all kinds.

The use of mesenchyme as a therapeutic substance arises from experiments conducted early in the 20th century by Dr. Alexis Carrel, 1912 Nobel Laureate in Biology, who demonstrated that organic tissues could be regenerated in vitro by the addition of fresh younger cells to the culture medium. In the 1930s, the Swiss endocrinologist Dr. Paul Niehans developed a technique for extracting cells from animals and injecting them into his patients to compensate for their bodies' deficiencies. One of the types of cells he found most beneficial was mesenchyme.

Mesenchyme, used in conjunction with other whole cells and cellular extracts, was popular in Europe during the1960s and 1970s. Many well-known celebrities and politicians visited reputable clinics and spas, including Dr. Niehans' Clinique La Prairie in Clarens, Switzerland, to receive live cell therapy. Notables such as Charles de Gaulle, Charlie Chaplin, and Sir Winston Churchill were just a few of the wealthy, powerful, and famous figures of the last century who went to these spas for live cell therapy, which included mesenchyme as a basic part of the rejuvenation process.

What makes mesenchyme so unique, special, and efficient is the fact that it is composed of multipotential cells, also known as mesenchymal stem cells, which have the ability to become almost any kind of tissue or organ. Embryologically, all connective and supportive tissues arise from mesenchymal cells. The versatility of these pleuripotetial cells allows them to form cartilage, bone, muscle, connective tissue, and organ tissue.

In all mammals mesenchyme eventually differentiates into three embryonic tissues - the endoderm, the mesoderm, and the ectoderm. During embryonic development, these three primitive cell types differentiate into all the body's organs and tissues. The endoderm forms the linings of the digestive and respiratory tracts. The mesoderm develops into muscle, connective tissues, bone, and blood vessels. The ectoderm differentiates into the epidermis and the nervous system. A portion of the mesenchyme remains in the placenta and the yolk sac surrounding the embryo in the fetus. It is this mesenchyme that is carefully separated to become the commercially available product."

Though the product can be obtained from many sources, I have found the following to provide a good product at a reasonable price at the time of this writing:

XtraCell CF Support by Douglas Laboratories
http://www.rockwellnutrition.com/XtraCell-CF-Support-by-Douglas-Laboratories_p_1289.html

XtraCell CF Support 24 vials by Atrium BioTechnologies

"Xtra-Cell™ CF Support provided by Douglas Laboratories® is an innovative frozen liquid extract consisting of selected proteins, peptides and other growth factors and signaling molecules obtained from porcine adrenal and mesenchyme tissues.

Features and Benefits:

- Nutritional support for a healthy adrenal function
- Helps regulation of the hypothalamic-pituitary-adrenal axis
- Increases cellular metabolic activity by 166% in vitro
- Organ-specific glandular substances
- Preservative free, 100% natural

Each vial contains:

- Porcine 5.5 ml
- Mesenchyme aqueous extract 125x
- Porcine adrenal aqueous extract 3.5 ml (enriched with Mesenchyme 125x)

Suggested use:

As a dietary supplement, take 1 bottle of Xtra-Cell CF Support per day or as directed by your healthcare professional.

Functions:

Xtra-Cell CF Support is manufactured and purified via a patented† low temperature process that involves homogenization, fractionation, and ultrafiltration of porcine adrenal and fetal mesenchyme tissue. The molecules present in this product are selected based on their size and molecular weight, and are isolated in their native state. The molecules present in this product are selected based on their size and molecular weight (less than 50,000 Daltons), and are isolated in their native state. Once the molecules are selected, the liquid is aseptically bottled and flash-frozen without preservatives to ensure optimal potency, freshness and bioavailability. This process can be applied to different starting materials, allowing for the creation of liquid extracts that are targeted for specific applications. The extracts created from these two tissues are highly bioavailable and of the highest quality available.

Adrenal:

Suboptimal adrenal function has been implicated in symptoms of fatigue, exhaustion and a reduction in the body's defenses against the stresses imposed by that fatigue. Enhancing adrenal function and maintaining cellular activity and energy are important factors in combating fatigue.* Supplementing with adrenal extract may help to stimulate the adrenal gland and promote homeostasis.*

Mesenchyme:

Mesenchyme is embryonic connective tissue composed of pluripotent cells, or cells that are undifferentiated and have the ability to evolve into almost any type of cell. The mesenchyme tissue used in Xtra-Cell CF Support is obtained from embryonic fetal porcine tissue from which cellular growth factors and other signaling molecules are extracted. In vitro data have shown that the components present in the mesenchyme extract can support cellular metabolism as demonstrated by an increase in fibroblast mitochondrial activity in the presence of unaffected cellular proliferation (figures 1 and 2). The combination of adrenal and mesenchyme extracts in Xtra-Cell CF Support synergistically provides nutritional support for fatigue, and helps to promote healthy adrenal function and improved cellular activity.*"

One vial should be taken 30 minutes before bedtime or as recommended by the manufacturer. No food or excess liquids should be consumed two hours before taking the product, and nothing should be consumed for eight hours afterward. Take one vial per day for 20 days. Take the remaining four vials on a weekly schedule, one per week. Repeat the procedure if your degenerative heart valve damage is severe or your response is slow. Elderly people respond more slowly because they lack natural human growth hormone.

The high-protein, high-fat, low-carbohydrate diet described in **Steps 1, 2, and 3** above must be started at least four weeks in advance of ordering the XtraCell™ liquid mesenchyme stem cell therapy. This therapy is believed to be very beneficial, but it will not overpower the highly destructive catabolic adrenalin and cortisol hormones created by eating carbohydrates.

Chapter 6

Step No. 6

Expectations, Starting Journal, and Follow-up Program

The expectations and measurements of progress are very important in the process of healing delicate heart valves. The following will help you to plan and measure your progress. Success always builds confidence and leads to further success.

Expectations

This program will show weekly progress that you can measure by comparing your heart rhythm, blood pressure, energy, pain levels, activity restrictions, sleep patterns, and overall comfort with that of the previous week.

Journal

Write a *Starting Journal* before you begin anything else. The journal should describe your present condition in great detail. Update your journal weekly during the first four weeks in order to compare your condition with your previous and starting entries. In this way, you can accurately measure your progress. Your journal should include the following topics.

- Enter facts such as the date, existing diseases, previous diet philosophy, current prescription drugs, etc.

- Enter detailed descriptions of your heart rhythm, blood pressure, energy level, pain level, activity restrictions, sleep patterns, and overall comfort levels experienced during typical daily activities such as walking, climbing stairs, job, recreation, and sleeping.

- Enter a number from 0–10 to describe the level of discomfort. Ten represents severe physical limitations, and zero represents feeling wonderfully normal without any restrictions in ordinary daily activities whatsoever.

- Enter symptoms that can include chest pains, angina (heart pain), heart palpitations, cardiac (heart) arrhythmias, rapid heart rate, lightheadedness, fainting spells, fatigue, shortness of breath, heavy breathing, breathlessness while lying down (orthopnea), severe shortness of breath during the middle of the night (paroxysmal nocturnal dyspnea), sweating without activity, symptoms of heart failure, leg swelling, and leg pain.

Follow-up Program

Write a new journal entry every month with all of the detailed information listed for the Starting Journal. The *Monthly Journal* will help to prevent slipping back into your old lifestyle. Compare these entries with the previous month and with the Starting Journal entries in order to measure your progress. You must not revert back to your old way of life simply because you begin to feel better. Doing so will cause your pain, discomfort, and physical limitations to return. Staying healthy and active requires a lifelong commitment and control of your treatment program. The following are a few follow-up guidelines and restrictions.

- The high-fat, high-protein, low-carbohydrate diet required on this program is an absolute lifelong necessity. Health will suffer in direct proportion to the percentage of carbohydrates reintroduced into the diet.

- Insulin, adrenalin, and cortisol hormones must be strictly controlled by the diet program presented here.

- Prescription drugs should be discontinued only upon your doctor's approval, but taking unnecessary drugs presents other health risks because of side effects.

- Review your initial Starting Journal entries and the other Monthly Journals to measure and understand the changes in your condition. This review builds confidence and keeps you on a healthy program.

Summary

Heart problems are very disturbing and life-threatening. The diet therapy program in this chapter has been shown to heal the cardiovascular system without presenting any harmful side effects that are common with pharmaceuticals, surgery, electrical shocks, pacemaker electronic heart devices, and other radical approaches. The best approach is to follow the diet therapy before the problem becomes severe or life-threatening.

The diet therapy can be followed in addition to other standard medical approaches. Talk to your doctor before beginning this or any other diet therapy program. Unfortunately, your doctor will most likely be opposed to or harshly critical of the diet therapy I present in this book. Let me give you a vote of confidence. My cardiologist supports my diet therapy 100%. He insisted that I stay on this diet, supplement, and pharmaceutical regime. If your doctor does not agree, perhaps you should discuss this approach with other doctors before dismissing my diet therapy. This is a scientific approach based on scientific investigation, personal experience, and comments by others who have tried it.

Reversing Heart Disease and Preventing Diabetes

Chapter 7

Learn When Exercise Can Kill You

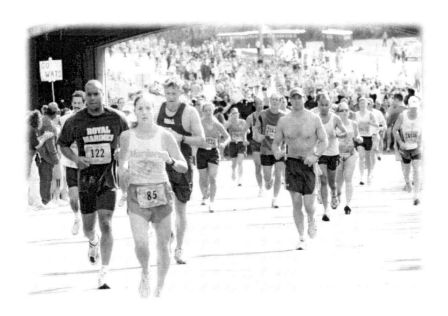

USMC Marathon in Washington, D.C., 2004
Marathon and Triathlon Races Are Often Deadly

Exercise is not the awesome health panacea as nearly everyone claims. Almost without exception, health and diet books rave on and on about the importance of exercise and claim that intense physical exertion is healthier than moderate activity. I cannot cite any book that is critical of exercise because there are none. Science and actual experience tell a far different story, proving that exercise can lead to numerous diseases—several that will bring early death. I'm not suggesting that you sit and do nothing all day like a couch potato. I am saying there are good exercises that produce excellent health benefits, and there are other exercises that can severely damage your body—even cause your death. The facts are presented here.

Skinny people who exercise and eat a low-fat diet are lulled into a false sense of security. They falsely think they have achieved optimum health because they are thin. I know two skinny people who exercised daily, ran 10k races, and ate a low-fat diet; they recently required open heart surgery to save their lives. Three out of four people I knew who recently died from cancer were skinny, exercised daily, and ate a low-fat diet. Cancer is now the leading cause of death, and the public is being bombarded with advice to exercise more, reduce dietary fats, and shun red meat. They are told to eat organic whole grains, fruits, and vegetables and to abstain from saturated animal fats and dairy products. This advice is totally wrong because it promotes carbohydrates that all digest into sugars in the body—the true cause heart disease, cancer, and diabetes.

In past centuries and prior to 1956, hard physical work and exercise were considered to be unhealthy. Obese children were rarely seen, perhaps only one or two in the typical high school. Obesity among adults was not a serious problem either. Diabetes was not the epidemic we see today. On July 16, 1956, President Dwight D. Eisenhower initiated a nationwide fitness campaign for the children of the United States because he had heard that European children were more fit. The program was known as the President's Council on Youth Fitness. In 1963, President John F. Kennedy changed the name of the program to the President's Council on Physical Fitness.

Government involvement in physical fitness has resulted in a steady decline in health.

President John F. Kennedy's health was a disaster because his low-fat, high-carbohydrate diet gave him autoimmune inflammatory bowel disease. His doctors placed him on immunosuppressant drugs, but the drugs wiped out his spine (a common side effect). At the time of his death, he was wearing a back brace that kept him upright in the seat of the car.

Health authorities in all English-speaking countries also began recommending a major switch from meat and animal fats to low-fat, low-cholesterol diets that were high in whole-grains, fruits, and complex carbohydrates. Saturated fat was labeled as the scourge of mankind. President John F. Kennedy strongly promoted the "get healthy" program that emphasized exercise and jogging. Kids were forced to run around the block during physical education classes instead of playing on the school playground. We were told that if we stopped smoking, exercised, and ate a low-fat diet we would achieve awesome health benefits.

Health clubs, yoga classes, jogging, biking, and running events are now on every street. One must be constantly on the lookout for runners and bikers who compete with automobile traffic for road space. Street signs with the image of a jogger or biker can be seen displaying the words, "Share the Road." Lines are painted on the streets to show the lanes for bikers and joggers. Low-fat diet programs abound with seminars and support groups. Smoking is now against the law in public places in most cities. Well, how did all of these new health programs work for the people in English-speaking countries?

The new obesity epidemic is literally off the charts. People stopped smoking and began running, but heart disease and lung cancer have actually increased. Lung cancer is now very common among athletes who have never smoked. Middle-age or younger marathon runners are dropping dead during the run. Diabetes is now epidemic with 65% dying from heart disease and 25% from cancer. The escalation of Alzheimer's is off the chart, and just the thought of the disease creates panic among the elderly when they forget a telephone number. Alzheimer's treatment centers are commonplace. Fitness clubs, books, seminars, and education programs have resulted in a decline in health.

Fitness clubs, books, seminars, and education programs have resulted in a decline in health.

Babies, infants, and children are not immune to the upturn in obesity and diseases. Children are now developing adult onset diabetes at an alarming rate. Autism has skyrocketed to about 1% of the infant population. Pregnant women are told to eat lots of fruits, vegetables, low-fat yogurt, and whole grains and to shun red meat, saturated fat, and cholesterol. But the scientific facts show that baby brains are made from protein, saturated fat, and cholesterol. Baby brains are not made from lettuce and fructose. The mothers of autistic children become irate and explode in anger at me when I say that their diet of fruit and vegetable salads, low-fat yogurt, and organic, zero-cholesterol whole grain cereals prevented their babies' brains from developing properly. Get a clue, Mommies! Baby brains are not made from lettuce.

Baby brains are not made from lettuce.

The United States' government health propaganda that is now the President's Council on Physical Fitness and Sports has been a disaster for the health of people in the United States and elsewhere in the world because it promotes exercise and nutrition myths that are not based on scientific facts. The following are a few of these myths:

Myth No. 1 - Exercise Will Make You Lose Weight and Cure Obesity.

This myth is so widespread and often repeated that most people believe it without question. The new *2010 USDA My Plate* health guidelines stress that exercise is the cure for the ever-expanding obesity problem in all English-speaking countries. The obese are told they can achieve normal weight and become healthy simply by moving the body. "Move the body - move the body," they are told. The obese are instructed to "get out there and work that fat off." The government health authorities claim people are obese because they are lazy gluttons, but the obese know it's a lie. Most have tried exercise to no avail. Exercise will not make an obese person thin. This is a slick trick to shift the blame for the failures of the past Food Guide Pyramids from the USDA to the obese who now suffer because they have followed the previous advice they received from these same government health authorities.

The fact is that the obese get a lot of exercise simply by hauling around extra pounds of fat. They huff and puff simply to haul the extra 100 pounds up a flight of stairs. Thin people who are screaming at fat people to exercise more would see how it feels if they strapped on 100 pounds of lard and carried it around 24 hours a day. Exercise will not make obese people thin.

Exercise will not make an obese person thin.

Exercise burns very few calories. A person who does grueling exercise for 60 minutes can then eat a snack in one minute that contains all the calories he just burned. To make matters worse, people are told they need to eat more carbohydrates for energy. This is another big lie. Carbohydrates are not needed for energy. The scientific minimum daily requirement for carbohydrates is zero.

United States government health and fitness programs have created an obesity epidemic.

The obese will never become thin and healthy by eating the high-carbohydrate diet as recommended by the *2010 USDA My Plate* no matter how much they exercise. We are told that carbohydrates are the primary source of energy and must be 50-60% of our daily caloric intake. The myth that carbohydrates are essential is stated over and over in health and diet articles, books, websites, and government guidelines, yet every person who goes on the low-carbohydrate diet quickly proves the fallacy of this myth. The lower the amount of carbohydrates in the diet the healthier one becomes. Carbohydrates cause many diseases that take years to develop and have come to be known as *age related diseases*—a convenient excuse.

Overweight people should never run or jog. The extra weight quickly crushes the knees and smashes the ankles. This is why we rarely see overweight people running. They simply can't endure the physical trauma. It is illogical to encourage overweight people to run and then criticize them when they are forced to stop. Trim runners who complain about an obese person not running should put a 50-lb. (23 kg) bag of wheat over each shoulder and try it. Thin people can run only because they don't have the extra weight to carry. Running did not make them thin. They were thin before they started running. More than likely, they are thin because their high-carbohydrate diet has given them a gastrointestinal disease as discussed in my previous book, *Absolute Truth Exposed - Volume 1*.

Mommy's diet of fruits, whole grains, and starchy vegetables during pregnancy can destine the child to a lifetime of obesity.

Many obese people are doomed in their struggle with obesity from the day they are born because of the diets their mothers ate. A woman who has developed insulin resistance as a result of her high-carbohydrate diet will blast the fetus with an onslaught of glucose and insulin. This attack will fry the metabolism of the fetus and transfer the insulin resistance to him. The child may appear to have inherited the obesity from Mommy, but actually it was a diet-caused condition for both of them. The only healthy option for the baby and child is to eat a low-carbohydrate diet that will not raise his insulin level.

Chapter 7

On December 5, 2009, Michel wrote from Sweden about his awesome improvements in health and athletic performance after eating the low-carbohydrate diet for only a few weeks.

Recent Testimony from an Athlete

"Hi,

I have to agree with everything you say! I switched to a low-carb high-fat diet a couple of months ago and I am free from the problems I had. Discovered that I was gluten intolerant and could quit my Omeprazol medication and found out that a lot of other minor issues went away by just cutting out carbs. I'm an ambitious athlete aiming to try to reach elite, but because I got very sick with flus, colds, and respiratory infections for nearly two months and all of my hard training was lost. When I switched to your diet my health got better already after two weeks. I have also discovered that I have almost doubled my endurance just by not eating carbs at all - which is the opposite of what athletes have been told the world over. Now I can run and ride the bike forever without hitting the wall, all I need is water. I haven't felt any lactic acid either, it's gone. My recovery time is faster than before. I run much better when burning fats for energy than I did on carbohydrates.

Michel"

Myth No. 2 - Exercise Will Prevent Heart Disease.

Running for hours day after day does not prevent heart disease. Excessive exercise will likely increase the risk for heart attack. Runners tend to eat a high-carbohydrate diet because they think they need extra glucose for energy. This is not the healthiest approach. Glucose causes insulin resistance and raises the blood insulin level, which alone is a heart disease risk. The heart muscles can easily burn fatty acids for energy instead of glucose. The following two marathon runners are prime examples of those who exercised excessively but still developed heart disease at a relatively young age.

The often-heard statement that exercise will prevent heart disease is totally false. Nothing could be farther from the truth. Professional and non-professional athletes die from heart disease at an alarming rate every year. James F. Fixx was a marathon runner, vegetarian, and author who stated in his 1977 book, *The Complete Book on Running*, that his university alumni who were couch potatoes lived longer than the athletes. He finished his book just in time because he died in his running shoes in 1984 from cardiac arrest while *exercising.*

The vegetarian diet and running
are a deadly combination.

Professional athletes die young. The major factor contributing to Mr. Fixx's heart disease was his vegetarian diet, severely deficient in protein and very high in carbohydrates, which produce the three heart disease-causing hormones—insulin, cortisol, and adrenaline.

Chapter 7

Dead Marathon and Triathlon Competitors

There was recently a great fanfare in the marathon runners' world because one ex-runner has survived to the century mark. Running marathons doesn't sound like a good way to live to be a hundred because an estimated 70,490 people in the United States have achieved this longevity without running a marathon. The astonishing news is the number of young marathon runners who collapse and die during competition.

> "United States currently has the greatest number of centenarians in the world, estimated at 70,490 on September 1, 2010."

Below is a partial list marathon or triathlon competitors who recently died. This is just a sampling of the cases because there are so many. Is this healthy exercise or mass deception?

These examples do not include the hundreds of professional athletes in other sports, such as basketball, football, hockey, and soccer, who simply collapsed and died from heart attacks. You've heard the story about marathon runner, James Fixx, but you may not know about Edmund Burke, Ph.D., a serious endurance cycling competitor. Dr. Burke died on a training ride on November 7, 2002, at age 53. You almost certainly haven't heard of Frederick J. Montz, M.D. (1955-2002), David A. Nagey, M.D. (1950-2002), or Jeffrey A. Williams, M.D. (1951-2002), three brilliant physicians at Johns Hopkins University who died while running. The oldest of the three was 51. These doctors certainly prove they did not understand what constitutes a healthy diet.

The mass media's cover-up and whitewashing of competitors' deaths during marathons and triathlons is rampant. Some media outlets that you would expect to cover the story don't say a word. Others may report the death or deaths in a vague manner the day after the race but scrub it from the records soon afterward. The Internet is thought to be the source for historical records, and many obscure facts from past decades can easily be found. I found a document relating to my grandfather's irrigation schedules for his farm nearly 100 years ago, but stories about dead marathon and triathlon competitors turn cold almost as quickly as their bodies.

News stories about dead marathon runners turn cold and are buried faster than their corpses.

A competitor may die during a race, but all of the many thousands of spectators will be just fine. The waiting ambulances are not for the spectators.

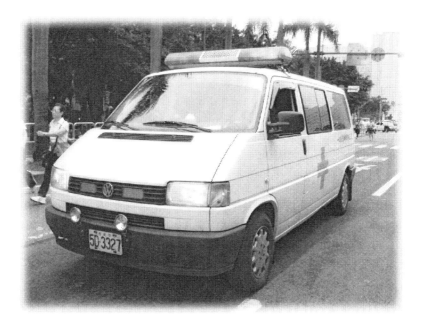

Ambulance at the Taipei, Taiwan Marathon, 2007

Chapter 7

The Athens Marathon is named after a town in Greece where the first runner died.

History of the Original Marathon
www.athensmarathon.com

"The modern Athens Marathon commemorates the run of the soldier Pheidippides from a battlefield at the site of the town of Marathon, Greece, to Athens in 490 B.C., bringing news of a Greek victory over the Persians. Legend has it that Pheidippides delivered the momentous message "Niki!" ("victory"), then collapsed and died, thereby setting a precedent for dramatic conclusions to the marathon."

The following are a few recent news stories about the deaths of competitors at marathons and triathlons. I'm sure the death rate would be much higher if it were not for the professional trainers, special diets, and extensive medical check-ups.

Philadelphia Marathon: Two Runners Dead After Collapsing During Race
HuffPost Chicago, November 20, 2011

"PHILADELPHIA -- Authorities say two who ran in the Philadelphia Marathon collapsed during the race and died of apparent heart attacks.

Philadelphia police Officer Jillian Russell, a spokeswoman, says a 21-year-old man collapsed at the finish line. She says a 40-year-old man collapsed about a quarter-mile before the finish line.

Russell says both were taken to a hospital, where they were pronounced dead."

Chicago Half-Marathon Runner Dies: Zachary Gregory Collapsed During Steamy Saturday Race

HuffPost Chicago, June 6, 2011

"Zachary Gregory, a 26-year-old physical therapist, died on Saturday after participating in a half-marathon in the sweltering heat that day.

Gregory went to the hospital in very serious condition, and was pronounced dead there at 9:52. An autopsy on Sunday was unable to conclusively determine the cause of Gregory's death."

Oshkosh Woman's Triathlon

Chicago Tribune, August 6, 2010

"OSHKOSH, Wisconsin
The family of an Oshkosh woman who died during a triathlon last summer has filed a lawsuit against the organizers. The lawsuit alleges that Midwest Sports Events and its executive director were negligent by failing to train lifeguards or provide adequate emergency care. Forty-three-year-old Kim M. Schmidt died while competing in the Oshkosh Area Triathlon. She was unresponsive when she was pulled from the water during the quarter-mile swim. She was later pronounced dead."

United Kingdom

Telegraph.co.uk, May 26, 2010

"RAF's second in command dies during triathlon. Air Chief Marshal Sir Christopher Moran, 54, who held the second most senior job in the Air Force, is thought to have suffered heart failure during the 5km run at the end of the race around RAF Brize Norton, Oxon."

Tel Aviv Marathon Runner Dies as a Result of Severe Dehydration

By Dan Even and Haaretz Service Tags: Israel news
April 11, 2011

"A 42-year-old man who participated in Friday's Tel Aviv marathon died Monday after being hospitalized for severe dehydration. The man collapsed of dehydration during the marathon on Friday and was brought to the emergency room in Ichilov Hospital in Tel Aviv. His condition continued to deteriorate and on Monday morning he died due to liver damage as a result of dehydration. During the marathon, 45 runners were hurt, most of them lightly. Two of those injured were still hospitalized in serious condition."

Man Dies in Hayden Triathlon

The Spokesman-Review, July 31, 2010

"A 60-year old man suffered cardiac arrest and died early this morning while participating in the Hayden View Triathlon. Leslie Chariton was swimming just after 7:30 a.m. when he was pulled from the race for treatment on Honeysuckle Beach, the Kootenai County Sheriff's Office said. He was transported to Kootenai Medical Center, where it was confirmed he died from cardiac arrest. His wife and son were at the race, a Kootenai officer said."

Coach Who Died at Triathlon

NWFdailynews.com, June 21, 2010

"The 40-year-old Shalimar Elementary School physical education teacher collapsed during the run portion of Eglin's My First Tri on Saturday. First responders assisted at the scene and transported her to the base hospital, where she was pronounced dead. 'She was perfectly healthy,' Ziegenhorn said. 'Bernie's whole life was physical education. She trained a year to do this and was perfectly healthy.'"

Learn When Exercise Can Kill You

Little Rock, Arkansas
March 2, 2008

"A 27-year-old Wisconsin man collapsed and died Sunday after completing the Little Rock Marathon. Adam Nickel, of Madison, Wis., was pronounced dead late Sunday morning near the finish line of the race, which attracted about 9,000 entrants, race officials said. Emergency personal used mouth-to-mouth resuscitation to try to revive Nickel until an ambulance arrived with a defibrillator. He could not be revived and was pronounced dead after being taken to the University of Arkansas for Medical Sciences Hospital."

Three Marathon Runners Suffered Heart Attacks in the Los Angeles, California, Marathon
Independent News and Media
www.iol.co.za - March 19, 2006

"Two men suffer fatal heart attacks along the 26.2-mile route. Another who collapsed is hospitalized in critical condition. The weather was perfect, the field enthusiastic, the times respectable, but Los Angeles' annual street party masquerading as street race was marred Sunday by the deaths of two runners and the collapse of an elderly man who was hospitalized in critical condition. Two retired law enforcement officers died after collapsing on the route. Det. Raul Reyna, 53, suffered a heart attack at mile 24 near Olympic Boulevard and Westmoreland Avenue, two miles short of the finish line. He died at Good Samaritan Hospital. The 28-year Los Angeles Police Department veteran had worked on the use of force investigation team at Parker Center, officials said. "His face was covered with blood and his eyes were open, but we never really got a pulse," said Lawson, a private pilot who volunteers part time on a ski patrol team. He and another runner, a physician, spent several minutes trying to revive Leone before paramedics arrived, said Lawson, who then resumed his run. Leone was

539

pronounced dead upon arrival at California Hospital Medical Center. Just nine blocks into the race Sunday, a third runner, believed to be in his 70s, suffered a heart attack near the intersection of Figueroa and 15th streets. The man, whose name was not released, was taken by paramedics to California Hospital Medical Center, where he was in critical but stable condition Sunday night."

San Francisco Marathon Racer Dies near the End of the Race
San Francisco Chronicle, July 31, 2006

"Friends say man, 43, was 'fit as a fiddle'. William Goggins, 43, of San Francisco, collapsed from apparent heart failure after he passed the 24-mile mark of the 26.2 mile race, authorities said."

Runner Dies during Marine Corps Marathon
October 30, 2006

"Earl Seyford, 56, of Olney, collapsed just before Mile 17 of the 26.2-mile course at approximately 12:20 p.m. He was airlifted from the 14th Street Bridge to Washington Hospital Center, according to race spokeswoman Beth Cline. A hospital spokeswoman confirmed that Seyford died at 1:10 p.m. but would not provide more details. A D.C. police spokesman said Seyford suffered what appeared to be "a heart attack or a stroke.""

Veteran Runner Dies in First Half of Pikes Peak Marathon
August 22, 2005

"A veteran marathon runner with no history of heart problems collapsed and died Sunday while competing in the Pikes Peak Marathon. Gary P. Williams, 59, of Norman, Okla., died of a suspected heart attack despite attempts by fellow competitors to save him shortly after he collapsed a little more than two miles from the 14,115-foot summit."

Runner in the Hong Kong Marathon has Died
February 14, 2006

"A 53-year-old runner who collapsed during the weekend Hong Kong marathon has died, a government spokeswoman said on Tuesday, February 14, 2006. The condition of a 33-year-old man who also collapsed during Sunday's race had improved from critical to serious, she added without giving the cause."

Competitor Dies in the Australia Day Triathlon
www.triathlon.co.nz, January 28, 2005

"A highly respected former teacher died in searing heat during an Australia Day triathlon. Neil Williams, 49, collapsed during the 2km run on January 28, 2005. He is believed to have suffered a heart attack."

Competitor Dies in the Noosa, Australia, Triathlon
www.smh.co.au, November 7, 2004

"A 37-year-old Sunshine Coast competitor died at the Noosa, Australia triathlon on November 7, 2004, after suffering a heart attack near the finish. Peter Semos was pronounced dead on arrival at Noosa Hospital, according to a statement from race medical director Richard Heath. He was competing in the 35-39 age category of the 1.5km swim, 40km cycle and 10km run triathlon and was apparently near the end of the run when he collapsed. Event staff reached Semos soon after the incident, but could not revive him. It is understood Semos' wife was a spectator at the race. According to race officials, there has been one other death in the event's 22-year history. Several years ago, a man suffered a heart attack during the swim. Noosa is billed as the world's second-largest triathlon and the event attracted about 5000 competitors."

Competitor Dies in Green Lake Triathlon, Spicer, MN
August 15, 2004

"Fifty-year-old Patrick Owen Boros was near the end of the swimming leg of the triathlon race on the morning of August 15, 2004, when he went under the water on Green Lake. Rescuers were able to quickly find Boros in about five feet of water, but efforts to revive him failed."

Competitor Dies in the Honolulu, Hawaii
www.honoluluadvertiser.com, December 10, 2002

"On Sunday afternoon, December 10, 2002, Grant Hirohata-Goto, 33, was pronounced dead at The Queen's Medical Center after he failed to respond to life support treatment at the marathon medical tent next to the finish line at Kapi'olani Park."

Mystery of Marathon Proportions in Ethiopian Runner's Death
www. scotlandonsunday.scotsman.com, January 9, 2005

"Alem Techale was expected to be the next great distance talent off the Ethiopian production line. Two years ago she won the world youth title at 1500m. In three months, she was to marry her boyfriend, Kenenisa Bekele, probably the greatest distance runner of the moment, with an Olympic gold medal and world records at 5,000m and 10,000m to prove it. Yet the girl who died was a world champion runner only 18 years old, who inexplicably dropped dead while on a routine training run with her fiancee."

Woman Dies in Bath Half Marathon
British Journal of Sports Medicine, March, 1998

"The dramatic death of Anna Loyley, age 26, in the Bath half-marathon in March, 1998, and the subsequent campaign of her parents has been covered in many national newspapers as well as by American internet journalism and short pieces and letters in the *British Medical Journal*. It led indirectly to a small conference on sudden cardiac death in sports. Organized by the National Sports Medicine Institute in March, 1999, with support from the British Heart Foundation, many of these issues were addressed."

Two Runners Die in the Beijing Marathon
www.english.people.cn, October 18, 2004

"October 17, 2004, in the Beijing Marathon, two persons running the marathon died. One of the victims was a fit young university student who started feeling ill around the 10km marker. Soon after the 19km marker, he fell unconscious and was pronounced "brain dead" at the Beijing hospital."

World-class Runner, Andy Palmer, Dies After a Run at Age 48
www.data-yard.net/10/palmer.htm, February 3, 2002

"February 3, 2002, Andy Palmer, an all-around athlete and passionate runner, collapsed and died after a long run at age 48. He placed in several marathons and set an American record in the 30K run in 1984."

Competitor in the Toronto Marathon Dies 1K from the Finish
www.toronto.cbc.ca, October 18, 2004

"October 18, 2004, a 43-year-old man participating in the annual Toronto Marathon Sunday collapsed and died just one kilometer from the finish line. Race officials said the unidentified male collapsed around 10:45 a.m. just short of the finish line at Queen's Park. He was taken to Mount Sinai Hospital where he was pronounced dead. "He stumbled, he said he wasn't feeling well and then he just collapsed," said Dr. Chris Woollam medical director of the Toronto Marathon."

Competitor Dies in the Beijing Marathon
October 17, 2005

"October 17, 2005, a runner dies in Beijing Marathon. The man, surnamed Wang, collapsed unconscious about 27 km (17 miles) into the race and was rushed to hospital, but doctors were unable to save him."

Marathoner Dies after Crossing the Finish Line
Fort Francis Times, October 17, 2005

"October 17, 2005, a marathoner dies after crossing the finish line. For the second year in a row, a runner has died in the Toronto Marathon. The unidentified 36-year-old man from Oakville, Ont. was running in the half-marathon yesterday morning with thousands of others and collapsed moments after crossing the finish line. Three people have died in the event in the last four years. Medical personnel working with the race rushed to his aid, first trying CPR, then a defibrillator. As an ambulance tried to get through the crowd, he was placed on a stretcher while health workers continued trying CPR and administering oxygen. He was taken to hospital with no vital signs."

Marathon Running Cardiologist and His Star Basketball Patient Both Die of Heart Attacks
New York Time Obituaries, January 25, 1995

"January 25, 1995, marathon running cardiologist and his star basketball patient both die of heart attacks. Dr. W. Thomas Nessa, a cardiologist for the Boston Celtics since

1987, died on Saturday. He was 48. The cause was a heart attack, his family said. In 1993, Dr. Nessa contributed to initial evaluations of Reggie Lewis, the Celtics' captain, who had collapsed during a game. Dr. Nessa helped convene a team of 12 heart specialists who began evaluating Mr. Lewis's heart condition. But Mr. Lewis abruptly got another medical opinion from a specialist who told him he had a benign fainting condition. He collapsed on the basketball court and died on July 27, 1993. Dr. Nessa was on the staff of New England Baptist Hospital and also cared for runners in the Boston Marathon, a race he completed several times."

Endurance racing kills heart muscles cells.

Marathon runners would be diagnosed positive for a heart attack if they visited a hospital emergency room directly after the race. Creatine phosphokinase (CPK) or creatine kinase (CK) is an enzyme that catalyzes the breakdown of phosphocreatine to phosphoric acid and creatine. CPK is a measurement of the breakdown of muscle tissue (muscle wasting) and is the first to be elevated after a heart attack (3 to 4 hours). The emergency room physician will measure the CPK enzyme in patients who are suspected to have had a heart attack. It is very likely that CPK will be elevated if blood is drawn a day or two after a weight-bearing workout or after an endurance race. CPK could also be elevated in cases of severe catabolism in which something is attacking heart tissue. CPK is elevated in people involved in earthquakes or industrial accidents who receive crushing injuries that damage and kill muscle tissues.

Chapter 7

Peak Performance Online
www.pponline.co.uk

"The truth is that marathon runners, ironman triathletes, and long-distance cyclists, swimmers, rowers, and cross-country skiers are all in the same boat. In fact, any athlete who participates in a strenuous test of endurance lasting about three hours or more has an increased chance of dying during - and for 24 hours following - the exertion, even when the athlete's chance of a death-door knock is compared with the risk incurred by a cigarette-smoking, sedentary layabout who spends the same 24 hours drinking beer and watching TV.

About 1 in 50,000: if you run marathons or participate in other forms of exercise which last for three hours or more, that's your approximate risk of suffering an acute heart attack or sudden cardiac death during - or within 24 hours of - your effort. For every 50,000 athletes, one will be stricken during such prolonged activity (1). Running a marathon or cycling intensely for three hours is riskier than taking a commercial airline flight, even in these troubled times!"

Every year we hear of several athletes wobbling on their feet during a game and collapsing in a heap before dying from a heart attack. The fans in the same age group are not dying from a heart attack, and they outnumber the athletes 1000 to 1. We would see several fans being hauled out of the bleachers on gurneys during every game if they had the same cardiac risk as the athletes.

Myth No. 3 - Exercise Will Prevent Metabolic Syndrome.

New studies are now proving that exercise does not benefit some people. This truth is surprising because most studies are fraudulently deceptive. The myth that exercise will prevent metabolic syndrome is scientifically unfounded and proved to be false in actual experience. Most medical doctors, professional nutritionists, and authors of diet books still believe the exercise myth. The following study, published in 2005, tries ineffectively to prove that exercise prevents metabolic syndrome:

Exercise and Risk Factors Associated with Metabolic Syndrome in Older Adults
Johns Hopkins School of Medicine
Baltimore, Maryland, USA, January 8, 2005

"A total of 51 men and 53 women completed the trial. Exercise significantly increased aerobic and muscle fitness, lean mass, and high-density lipoprotein cholesterol and reduced total and abdominal fat. DBP was reduced more among exercisers. There were no associations among changes in fitness with risk factors. Reductions in total body and abdominal fat and increases in leanness, largely independent of weight loss, were associated with improved SBP, DBP, total cholesterol, very low-density lipoprotein cholesterol, triglycerides, lipoprotein(a), and insulin sensitivity. At baseline, 42.3% of participants had metabolic syndrome. At 6 months, nine exercisers (17.7%) and eight controls (15.1%) no longer had metabolic syndrome, whereas four controls (7.6%) and no exercisers developed it (p =0.06)."

The study's dirty little secret is that the people were placed on diet restrictions in addition to an exercise program. This is why eight of the controls no longer had metabolic syndrome. Are we to believe that simply by being the control and making no changes in lifestyle will correct metabolic syndrome? The diet restrictions were responsible for the reduction in metabolic syndrome, not the exercise. The diet must have reduced calories and carbohydrate consumption by restricting foods such as sugar, potatoes, white bread, and white rice. Metabolic syndrome is reduced when carbohydrates are reduced. People who begin an exercise program without any changes in diet quickly learn their obesity, diabetes, heart disease, and other symptoms remain unchanged. It has been proven in Myth No. 2 that people like marathon runners still develop metabolic syndrome and heart disease even though their exercise programs could not be more intense.

Metabolic syndrome, also called *Syndrome X*, is the result of insulin resistance in cells caused by the continuous over consumption of carbohydrates for many years. The symptoms that identify the condition are obesity, high blood pressure, and blood sugar problems. Obesity can be misleading because many thin people with normal blood pressure develop insulin resistance. The five-hour glucose tolerance test is the best method for diagnosing metabolic syndrome and diabetes. The fasting patient is given a drink containing 100 grams of glucose followed by hourly measurements of blood glucose and insulin. Insulin resistance is confirmed when the insulin level continues to rise without a significant corresponding drop in glucose level. The glucose will become abnormally high. The degree of insulin resistance can be seen by the amount of lag time between the insulin level and the glucose response. The peak in glucose in insulin resistant patients can be followed by hypoglycemic symptoms where the blood glucose plunges below normal with a high insulin level remaining. A test using glucose readings only without insulin measurements is not as definitive. Results are abnormal when the glucose reading exceeds the following:

- Fasting blood glucose level ≥95 mg/dl (5.33 mmol/L)
- 1 hour blood glucose level ≥180 mg/dl (10 mmol/L)
- 2 hour blood glucose level ≥155 mg/dl (8.6 mmol/L)
- 3 hour blood glucose level ≥140 mg/dl (7.8 mmol/L)

Learn When Exercise Can Kill You

The following study shows that some people receive no health benefits from exercise. This frank admission is very rare in discussions about the benefits of exercise.

Exercise 'may benefit some less'
BBC News – Health – December 2, 2004

"Louisiana University researchers put 742 people through a strenuous 20-week endurance training programme.

The researchers selected the volunteers from 213 families, none of the participants had undertaken regular physical activity for the previous six months.

All were asked to use exercise bikes. By the last six weeks of the study, they were exercising for 50 minutes, three times a week, at 75% of the maximum output they were capable of before the study.

In this study, the researchers found training improved maximum oxygen consumption, a measure of a person's ability to perform well, by an average of 17%.

But the most "trainable" participants improved by 40% - and the least showed no improvement at all.

Claude Bouchard, who led the research, said: 'There is an astounding variation in the response to exercise. The vast majority will benefit in some way, but there will be a minority who will not benefit at all.'"

Metabolic Lockup

I have coined the term *metabolic lockup* to describe a condition encountered by some avid runners and bicyclists. The body literally enters a period of metabolic fatigue. It locks up. The continuous onslaught of dietary carbohydrates combined with a deficiency of healthy animal protein and fats simply fatigues the metabolic system. The leg muscles in runners and cyclists refuse to function to the desired degree. People can walk around and appear healthy, but heavy exertion is simply impossible because the leg muscles feel as if their strength has vanished. This condition does not occur in those on a low-carbohydrate diet who burn animal fats for energy.

The competitive runners and bicyclists seek to carry as little extra weight as possible. They are very thin and few have substantial muscle tone. They abhor body fat and their legs look like skin-covered bones and tendons. The gastrocnemius muscles above the Achilles tendons look like knots. I see the bikers training in my neighborhood by riding in a pack of 10 or more and clustered dangerously close to each other for some reason that I don't understand. Identical outfits and skull caps make them look like clones. I refer to them as *skeletons* as I drive by, hoping one will not make a mistake that will cause the whole group to become a big pile in front of my car.

Watch out for the skeletons on bikes.

Bicyclists riding on roadways in traffic are especially hazardous to themselves and others. Sometimes they ride several abreast and spill over from the shoulder into the traffic beyond the bike lane. Others deliberately ride in the traffic lane where they intentionally block traffic because of their slow speed. They seem to have chips on their shoulders and become nuisances and safety hazards in violation of roadway laws. They are frequently seen running red lights and stop signs as well as making illegal turns. This kind of activity is certainly not healthy. The worst offenders seem to be the ones dressed in professional riding clothes and acting like they are going win the Tour de France next year. They proliferate in college towns like Boulder,

Colorado, where the police are very lenient about enforcing bicycle laws.

Many have been told by professional trainers that eating animal protein and fats will increase their weight and make them less competitive; therefore, they should eat a high-carbohydrate diet because carbohydrates are "the primary fuel for the body." As a result, they have poor muscle tone, very little body fat, and have trained their bodies to perform on glucose instead of dietary fat. This makes them prime candidates for metabolic lockup when the glucose burns off in the middle of the race and leaves them with no energy. Marathon runners describe this condition as *hitting the wall.*

Sherrie was a good example of metabolic lockup. She was addicted to running marathons. Yes, the adrenaline rush from intense running and bicycling can easily become an addiction. I suggested she eat more protein and fat in the form of fatty meats and greatly reduce her carbohydrate intake. She instantly rejected this idea, claiming she couldn't run if she "bulked up" on the diet I suggested. A few months later, she had muscle cramps in her legs while training for an upcoming marathon. She tried everything that her trainer and running friends suggested, but nothing they advised relieved the leg pain and extreme weakness. She allowed her body to rest and recover for a few weeks until she felt she was strong enough to run in the marathon, but she collapsed less than half way through and was barely able to walk. Now she works in a store and sells special shoes to runners. Her marathon running career is over, but she still doesn't understand why.

Chapter 7

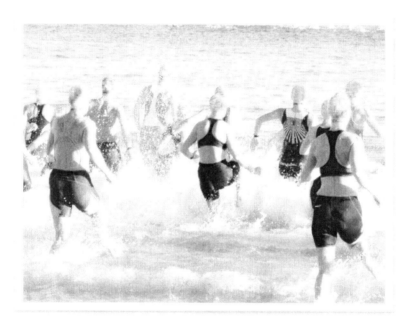

**Water Start at the Women's Triathlon
Mooloolaba, Queensland, Australia**

Myth No. 4 - Running is Healthy Exercise.

Don't believe this myth. Running is not a healthy way to exercise for many reasons. It has been solidly proven that running destroys the knees, ankles, and feet. The typical runner will develop knee problems within 20 years at best and within months for some individuals. Runners often have knee damage that eventually requires surgery and forces them to discontinue all running.

- Approximately 40–50% of runners or joggers will be injured in any one-year period.

- Approximately half to three quarters of these will be overuse injuries directly related to the impact of repetitive stress on the ligaments, tendons, joints, and lower back.

- Running puts a force on ankles is three to five times the body weight.

- The human anatomy is simply not designed for long-distance or frequent running.

Female runners are particularly prone to health damage. Women in their late teens or twenties can be seen running along highways and in the parks because they believe that this will make them healthier. This is certainly not the case. Damage to the female hormonal system is the first noticeable health problem, and a complete cessation of the menstrual cycle is common. Body fat produces estrogen, and women with very low body fat have hormonal imbalances as a result. These women can become temporarily infertile or suffer a miscarriage if they do become pregnant.

Young women who are able to conceive and give birth can be seen running behind baby strollers close to highway traffic, thereby placing their babies and themselves at great risk. Women should not be doing this sort of exercise. What are they thinking? Do they seriously believe that running at age 16 or 25 will prevent heart disease when they are 60 or 70? The answer is, "No." They will stop running long before they're 50 because of the damage done to their bodies. While on my daily bike ride, I see many young women jogging. I also see a few older women walking but none jogging or riding a bike.

Recent Testimony from the Mother of a College Coed

"By the way, my daughter is much better... she's stopped being a vegetarian (yay!), cut way back on the jogging, got her period back (after 8 months!), and her bowels seem better too. Thanks for all your encouragement."

I know two vegetarians who exercised a lot but still died in their early 50s. I mentioned Scott and Nancy in my first book, *Absolute Truth Exposed – Volume 1*, but their stories are worth repeating. Oh, no, they didn't die from heart disease. Both died from cancer. Here are their stories:

Scott was a 50-year old, healthy-looking landscaper. He was trim, and his weight was perfect for his size. When we discussed health and diet in 2002, he rejected my low-carbohydrate diet comments and stated he was a vegetarian. He had just formed a vegetarian support group, but his diet and extensive daily exercise did not treat him well. Scott was diagnosed with inoperable colon cancer in 2005. He died in June 2006.

Nancy found that the vegetarian diet and extensive exercise will not eliminate the risk for cancer but will most likely increase the risk. Avoiding red meat and animal fats will not eliminate the cancer risk. She was a vegetarian triathlon competitor who sadly discovered this fact. Nancy participated in triathlon and marathon events even though she was 49 years old. She developed a persistent cough that her doctor said was due to post nasal drip. When the cough became worse, she visited another doctor. Her chest x-ray revealed tumors in her lungs that proved to be cancerous.

Extreme exercise can cause many types of cancer.

Her chemotherapy seemed to place the cancer well into remission. The tumors shrank for a while but recurred. She was given every new experimental cancer drug available, but nothing worked and the side effects were horrible. She had chemo a second time, although doctors rarely perform it. It didn't help. Nancy didn't realize that excessive exercise literally wipes out the immune system, but it is common knowledge that marathon runners get sick easily after a race because their immune systems are shot. A strong immune system is necessary to prevent cancer. She was a vegetarian and didn't understand that all immune cells are made from amino acids such as those found in meat. Nancy had an unprecedented third round of chemotherapy. She died in December 2006, approximately two years after her original diagnosis.

Ex-NYC Marathon Champ undergoing Cancer Treatment
USA Today – June 20, 2005

"NEW YORK (AP) — Nine-time New York City Marathon champion Grete Waitz has been diagnosed with cancer and is undergoing treatment in her native Norway.

Waitz, 51, won the New York City Marathon from 1978-80, 1982-86 and 1988, the London Marathon twice (1983, 1986), was world marathon champion in 1983, a five-time world cross-country champion and won silver in the marathon at the 1984 Olympics."

Thankfully, Grete Waitz has survived her cancer diagnosis and treatment, but many professional athletes do not. Professional marathon runners and endurance bicyclists place themselves at increased risk for cancer because all of the body's cancer-fighting immune cells are made from polypeptides—complex molecules of amino acids. The best source for obtaining the essential amino acids is the meat of animals.

Woman who got Engaged at Finish of Marathon Dies of Cancer
www.burlingtonfreepress.com – November 20, 2010

"Jessica Pasquarello Vashaw, a former Fletcher Allen Health Care nurse who had a diamond-and-sapphire engagement ring slipped on her finger after crossing the finish line of the KeyBank Vermont City Marathon in 2007, has lost her five-year battle with breast cancer. She was 26."

Marathon Champion McCann Dies of Cancer
www.guardian.co.uk – December 8, 2008

"Kerryn McCann, the Australian marathon gold medallist at the last two Commonwealth Games, has died of cancer at the age of 41. McCann was surrounded by her family when she died at home overnight, Athletics Australia's president, Rob Fildes, said today."

Montgomery Runners raise More Than $35K in NYC Marathon in Coach's Memory
www.gazette.net – November 26, 2010

"When Julie Sapper crossed the finish line at the ING New York City Marathon Nov. 7, she wanted to feel happy and proud of her accomplishment, but could not.

Her friend and running coach, Mike Broderick, died just two days before the marathon and one day before his 54th birthday. He was diagnosed with stage 4 lung cancer in early October, Sapper said.

Broderick was a fixture in the Montgomery County running scene, Sapper and others said. He worked as a coach and headed up the Montgomery County Road Runners Experienced Marathoner's Training Program." He was running a half marathon with a cough that turned out to be cancer," said Sapper, a lawyer and running coach. "We were devastated.""

Melanoma Risk for White Marathon Runners
Medical News Today - November 21, 2006

"If you have white/fair skin and do a lot of marathon running you should be aware that your chances of developing melanoma might be higher, say researchers from the Medical University of Graz, Austria. Dermatologists there found that a noticeable number of their melanoma patients were ultra-marathon runners.

In fact, two of the authors of this study were enthusiastic marathon runners and wondered whether their activity might be linked to an increased risk of developing skin cancer.

The researchers looked at 420 people, half were marathon runners while the other half were not. All were checked by a dermatologist (skin doctor). They found more abnormal moles and lesions among the marathon runners. 24 of the runners required surgical treatment, compared to 14 from the non-marathon group."

The researchers investigating melanoma among marathon competitors have made a very common mistake. They flippantly assume the cancer was caused by the sun, but there are many variables between the marathon runners and the non-marathon group, such as the extent of extreme physical activity, diet, mineral depletion from sweating, and hormone levels. Studies are not valid unless they have only one variable, not dozens. The conclusion that sun exposure caused the higher incidence of melanoma is pure conjecture.

People who play golf often get long hours of sun exposure, but they are not engaging in extreme physical activity as are marathon competitors. Yet the researchers did not use golfers or other similar groups with equivalent sun exposures in the comparison with the marathon runners. This story is actually additional proof that too much exercise suppresses the immune system and leads to increased cancer risk.

Beware of studies that are pure conjecture.

The theory that sun causes skin cancer is simply false. People often get melanoma in areas of the body that have been completely covered by clothing, and the elderly who are confined to indoor living have a higher incidence of melanoma than those who are outdoors golfing, boating, or fishing. Actually, vitamin D that we receive from sun exposure has been scientifically proven to prevent cancer.

Vigorous exercise raises the levels of free radicals, which cause aging, cell damage, cancer, and other diseases. This type of exercise has the same effect as smoking three packs of cigarettes a day. Jogging in smoggy cities or along highways makes exercise unhealthier than smoking. Marathon and triathlon competitors are combining free radicals, suppressed immune cells, glucose, and disease-causing hormones like insulin, cortisol, and adrenaline to produce a poisonous cocktail that gives them cancer.

Dietary supplements will not kill cancer cells. Wild claims made by those selling herbal products are simply not true. Herbs will not kill cancer cells. Chinese medicine will not kill cancer cells. Homeopathic products will not kill cancer cells. Acupuncture will not kill cancer cells. Magnetic therapy will not kill cancer cells. All of these treatments are frauds.

The high-fat, low-carbohydrate ketogenic diet I present in this book will prevent cancer and heart disease. It will slow and restrict cancer cell growth in existing cancers and will slow or kill fungal cells that grow in association with cancer cells. Normal body cells that are infested with a fungus are sometimes mistaken for cancer cells. In order to kill the fungus, anti-fungal medication should be taken in addition to this high-fat, low-carbohydrate ketogenic diet. The following study shows that a ketogenic diet of 80% fat will eliminate cancerous tumors, but reintroducing carbohydrates causes the tumors to grow again.

Metabolic Management of Glioblastoma Multiforme Using Standard Therapy Together with a Restricted Ketogenic Diet:
Case Report - 22 April 2010 Nutrition & Metabolism 2010, 7:33doi:10.1186/1743-7075-7-33
http://www.nutritionandmetabolism.com/content/7/1/33

Background

"Management of glioblastoma multiforme (GBM) has been difficult using standard therapy (radiation with temozolomide chemotherapy). The ketogenic diet is used commonly to treat refractory epilepsy in children and, when administered in restricted amounts, can also target energy metabolism in brain tumors. We report the case of a 65-year-old woman who presented with progressive memory loss, chronic headaches, nausea, and a right hemisphere multi-centric tumor seen with magnetic resonance imaging (MRI). Following incomplete surgical resection, the patient was diagnosed with glioblastoma multiforme expressing hypermethylation of the MGMT gene promoter."

Methods

"Prior to initiation of the standard therapy, the patient conducted water-only therapeutic fasting and a restricted 4:1 (fat: carbohydrate + protein) ketogenic diet that delivered about 600 kcal/day. The patient also received the restricted ketogenic diet concomitantly during the standard treatment period. The diet was supplemented with vitamins and minerals. Steroid medication (dexamethasone) was removed during the course of the treatment. The patient was followed using MRI and positron emission tomography with fluoro-deoxy-glucose (FDG-PET)."

Results

"After two months treatment, the patient's body weight was reduced by about 20% and no discernable brain tumor tissue was detected using either FDG-PET or MRI imaging. Biomarker changes showed reduced levels of blood glucose and elevated levels of urinary ketones. MRI evidence of tumor recurrence was found 10 weeks after suspension of strict diet therapy."

Conclusion

"This is the first report of confirmed GBM treated with standard therapy together with a restricted ketogenic diet. As rapid regression of GBM is rare in older patients following incomplete surgical resection and standard therapy alone, the response observed in this case could result in part from the action of the calorie restricted ketogenic diet. Further studies are needed to evaluate the efficacy of restricted ketogenic diets, administered alone or together with standard treatment, as a therapy for GBM and possibly other malignant brain tumors."

The high-fat ketogenic diet requires restricting protein and severely limiting carbohydrates. If you have cancer, talk to your physician about the ketogenic diet containing at least 80% fat, 15% protein, and 5% or less of carbohydrates as shown in the following study. Calories were also severely restricted to prevent the body from converting dietary protein to glucose.

Famous Tour de France cyclist, Lance Armstrong, is another good example that proves excessive exercise causes cancer. He developed testicular cancer, but fortunately he appears to have survived the disease. In March 2006, the announcement was made that Lance Armstrong's ex-mate, Sheryl Crow, had been diagnosed with breast cancer. The big question remains, "What diet and lifestyle philosophy were they following that caused them both to develop cancer? They certainly did not eat a 100% meat diet like the Eskimos of the past century who were free of all cancers. The Eskimos no longer enjoy a cancer-free lifestyle since they began eating the high-carbohydrate diet introduced by the white man.

Government health, nutrition, and medical organizations tell us to eat multiple servings of whole grains, fruits, and vegetables each day to support a strong immune system. People consider these sources to be highly credible, but they are scientifically wrong. All immune cells are made from polypeptides, which are complex molecules made from amino acids. Fruits contain almost no amino acids. Vegetables contain very few amino acids, and whole grain products are lacking some of the essential amino acids. Red meat, fowl, fish, seafood, eggs, and cheese are natural, wholesome foods that contain an abundance of all of the essential amino acids needed to build a very strong immune system.

People with autoimmune diseases, such as rheumatoid arthritis, multiple sclerosis, lupus, Sjogren's dry eye syndrome, ulcerative colitis, Crohn's disease, inflammatory bowel disease, irritable bowel syndrome, and more than four dozen other diseases should not jog, hike aggressively, run marathons, or participate in endurance races. These kinds of activities will most certainly trigger a major autoimmune disease flare. This topic has been covered in great detail in *Absolute Truth Exposed – Volume 1.*

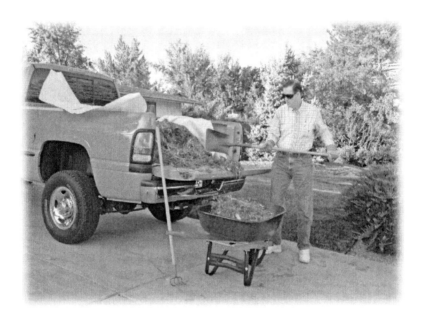

Yard Work Can Be Great Exercise

Yoga is not healthy exercise.

Testimony from an Ex-vegetarian who Practiced Yoga

"Hello,

I'm writing to let you know that as a recovering vegetarian and sufferer of degenerative spine disease, I love your information and have been reading it for days now.

I am especially interested in your section on exercise myths as I have been practicing yoga regularly for a few years and until very recently was considering training to become a yoga teacher. But Weston Price (and Lierre Keith, Sally Fallon, Gary Taubes, etc.) intervened just after I endured a two-hour workshop taught by militant vegans that offended me deeply with its attitude of rage and hypocrisy, and has left a sour taste in my mouth regarding the entire yoga world as a result.

Additionally and ironically, the gains I have experienced from changing my eating habits from high-carb (vegan) to low-carb (meat) has eclipsed any gains I've made practicing yoga (toned arms, temporary feeling of relaxation). I've since cut my practice way down as my taste for it has diminished, quit therapy, and have recovered from a lifetime of mood-swings, depression, anxiety, self-hatred, and PMS. Yoga could not touch any of those deep-seated pains. It's nothing short of a miracle. To think that

563

the answer to my suffering has literally been under my nose all these years fills me with awe every day. Of course, no one in the yoga community wants to hear that eating meat actually solves the problems of the mind that yogis spend hours on with little to no improvement.

So my question to you is this: Would you ever consider adding a page of yoga myths in the same way that you have with running? I would love to read it and cannot find anything on the internet that questions the benefits of yoga.

Thank you for considering this, and for your hard work. I look forward to reading more of your articles.

Sincerely,

Elise"

**Elise has a right to be angry.
Her health was damaged by dietary dogma.**

Myth No. 5 - Humans Are Natural Born Runners.

A popular nutrition and health website suggests that humans are designed to run. This claim doesn't stand the test of a detailed scientific analysis of human anatomy and physiology. Humans can certainly, run, but it is nothing to brag about. Compared to many animals, humans are poor runners.

Humans are not designed to be good runners.

As predators, humans are fairly inept at chasing down and capturing prey. Try chasing a deer sometime and see how successful you are. The deer can quickly run over three hills and disappear. A man is completely exhausted after running a few hundred yards up the first hill, but many animals are very long-distance runners. We humans must use our superior brain power to catch prey because we are ineffective runners. We hunt in packs, stalk the prey to get closer, and use weapons to kill from a distance. Running destroys the human body.

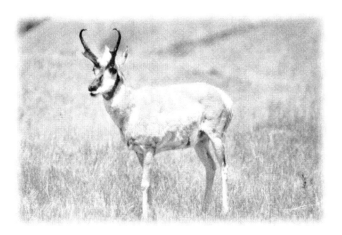

Pronghorn Antelope (Antilocapra Americana)
Fastest Animal in North America - 60 mph for Short Distances

Myth No. 6 - Carbohydrates Are Necessary for Energy.

This myth will never die. Athletes gulp down high-carbohydrate foods because they think glucose is the only available energy source. They are totally unaware of the dreadful damage they are doing to their bodies. Cells are literally being driven to exhaustion by the onslaught of excess fuel and insulin. This process is analogous to a top-fuel dragster burning nitromethane, which literally fries the engine during each race. Insulin is analogous to the turbocharger that stuffs the fuel into the engine. Carbohydrates will eventually fry your metabolism. On the other hand, eating fat for energy is analogous to a large truck burning diesel fuel, which allows the engine to last for a million miles.

Carbohydrates will eventually fry your metabolism.

Body cells can use either fat or glucose for energy. Insulin is required when glucose is used as fuel but is not needed to burn fat. Insulin forces the glucose into the cells like a supercharger on a race car. The glucose we eat and the oxygen we breathe burn in the cells just like in a little engine. The combustion is less than 30% efficient in producing work (running), and the rest must be expended as heat, i.e., sweating with evaporative cooling, conduction, and convection. The pre-race consumption of carbohydrates is nicknamed *carb-loading* and causes the surge of glucose and insulin. The body counteracts high insulin by secreting adrenaline and cortisol hormones that kick the body into overdrive. You can read more about adrenaline and cortisol below. I describe this harmful combination as the *Rieske Metabolic Supercharger Cycle (RMSC)*. The runner feels awesome in this hyped-up state because he is truly supercharged. Carb-loading will make you feel like power-woman, iron-man, or mega-manager blasting through the airport.

Excess adrenaline causes these supercharged reactions:

- Increased blood pressure
- Increased heart rate
- Contraction and constriction of the blood vessels
- Accelerated respiration rate
- Dilated respiratory passageways
- Decreased digestion rate
- Increased efficiency of muscular contractions
- Increased blood sugar level
- Stimulation of cellular metabolism

It's no wonder the adrenaline rush is addictive. An insulin, adrenaline, and cortisol rush may save one's life when being chased by a lion, but it will eventually cause death when it occurs repeatedly day after day during exercise, running, and bicycling. Insulin packs glucose into the cells for energy, but it is also doing silent damage. It is a super powerful anabolic hormone that packs small, dense LDL molecules, bad omega-6 vegetable oils, heavy metals, and free-radical molecules into the walls of the heart arteries. These undesirable molecules cause an inflammatory response that requires the body to patch up the damage. The patches become artery plaque and set the stage for a future heart attack.

This is the precise *Rieske Metabolic Supercharger Cycle* that killed marathon runners, James F. Fixx and Brian Maxwell. Saturated and monounsaturated fats from animal sources provide energy to the cells without stimulating insulin and do not cause heart disease. In his 1984 book, *Galloway's Book on Running,* marathon runner, Jeff Galloway, describes how he tried carb-loading before a marathon but as a result couldn't finish the race. He admits that runners should burn fat for energy.

People addicted to extreme physical exercise cannot easily give up carb-loading because it has become a daily routine. They may try to switch to fat for energy, but they feel a huge physical and psychological letdown from adrenaline withdrawal. They have become obsessive compulsive adrenaline addicts who can't stop powering up on sugars and running.

Exercise can become an obsessive compulsive adrenaline addiction.

Adrenaline and cortisol are produced in the adrenal medulla. The adrenal glands get tired of producing excessive levels of adrenaline and cortisol just as the pancreas gets tired of producing excessive amounts of insulin. Adrenal exhaustion or adrenal fatigue will eventually occur, and when the adrenal glands collapse, so will you. One day the runner is full of power. A couple of months later he is weak, exhausted, and aches all over. The doctor says he has chronic fatigue syndrome (CFS) or fibromyalgia and usually tells him that nobody knows what causes it. Well, the doctor may not know what causes it, but the answer is easy. Neither the doctor, marathon runner, nor the physical trainer suspects the carb-loading diet is the cause for the runner's collapse three quarters of the way through a race. They examine water consumption, vitamins, and minerals without finding the answer. Next, they consider viruses or some other pathological cause. If they find a problem with adrenal hormones, they will fail to make the connection to the high-carbohydrate diet.

The same thing happens to the obese from an excessive consumption of carbohydrates even though they may get very little exercise. The high insulin level stimulates the over production of adrenaline and cortisol that fatigue the adrenal glands. These steps describe how the high-carbohydrate diet causes the progression from normal weight to obesity, diabetes, and chronic fatigue syndrome.

Guides and promoters of Mount Everest climbing expeditions generally recommend and prepare food that is very high in carbohydrates. They have the misconception that the expedition members will perform better on a high-carbohydrate diet because they have been brainwashed to believe carbohydrates are needed for energy. Tim Medvetz, a 240-pound ex-Hells Angels' motorcycle rider, successfully climbed Mount Everest on his second attempt.

Tim commented in the television documentary that he felt much stronger, healthier, and climbed easier when he ate the Sherpa's diet of high-fat yak meat instead of the low-fat, low-protein, and high-carbohydrate foods used by the United States' expeditions. The yak is a domestic animal similar to a cow that is raised for meat and milk and routinely used as a beast of burden.

Tim's awesome success was achieved in spite of breaking two bones in one of his hands on the day he reached the summit. He had wrapped one of the anchor ropes around his gloved right hand in order to have a more secure grip, but his foot slipped and the loop tightened painfully around his hand, snapping the bones. His waist harness was clipped to another anchor rope, which prevented him from falling to his death. He kept his injury secret so the expedition leader would not force him to abandon his quest for the summit, after which he could only use one hand on the ropes and ladders during the descent. His achievement and determination were truly impressive.

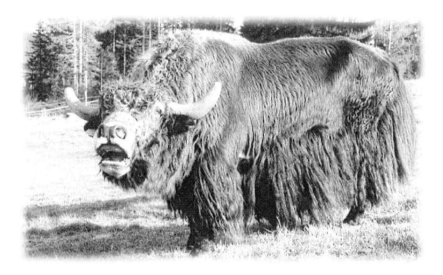

Sherpas' Diet on Mt. Everest Is Yak Meat and Fat

Another member of Tim Medvetz's expedition, Betsy Huelskamp, is a female vegetarian and professional trainer who failed in her attempt to climb Mount Everest. She was trim and healthy-looking at home in the city gym. Tim was, well, noticeably overweight. Okay, he was fat, but Betsy collapsed from exhaustion midway up the mountain and could not continue. She may have looked great in the gym, but her weak, skinny, vegetarian body completely failed under the harsh conditions of Mount Everest. Her diet gave her adrenal fatigue and failure.

Carbohydrates are not needed for energy! Don't believe this universal myth. The scientific and actual requirement for carbohydrates is zero. Athletes would be well advised to eat the high-fat, high-protein, and low-carbohydrate diet of the Sherpas to maintain a healthy body and prevent insulin resistance of the muscle cells. The harmful effects from adrenaline and cortisol do not occur when insulin is kept low. Adrenal gland exhaustion is caused by eating carbohydrates.

Another pair of more successful climbers, David Tait and his Sherpa, Phurba Tashi, wanted to set a new world record by climbing up and over Mount Everest, descending on the other side, and returning in what is called a *double traverse*. He and his Sherpa made it over the top and down the other side, but David voluntarily discontinued, stating that he did not want to achieve the world record while Sherpa Phurba Tashi, who was obviously a more superior and capable climber, was climbing next to him.

Sherpa guides are never skinny vegetarians.

Sherpa guides do more than climb the mountain. They carry the hardware, ladders, ropes, stakes, tents, oxygen bottles, food, heating fuels, and much more. The media, sports magazines, expedition leaders, professional nutritionists, athletic trainers, and the climbers from foreign countries all attribute the outstanding performance of the Sherpas to one thing—they were born and grew up at this high altitude. Yes, being born there does give them a slight advantage, but this excuse is accepted without the slightest challenge. The meat and animal fat diet of the Sherpas is the dirty little secret that Tim Medvetz let out of the bag. They climb well because their bodies are not insulin resistant, and their muscles are well trained to burn dietary fats for energy. The Sherpas' awesome performance results from a combination of diet and lung development.

Myth No. 7 - Runners Should Eat a Low-Fat Diet.

This myth seems so true, innocent, wonderfully healthy, and wholesome that most runners never question it. Marathon runners who eat a low-fat, carb-loading diet reach a point in the middle of the race where the muscles run out of glycogen (stored glucose) in what they call *hitting the wall*. The legs should have switched to burning lipids for energy but don't easily do so because this condition rarely occurs. Sudden leg fatigue is particularly true when a marathon runner trains at shorter distances by carb-loading without ever exhausting the glycogen stores in the muscles. The legs have never learned to burn lipids for energy, but they need to be trained to do so.

Fat-loading provides long-lasting energy for endurance competition.

Competitors should power the body with my diet therapy composed of animal protein, natural animal fats, essential fatty acids, vitamins, and minerals, particularly for long endurance races, marathons, triathlons, and mountain climbing. Dietary fat provides energy that never seems to run out. Professional athletes in the last century ate a high-fat diet called *fat-loading* before each competition, but the practice was discontinued when sprint racers convinced everyone to switch to carb-loading.

Sprint racers should train and compete differently from endurance racers. Sprint racers should eat a low-carbohydrate diet during daily routine and training. They could then eat carbohydrates for supercharged performance during the short contest. Eat pure glucose sugar minutes before the race to blast off the blocks like a nitromethane top fuel dragster.

Myth No. 8 - Exercise Prevents and Reverses Heart Disease.

No! Do not believe this common lie. Exercise neither prevents nor reverses heart disease. People who have partially plugged heart arteries or have had artery bypass surgery are immediately placed on an exercise program. They are told the exercise will open the plugged arteries and prevent new blockages. The poor patient believes this myth only to be severely disappointed by a diagnosis of new heart problems or another heart attack. The doctor may insist the patient's heart condition worsened because he didn't exercise enough or ate too much fat. It is always the patient's fault and never the fault of unscientific advice. When the patient has a heart attack and dies, the answer is simple—he had heart disease. In actual practice, bypass arteries can become completely plugged again in only one year because of the low-fat, high-carbohydrate diet recommended by the American Heart Association® (AHA).

Exercise does not prevent heart disease.

It is very dangerous to exercise with a heart that has partially plugged arteries. Don't do it! Heart pain is a signal that muscle damage is taking place because the heart muscle cells are being deprived of oxygen. The result could be a sudden heart attack and death. It is theorized that marathon runner James F. Fixx was running with severe heart pain before he was stricken and died. Perhaps he thought he could "run through" the problem and cure his heart disease. Nobody knows for certain why he continued to run with heart arteries that were virtually plugged, but it was certainly the wrong thing to do.

I shudder at the risks some people in my neighborhood take while jogging. They are well out into the street, running with the traffic because we have no sidewalks. Joggers should run against the direction of the traffic but many don't. To make matters worse, some runners are wearing earphones and audio devices that prevent them from hearing the traffic approaching from the rear. I have a little rearview mirror on my bicycle as a safety measure to check the traffic that is overtaking me from behind.

Young mothers like to run on the neighborhood streets while pushing their babies in jogging strollers. They certainly couldn't react quickly to a traffic situation to protect the child who is being placed at an unnecessary risk. Frankly, I don't understand what they're trying to accomplish. Will exercise prevent them from having a heart attack in their 60s or 70s? No! I rarely see women older than 50 jogging or riding bicycles. Nearly all men and women my age have stopped doing regular outdoor exercise, proving that the exercise they were doing 15 or 20 years ago has not provided the excellent health they were told to expect.

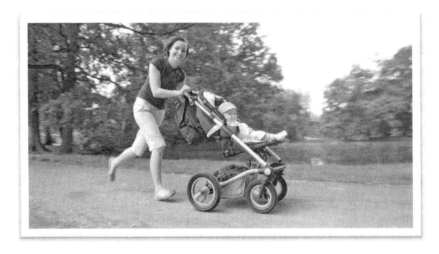

Jogging Baby Strollers Are Unhealthy Exercise and Can be a Danger to the Baby

Myth No. 9 - Exercise Builds the Body.

This assumption is false. Exercise tears down the body. The techniques used by bodybuilders will build up the body by first tearing down the tissues with high stress and then allowing them to heal and grow. Excessive exercise simply runs the muscles into exhaustion and fatigue. The phrase "no pain - no gain" is a concept that does not apply to endurance runners, and pain during competition or practice is an indication that damage is being done. Running through the pain is not a healthy practice.

Bodybuilders don't use endurance exercises.

Running can greatly damage the body. Sherrie, who was mentioned earlier, is a good example. She was addicted to marathon running because it produces an adrenaline/cortisol rush. Runners typically comment about the wonderful feeling of euphoria and become depressed when illness or a business trip prevents them from running. They can get so addicted to insulin, adrenaline, and cortisol that they insist on running under almost any condition—in dangerous traffic, at night, in the rain and snow, and on icy roads or jogging paths. They are truly hormone addicts.

Sherrie never won a marathon, and since she could never celebrate a victory, she was always under pressure to do better. She tried to improve her performance by avoiding red meat and animal fats so she would not "bulk up with extra muscle mass" that would slow her speed.

Sherrie's diet and extreme physical activity destroyed her body rather than making it healthier. Instead of getting faster, she developed severe leg cramps and spasms that prevented her from finishing the race. Soon her spasms were so bad she

575

couldn't walk normally. Sherrie was addicted to the catabolic hormone rush, and her body was literally consuming itself.

A doctor who had been jogging frequently for nearly 20 years is another example. He said that the knees can't continue to be pounded for much longer than that, and he knew he was reaching the end of his running career. Unfortunately, at age 55 he was entering a period of life in which exercise is strongly recommended by professional medical societies as the key to diabetes and heart disease prevention. It's difficult to get an effective total body workout without using the legs because they are by far the largest muscle group in the body. The doctor did not explain what he was going to do as the damage to his legs and knees increased.

Endurance exercise tears down the body.

A friend who is now 65 years old is another example. She jogged for many years but required knee surgery about five years ago. Now she gets very little exercise and has developed heart disease. Runners need to have a backup plan when running destroys their knees, ankles, and feet.

The carb-loading diet turns cyclists and marathon runners into skeletons of moving skin, tendons, and bones as a result of the catabolic depletion of muscle mass. Their bodies actually consume the muscles as an energy source during practice and competition; this is why they are extremely skinny. My high-fat, high-protein anabolic diet and exercise program builds muscles, tendons, ligaments, and vertebral discs to provide a strong, muscular, and healthy body.

Walking has been touted as an excellent form of exercise, but it too has several drawbacks. Walking is not aerobic enough, especially when the route is level or the pace is too slow. Walking can also damage the feet over a long period of time as occurs in the elderly when the fatty padding in the ball of the foot gradually moves forward, causing pain and tenderness. The following is a general guideline for healthy exercise for the average person who is not engaged in competitive sports.

Don't jump into a diet and exercise program the way most people do. Their doctors tell them to lose weight by cutting dietary fat, reducing calories, and exercising. Some patients take the challenge by going on a starvation diet and exercising vigorously. This can get old quickly, and after they see very little progress or none at all, they give up everything completely and quit.

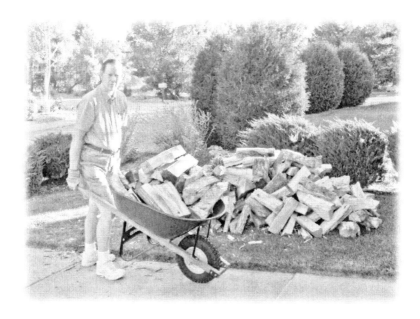

Kent Hauling Firewood, August 26, 2011

Guidelines for Healthy Exercise

The high-fat, high-protein, and low-carbohydrate diet in addition to healthy exercise as presented below will preserve health and heal the body. Healthy exercise should be thought of as variety of everyday activities plus a few extra activities. Some of the activities should be demanding enough to increase the heart rate to 70–80% of maximum for approximately 15 minutes. The exercise should not be strenuous for a long period of time so as to cause an unhealthy adrenaline spike. The maximum heart rate is considered to be 220 minus your age. Low-energy exercises like walking slowly for long periods of time do not produce the healthy cardiovascular effect but simply fatigue the body. Healthy exercise is strongly suggested for overall cardiovascular health. One doesn't have to join a club and pay money to get a healthy level of exercise.

Below are a few suggested "Do's and Don'ts."

Diet:

- Eat a high-fat, high-protein, and low-carbohydrate diet for healthy energy that doesn't damage the body with a glucose and insulin rush.
- Take supplements as outlined in previous chapters.

Activities to do:

- Hike hills and mountains but not to the point of exhaustion or an adrenaline rush.
- Swimming can provide excellent exercise.
- For an awesome cardiovascular exercise, ride a bicycle aggressively for 15 minutes where some of the terrain has uphill sections, but avoid riding in traffic This exercise does not stress or damage the knees, ankles, or feet.
- Get the heart rate up for 15 minutes but avoid exhaustion.

- Walk at a brisk pace for 30 minutes every day with some uphill sections. This may be hard on the feet for overweight people.
- Snow or water skiing can be healthy or extremely hazardous depending on risks taken.
- Park at the far end of the parking lot and walk the extra distance. You car will appreciate it also.
- Climb the stairs instead of taking an elevator.
- Wash the car instead of using a drive-thru car wash.
- Mow the lawn instead of paying someone else who gets the exercise instead of you.
- Play sports like tennis, racquetball, volleyball, and basketball but not to exhaustion.
- Exercise outside in fresh air rather than in the house, city smog, or near dirty and dangerous traffic.

Activities to avoid:

- Don't perform "extreme" sports. They are definitely not healthy and are often deadly.
- Don't exercise to the point of addiction from the adrenaline rush.
- Don't sit or stand longer than one hour without some activity that uses the legs. This will avoid blood clots.
- Don't pull one leg up under the other leg and sit on it.
- Don't eat carbohydrates for energy because they cause metabolic syndrome.
- Don't burn candles indoors and avoid chemicals that cause indoor pollution.
- Don't use electrostatic air cleaners because they give off lung-damaging ozone. Some new models have an ozone elimination section that may or may not be effective in reducing the hazard.
- Don't use electrostatic copy machines in a closed office with poor air circulation because they give off ozone.

These suggestions are more important as we age because older people just don't have the resilience that youthfulness provides. College students can be seen running all over town and pounding themselves into the pavement, but they bounce right back because they're young. I never see folks my age charging around town or in my neighborhood. I can run at a very brisk pace, but most people my age can't run at all, and many can't walk very far. We see them riding around the supermarket in battery-powered shopping carts. Perhaps you didn't notice that supermarkets didn't have battery-powered shopping carts before the start of the low-fat, high-carbohydrate craze.

Now we see severely obese shoppers filling their electric carts with boxes of whole grain cereal; 10 different types of fruits 365 days a year; low-fat, low-cholesterol yogurt and milk; whole grain bagels and bread; and boxes of pasta products each marked "low-fat and zero-cholesterol." And of course, each of the packages has a big red heart symbol and a check mark with the words *heart healthy*.

The healthy heart symbol found on many food boxes has caused a decline in health.

These products are actually a heart attack, cancer, and diabetes waiting to happen. Life expectancy in the United States is projected to decrease in future years as a result of the obesity, diabetes, heart disease, and cancer epidemics. These are occurring because the official dietary recommendations suggest that people avoid fats, especially saturated fats, and eat more carbohydrates in the form of fruits, vegetables, and whole grains. These diseases have become epidemic because people are trying harder and harder to comply with the government recommendations as evidenced in recent surveys. The official government dietary recommendations found in the *2010 USDA My Plate* are wrong.

Riding my bicycle and hiking hills and mountains are my preferred forms of exercises. Bicycling allows the rider to determine the intensity of the exercise. Simply pedal faster and shift into higher gears to reach any aerobic level desired. Bicycling is gentle on the feet, ankles, and knees as well as most other parts of the body. One area of concern, however, is the neck. Most bicycles are designed to place the rider in a severely head-forward position that requires him to pull the head back in order to look forward. The problem is exaggerated on my bike because I am 6'6" (2.00 meters) tall, and the handlebar stem did not have enough adjustment to reduce the head-forward position. I purchased a replacement set of handlebars that curve out and up to a higher level, which places me in a more upright position.

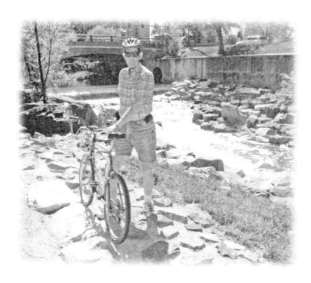

Kent on Cherry Creek Trail
Denver, Colorado, September 18, 2011

Chapter 7

Bodybuilding Diet and Exercises

Bodybuilders eat a high-protein diet and supplement with additional protein powder in order to build body mass, muscles, ligaments, tendons, and bones. Millions of bodybuilders have proved this over several decades of testing and refinement. The science behind the high-protein diet confirms the results found in actual practice. The goal of bodybuilders and most health conscious individuals is to preserve and build lean muscle while controlling body fat. This can be done by a combination of diet and exercise.

Diet and Exercise Step No. 1

Eat the ultra low-carbohydrate diet on a daily basis but particularly before engaging in the intense exercise program in Step No. 2 below. This caution is given because most exercise books recommend a high-carb diet before exercise in order to fuel the muscles. This is backward to what is needed to control body fat and build lean muscle. Meat provides the full complement of all essential and non-essential amino acids needed to build strong bones, tendons, ligaments, and muscles without adding undesirable carbohydrates.

Fruits, starchy vegetables, and whole grains do not build strong, robust, healthy bodies.

Vegetarian foods such as whole grains, soy, and legumes do not fulfill these requirements and are unacceptable substitutes. The diet should include a generous amount of healthy animal fats, and carbohydrates should be kept to a minimum. Polyunsaturated omega-6 vegetable oils should be avoided like the plague that they are. The healthy diet consists mainly of animal products such as red meat, fowl, fish, and seafood with the natural fats. Eating a diet that is 100% meat with its natural fat is perfect. It contains 100% of the required vitamins, minerals, essential fatty acids, and essential amino acids. Don't be fooled into believing that fruits and vegetables are requirements for a healthy diet. Those claims are scientifically false.

Diet and Exercise Step No. 2

Perform a high-intensity exercise program such as weight lifting, bicycling, swimming, or climbing hills or stairs. Do this program very aggressively for 15 minutes only. Longer programs are bad because they elevate adrenaline and cortisol, catabolic hormones that break down the body. The leg muscles are the largest muscle group, so concentrate on exercises that use the legs. The muscles will suddenly become weak because this program is intended to quickly burn glycogen (muscle glucose storage), but keep going for the full 15 minutes. The muscles will switch to burning fat for energy. If you don't feel any muscle weakness before the exercise is completed, it could be for either of the following reasons:

- You may not have been eating the ultra low-carbohydrate diet for several days prior to the exercise. Your muscles retained a full load of glycogen.

- Your muscles may have become accustomed to burning fat for energy because you have been on the low-carbohydrate diet for a long period of time.

Perform the high-intensity exercise program five to seven times per week.

- Lift weights with periods of intense effort and rest (called *reps*). Concentrate on the legs but use other body muscles as well for a full body workout, or

- Ride a bicycle in a circular course that has gradual uphill sections followed by downhill sections for resting. This functions like reps to build the body.

- Hike up and down flights of stairs. This functions like reps.

- Hike up and down a hill.

Diet and Exercise Step No. 3

Eat a high-protein, medium-fat snack with a small amount of carbohydrates after completing the exercise. You can also prepare a protein and glutamine drink to supplement a snack of meat or fish. Eat about 10–20 calories of carbohydrates to stimulate a low-level insulin rush. My recommendation is to eat two Dove® Dark Chocolate Silky Smooth Promise candies. They are delicious, so be careful not to overindulge. Insulin is an extremely powerful anabolic hormone that stimulates the body to use the amino acids to build muscles, tendons, ligaments, bones, vertebral discs, and virtually the entire body. The cholesterol in the meat is very beneficial because the body uses it to make hormones, and the carbohydrates restore the glycogen in the muscles.

I generally do not recommend carbohydrates, but I do recommend them for this special method of bodybuilding. Acceptable carbohydrates in very limited amounts are:

- Two Dove® Dark Chocolate Silky Smooth Promises
- Six tablespoons of potatoes, sweet potatoes, or yams
- Several fried pork skins with a little honey
- Three tablespoons of ice cream made with real cream and real sugar. Avoid ice cream that is labeled low-fat or contains artificial sweeteners or thickeners such as carrageenan and guar gum.

584

Scientific Facts That Support This Bodybuilding Program

The low-carbohydrate diet in **Diet and Exercise Step No. 1** causes the body to deplete glucose from the liver and carbohydrates from the digestive tract. This is opposite to the carb-loading technique that turns cyclers and marathon runners into *skeletons* of moving skin, tendons, and bones as a result of the catabolic depletion of muscle mass. The muscles that are used in competition are somewhat protected from being consumed. This program builds muscles, tendons, ligaments, and vertebral discs to provide a strong, robust, and healthy body.

Building a strong, robust, and healthy body requires a diet rich in animal protein and fats.

The exercise in **Diet and Exercise Step No. 2** further depletes the glycogen in the muscles. It also puts the muscles into a rebuilding mode because the exercise breaks down the muscle cells. This exercise must be short but strenuous as is typically done by bodybuilders.

The high-protein, medium-fat diet outlined in **Diet and Exercise Step No. 3** with a moderate carbohydrate intake will promote a modest insulin rush that promotes anabolic rebuilding of the body. The glucose produced from the carbohydrate digestion is used to restore the depleted stores of glucose in the liver and restore the glycogen in the muscles. The carbohydrates fill the empty glucose stores but are not converted to body fat because the quantity is limited. Therefore, the program rebuilds the body without adding body fat.

Bodybuilders typically eat a lot of meat as a high-quality protein source and supplement with protein powder drinks and shakes. Whey protein powder contains all of the essential and non-essential amino acids necessary to build a strong, healthy body. The product listed below is made from the whey protein from cows' milk and all of the lactose (milk sugar) has been stripped from the product during manufacture. It is pre-digested using special healthy bacteria to breakdown the protein molecules into the individual amino acids and branched-chain amino acids. The amino acids can pass through the intestinal-blood barrier to quickly become available for healing the body and building bone collagen, ligaments, tendons, and muscles. Extra glutamine amino acid is also recommended.

Protein and Glutamine Drink - Prepare a drink made with whey amino acid protein powder that is enriched with extra glutamine amino acid. BioChem® Low Carb® whey protein powder is an excellent choice. It consists of a full complement of amino acid isolates that heal the body and require no digestion. Prepare the drink by blending 8–16 oz of reverse osmosis with UV lamp water or unsweetened, low-sodium tomato juice with 1 heaping teaspoon (12 gm) of whey protein powder plus 1 rounded teaspoon (8 gm) of glutamine amino acid powder. Stir vigorously with the teaspoon. The whey protein must be specified as "isolates from cross flow microfiltration and ion-exchange, ultrafiltered concentrate, low molecular weight, and partially hydrolyzed whey protein peptides rich in branched-chain amino acids and glutamine peptides." The low-carbohydrate type at 1 gm per scoop or less is best, but it should not be more than 4–5 gm of carbohydrates per scoop. Do not substitute protein from soy, egg, casein, or any other source. Sugar or any other sweetener is unacceptable. Use the natural flavor without additives. This amino acid drink can be enjoyed anytime with or without a meal. **Keep in the refrigerator after opening. Old product should be discarded because it can support bacteria and become contaminated. Whey protein powder can cause some gas and an unusually full feeling.**

Strong, Healthy Bodies Require Essential Fatty Acids

Alpha-linolenic fatty acid (ALA), eicosapentaenoic acid (EPA), and docosahexaenoic fatty acid (DHA) are the three most nutritionally important omega-3 fatty acids. Alpha-linolenic fatty acid is one of two fatty acids traditionally classified as essential.

Carlson's® Lemon Flavored Cod Liver Oil is an excellent source for supplemental omega-3 fatty acids. However, the one-teaspoon daily serving listed on the label is not sufficient to meet the goal of providing optimal nutrition. Instead, take one tablespoon with breakfast and one tablespoon with dinner.

Essential omega-6 linoleic fatty acid is the precursor for arachidonic fatty acid that is often referred to as being essential. Meat has generous amounts of arachidonic fatty acid, and no additional dietary supplementation is required to achieve optimal health.

I received a letter from a bodybuilder who complained about the results he achieved when he followed the high carbohydrate diet suggested in books and magazines. He explained that he gained muscle mass on the program but also gained a considerable amount of body fat. He was very upset and considered himself to be a slob rather than a muscleman. He switched to my low carbohydrate ketogenic bodybuilding diet and had great results. He lost body fat and maintained his good muscular structure. In future workouts, he can continue to build strong muscles, ligaments, tendons, and bone collagen without adding body fat.

About 30% of the bone matrix consists of collagen (protein structure that provides the strength or tensile-bearing capacity of the bone). Bones generally break from tensile fractures, not compression failure as is commonly thought. Weak bones are the result of a protein-deficient diet. Yes, red meat builds strong bones—calcium supplements don't. Women are prone to bone and hip fractures because they believe the mass media and professional nutrition societies that tell them to shun red meat and take calcium tablets. It hasn't worked because it's scientifically false. Hip fractures are becoming more common because women are trying even harder to comply with erroneous recommendations. Remember, if it's common mass media hype, it's most likely wrong.

Red meat builds strong bones.

My wife, Marti, took a serious fall on her bicycle when she accidently clipped a garbage can that had been placed in the street. She crashed hard on the pavement, landing flat on her hip and side. Her hip was bruised, and she had abrasions on her arm and palm of the hand. She had an annual checkup with her doctor two weeks later, and the doctor was irate when Marti told her she would not take the bone density test typically given to all senior and even middle-aged women. Marti told the doctor she had already given herself a bone density test two weeks earlier when she crashed her bike. The doctor still wasn't pleased with her refusal to take the test.

Most women Marti's age no longer ride a bicycle, let alone survive a serious crash with only bruises and abrasions. Medical and nutritional experts seem to have a very misguided understanding of human physiology because they are continually giving advice that is directly opposite to the scientific truth. Protein builds strong bones, not calcium.

Reversing Heart Disease and Preventing Diabetes

Chapter 8

Scientific Proof Feedlot Beef Is Awesome Food

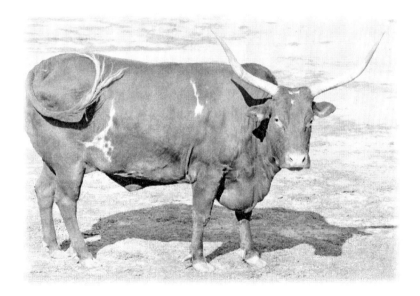

Texas Longhorn Steer

There have been no independent studies or tests to show that grass-fed beef steaks taste better than feedlot beef steaks. The opposite is true. Feedlot beef steaks generally receive a higher grading because they have fattier marbling. In a blind taste test, feedlot beef will be rated as tasting better than grass-fed beef. The organic and grass-fed beef producers' claim that their meat tastes better and is healthier is simply false, and gullible consumers believe it because they are psychologically brainwashed. If you tell lies often enough, people will believe them.

A generous amount of marbled fat in meat gives the delicious flavor people enjoy.

Grass-fed beef producers generally claim their meat is leaner, and this is true. However, lean meat always gets a lower USDA grading than fatty meat with good fat marbling. Grass-fed beef producers speak of beef fat as if it were unhealthy. Feedlot operators give the cattle the optimal fortified nutrition to build healthy muscle and fat. Remember, beef fat is very healthy food as I have proved in previous chapters. They also claim their beef has a higher omega-3 fat content. Both of these claims are false. All beef fat, including the saturated fat, is very healthy, and the omega-3 content is the same as found in feedlot beef. Your health and healing could suffer if you depend on grass-fed beef for the essential omega-3 fatty acids. Eat fresh salmon at least once a week and take Carlson's® lemon flavored cod liver oil as recommended in Chapters 4 and 5.

The beef industry is its own worst enemy. Hoping to increase sales of its product, the smaller grass-fed beef industry criticizes the larger feedlot producers, but by doing so they turn people away from eating beef entirely. Few people are willing to pay the outrageous price for grass-fed beef because regular supermarket beef is expensive compared to pork, chicken, and turkey.

Scientific Proof Feedlot Beef is Awesome Food

I receive numerous letters from grass-fed beef promoters who falsely claim that grain fed to feedlot steers somehow makes the meat less nutritious, but they never provide scientific support for their claim. Cows are herbivores. They eat grain because it is their natural food. Grain does not make the steers unhealthy. It promotes weight gain consisting of both lean meat and fat in the same way as the high-carbohydrate diet promotes obesity in humans. The meat producer desires to have fat-laced meat because it has better flavor and is actually healthier for the consumer, contrary to the false claims from people with fat phobias.

The beef industry is its own worst enemy.

The beef industry falsely emphasizes that cuts which are naturally low in fat are healthier. The industry does very little to defend its own product from misrepresentation. This chapter presents the truth about beef because the beef industry won't.

Beef contains heme iron that is essential for good health. Whole grains contain free elemental non-heme iron that is unhealthy. Elemental iron promotes the oxidation of LDL cholesterol within the endothelial layers of the blood vessels. Some researchers have implicated free elemental non-heme iron as a risk factor for heart disease. Therefore, the iron in whole grains and other vegetable foods can be a risk factor for heart disease, but the heme iron in beef and other meat is not. Vegetarians often have iron deficiency anemia because elemental iron from grains and vegetables is not well absorbed. Heme iron found in meat, poultry, and fish is absorbed more easily than the non-heme iron found in plant foods. For example, your body absorbs four times as much iron from a 6.4 ounce (180 gram) serving of cooked beef sirloin steak than from a 1½ cup (350 ml) serving of bran flakes.

591

Heme iron is also better than non-heme iron because it does not accumulate in the body to cause an unhealthy overdose. The body can easily secrete the extra heme iron obtained from eating red meat to maintain a healthy balance, but the body has a difficult time getting rid of excess non-heme iron obtained from eating whole grains and vegetables. The body regulates heme iron in a natural manner, but elemental iron tends to promote a deficiency or excess, generally a deficiency.

Eating red meat prevents iron deficiency anemia.

Do not buy any beef that is labeled as containing "natural flavors." Yes, the additives are naturally bad for you. Typical additives are sugar and monosodium glutamate (MSG), a nerve toxin that makes cancers incurable. In some countries, this practice is widespread and the meat has been given the nickname *sweet meat*. Do not buy any meat labeled as containing natural flavors—period.

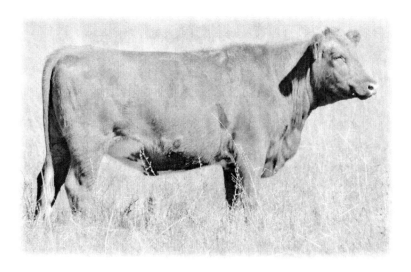

Red Angus Cow in Winter Grass Pasture

Scientific Proof Feedlot Beef is Awesome Food

Is Beef Safe to Eat?

Beef is one of the healthiest foods you can eat. Beef is naturally loaded with protein, fats, vitamins, minerals, enzymes, and a multitude of other nutrients that are essential for optimal health. All of the negative claims about red meat are untrue, and upon close examination, the negative studies are always found to be falsified in some manner. A diet consisting of 100% red meat provides wonderful health.

The claims that supermarket beef contains harmful antibiotics, hormones, insecticides, toxins, diseases, and bad fats are simply false. I will expose these myths, distortions, and lies propagated by vegetarians, grass-fed beef salesmen, and carbohydrate food manufacturing companies.

Feedlot beef is safe to eat. Don't believe the lies.

The responsibility for assuring the safety of our meat supply is on the shoulders of the United States Department of Agriculture (USDA). This is reason enough to be highly suspicious of our meat. The USDA does not promote meat as healthy food, so I will. Our supermarket beef is a safe, wholesome, and very healthy when it isn't processed or contaminated with unhealthy additives as mentioned. I am not suggesting that you eat meat containing pesticides, antibiotics, and synthetic hormones. I am saying that supermarket feedlot beef does not contain pesticides, antibiotics, and synthetic hormones. I will address these issues in great detail later in this chapter. If supermarket beef were not healthy, I would be the first to condemn it. I reversed my heart disease while eating high-fat cuts of supermarket beef along with the fat.

593

Chapter 8

Are Humans Designed to Eat Meat?

In Chapter 2, I presented detailed scientific proof that meat is an ideal food. The design of our digestive organs and digestive enzymes shows that mankind is basically a carnivorous species with the ability to digest carbohydrates from grains, nuts, legumes, fruits, and vegetables. Health is damaged and declines in proportion to the amount of carbohydrates consumed. As discussed in previous chapters, the high-carbohydrate diet causes many diseases.

Meat does not putrefy in the gut as vegetarians falsely claim. The stomach secretes a large amount of acid and enzymes to break down the protein into individual amino acids for absorption in the small intestine. The body was designed to digest meat and does so without the need for bacteria.

Does Meat Contain Genetically Modified Organisms?

I do not recommend eating foods containing genetically modified organisms (GMO or GM), but they are almost impossible to avoid in the United States. Buying foods labeled "GMO-Free" is not only a waste of money but encourages corruption in the food industry that rakes in huge profits.

The diet therapy program I present in this book will help to protect you from GMO risks. The reason is scientific. This program is based largely on animal protein and natural animal fats. The GM organisms are commonly found in grains, legumes, vegetables, and fruits. Pasture grasses and hay fed to feedlot steers are rarely contaminated with GM organisms. Animals, birds, and fish digest vegetation that can contain GMOs, but their digestive systems and livers will breakdown most of the GM molecules before they can be incorporated into the flesh. Their kidneys discharge some of the undesirable molecules in the

594

urine, and additional GM molecules will be discharged in the feces. Therefore, animal protein and fats give us protection from GMO molecules. On the other hand, the vegetarian diet provides direct exposure to GMO molecules in whole grains, fruits, and vegetables.

Soybean plants are the most genetically modified organism (GMO) in the food supply of the United States. As of January 2006, the percentage of soybeans that have been genetically modified is estimated to be 75% and climbing fast. Virtually all soy products on supermarket shelves have been contaminated. Just because a soy product is labeled as organic does not mean it is GMO-free. Vegetarians gorge themselves on soy milk and soy burgers. In a frantic effort to provide amino acids in the diet, vegetarian foods such as breads, bagels, cereals, crackers, pastas, snack bars, and energy drinks have been fortified with soy protein made from GMO contaminated soybeans.

Vegetarians have a high exposure to GMO foods.

Virtually all grains and seeds that are thought to be natural have been GM or GMO contaminated by unintentional cross breeding. This applies to grains such as wheat, maize (corn), oats, spelt, barley, rice, millet, rye, amaranth, quinoa, and buckwheat. Seed foods, including flax, mustard, rapeseed, sunflower, hemp, and poppy are contaminated with GM organisms. Buying GMO-free grains and seeds is a waste of money because you are simply purchasing a fraudulent product at an exorbitant price and encouraging corruption within the food supply chain. The only way to escape GMO contaminated vegetarian foods in the United States is to not eat them.

Is Raw Meat Healthier Than Cooked Meat?

Raw meat is not healthier than properly cooked meat. Rare steaks taste better to me, and I have never gotten ill from eating them. However, the surface must be seared enough to kill all pathogens, Ground beef must be thoroughly cooked until the center does not show any pink, but overcooked meat is unhealthy because the fats become rancid from oxidation. Recent claims that raw meat is healthier than cooked meat are false and dangerous. Eating raw ground beef could give you food poisoning and kill you.

Steaks grilled and served rare are perfectly acceptable if they have never been stabbed with a fork before cooking. A fork stabbed into raw meat will push the surface contamination into the center where bacteria will not be killed unless the meat is thoroughly cooked. If in doubt, cook the meat until the center is not pink—a point where the temperature above 160 degrees F. (70 degrees C.).

Raw fish and other raw seafood present a risk for parasitic infection as is the case with raw pork. Eating raw chicken or turkey presents a risk for deadly salmonella or pathogenic infection. Laws in the United States allow food to be treated with high-energy gamma radiation in order to destroy most pathogens. I know one restaurant that does not hesitate to serve expensive ground beef burgers cooked rare. I have never ordered mine rare because I don't know if the beef has been irradiated. On my recent visit, I asked the waitress about it, and she reluctantly admitted it had been irradiated. She felt better when I told her I preferred it that way. The risk for E-coli poisoning is much more serious than the risk from gamma radiation. I don't go there often because the meat is too lean, and they cater to the public's fat phobia.

What is food irradiation?

http://digestive.niddk.nih.gov/ddiseases/pubs/bacteria/#9

"Food irradiation is the treatment of food with high energy such as gamma rays, electron beams, or x rays as a means of cold pasteurization, which destroys living bacteria to control foodborne illnesses. The United States relies exclusively on the use of gamma rays, which are similar to ultraviolet light and microwaves and pass through food leaving no residue. Food irradiation is approved for wheat, potatoes, spices, seasonings, pork, poultry, red meats, whole fresh fruits, and dry or dehydrated products. Although irradiation destroys many bacteria, it does not sterilize food. Even if you're using food that has been irradiated by the manufacturer, you must continue to take precautions against foodborne illnesses—through proper refrigeration and handling—to safeguard against any surviving organisms. If you are traveling with food, make sure perishable items such as meats are wrapped to prevent leakage. Be sure to fill the cooler with plenty of ice and store it in the car, not the trunk. If any food seems warmer than 40°F, throw it out."

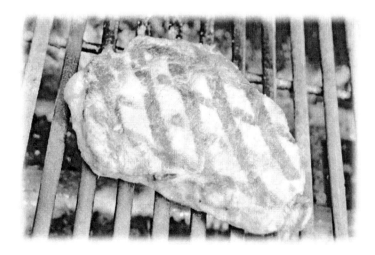

Beef Steak on a Barbeque Grill

597

Chapter 8

Does Supermarket Beef Contain Antibiotics?

This may surprise you, but the answer is, "No." Animals are given antibiotics at times, but the residue is not permitted in the final meat that you buy at the supermarket. Antibiotics are removed over time by the animals' bodies just as they are in humans. The administration of antibiotics is stopped in advance of slaughter to allow them to be removed naturally by the animals. The clearing time is approximately two weeks but varies according to the manufacturer of the antibiotic or drug. Therefore, we should have very little concern about the presence of antibiotics in the meat we purchase at the supermarket.

Meat from feedlot beef does not contain antibiotics.

Myth: The use of antibiotics and growth hormone implants in livestock production is causing hazardous residues in beef and contributing to the development of health problems in humans.

Fact: No residues from antibiotics or growth hormones are found in supermarket feedlot beef, and there is no valid scientific evidence that antibiotic use in cattle causes any illness or results in the development of antibiotic-resistant bacteria.

The following reference explains the procedure for the administration of antibiotics and other drugs to animals intended for human consumption.

> **Focus on Beef – USDA**
> http://www.fsis.usda.gov/Fact_Sheets/Beef_from_Farm_to_T
> able/index.asp
>
> "Antibiotics may be given to prevent or treat disease in cattle. A "withdrawal" period is required from the time antibiotics are administered until it is legal to slaughter the animal. This is

> so residues can exit the animal's system. FSIS randomly samples cattle at slaughter and tests for residues. Data from this Monitoring Plan have shown a very low percentage of residue violations. Not all antibiotics are approved for use in all classes of cattle. However, if there is a demonstrated therapeutic need, a veterinarian may prescribe an antibiotic that is approved in other classes for an animal in a non-approved class. In this case, no detectable residues of this drug may be present in the edible tissues of the animal at slaughter."

I have not found any study from a reliable source which shows that supermarket feedlot beef contains unhealthy antibiotics, hormones, pesticides, herbicides, or any other toxins. I have not found any study from a reliable source which shows that eating supermarket feedlot beef causes any disease, ailment, or health concern. Statements that claim otherwise are simply propaganda.

Eating organic vegetables could increase the risk for ingesting antibiotics when the plants are fertilized with manure from animal feedlots. Approximately 90% of the antibiotics given to animals are excreted in the feces and urine. Organic farmers spread the manure on the soil where the plants can then absorb the antibiotics. Organic vegetables are more likely to contain antibiotics than supermarket meats.

Does Supermarket Beef Contain Unsafe Hormones?

This may surprise you, but the answer is, "No." Animals are given hormones to increase growth and to correct the deficiencies caused by castrating young bulls. However, these animals have naturally occurring hormones that are also found in humans and other animals. These hormones are not permitted to be of a nature or quantity that would present any health hazard when consumed by humans.

> **Beef - From Farm to Table – USDA**
> http://www.fsis.usda.gov/Fact_Sheets/Beef_from_Farm_to_T able/index.asp
>
> "Hormones may be used to promote efficient growth. Estradiol, progesterone, and testosterone (three natural hormones), and zeranol and trenbolone acetate (two synthetic hormones) may be used as an implant on the animal's ear. The hormone is time released, and is effective for 90 to 120 days. In addition, melengesterol acetate, which can be used to suppress estrus, or improve weight gain and feed efficiency, is approved for use as a feed additive. Not all combinations of hormones are approved for use in all classes of cattle. Hormones are approved for specific classes of animals only, and cannot be used in non-approved classes."

Hormones are naturally present in infinitesimal amounts in all meat regardless of whether or not the animals have been implanted. There is more estrogen in plant-source foods (especially soy) than in meat. The human body produces hormones in quantities much greater than would ever be consumed by eating beef or other foods. Hormones in beef from implanted steers have no physiological significance for humans whatsoever. The estrogen level in a 9 oz. serving of beef from an implanted steer is 5.55 nanograms where one nanogram is one billionth of a gram. The level in the same size portion of beef from a non-implanted steer is 3.9 nanograms. By comparison, a non-pregnant woman produces 480,000 nanograms of estrogen daily.

Meat from feedlot steers does not contain unhealthy hormones.

It is interesting that so many women are in a panic about hormones in beef when they are taking massive doses of synthetic hormones for birth control and hormone replacement therapy after menopause. They also eat food and drink water from plastic bottles that contain esters that are chemically similar to estrogen. All meat for human consumption contains natural hormones, but these do not produce any illnesses or diseases.

Those with an agenda have brainwashed people to believe they should avoid eating supermarket feedlot beef because it is full of dreadful hormones, yet they jump headlong into the soy mania as they consume mega doses of phytoestrogens that seriously disrupt healthy hormones levels in both sexes. A phytoestrogen is a molecule that appears very similar to the human estrogen molecule, but it is not the same. The phytoestrogens enter receptor sites that are intended for estrogen. Since phytoestrogens are not the same as estrogens, they disrupt the normal function and cause long-term illnesses and diseases. The panic over beef hormones is totally unwarranted.

Soy products should be outlawed for human consumption, but soy continues to be used as a protein replacement for meat. Phytoestrogens from soy products are believed to contribute to the early maturation of females and the late maturation of males.

Does Supermarket Beef Contain Pesticides?

This may surprise you, but the answer is, "No." Cattle and other animals could possibly get pesticides from corn, grain, and hay but this is unlikely. Pesticides that are presently approved in the

United States are highly biodegradable and are not likely to be on the animals' food supply at the time it is eaten. In addition, the animals remove the pesticides the same way humans do—through the liver. Very little pesticide residues remains in the flesh and fat.

Meat from feedlot beef does not contain pesticides.

The United States Department of Agriculture (USDA) has regulations that list each pesticide and the corresponding limit of residue allowed in meat, poultry, and eggs. The following reference is available for those wishing to see the details.

> **U.S. Residue Limits For Pesticides In Meat, Poultry, and Egg Products 2001 FSIS National Residue Program**
> http://www.fsis.usda.gov/OPHS/red_book_2001/2001_Resid ue_Limits_Pesticides_App5.pdf

Amino acids found in red meat are natural detoxifiers. They protect against radiation, pollution, ultra-violet light, chemicals, and other sources of free radicals. Aspartic and glutamic amino acids found in red meat protect the liver by helping to remove ammonia from the body.

Does Supermarket Feedlot Beef Contain Bad Fats?

This may surprise you, but the answer is, "No." The national and state beef associations in the United States are their own worst enemies because they propagate the false notion that beef fat is unhealthy by suggesting you eat the low-fat cuts. Beef contains very healthy fats that are essential in the human diet in order to grow, heal, and thrive. Yes, beef contains saturated fats, but saturated fats are not the villains described by the politically correct nutrition groups. Saturated fats are very healthy foods.

Does Beef Have a Poor Essential Fatty Acid Ratio?

The ratio of essential omega-6 to omega-3 fatty acids is very good for some cuts of beef but a little higher in others. The difference is negligible. The ratio for venison and elk meat can be higher than in some cuts of beef. The claims that supermarket feedlot beef has an unhealthy ratio are pure fantasy and propaganda. Dr. Mary G. Enig's research found in her book, *Know Your Fats*, shows that all meat is healthy.

Type of Meat	Omega-3 fat, g	Omega-6 fat, g	Omega-6/3 Ratio
Deer/Venison Roasted, 3.5 oz.	0.09	0.53	5.9
Elk Meat Roasted, 3.5 oz.	0.06	0.34	5.7
Buffalo Meat Roasted, 3.5 oz.	0.06	0.14	2.3
Beef Steak, Club Broiled, 1/4" Trim, 3.5 oz.	0.02	0.28	14.0
Beef Roasted, Bottom Round, 1/4" Trim, 3.5 oz.	0.17	0.47	2.8
Lamb, Shoulder Roast, 1/4" Trim, 3.5 oz.	0.34	1.27	3.7

Chapter 8

Is Grass-Fed Beef Better Than Supermarket Beef?

Feedlot beef can technically be said to be organic if the animal is never given antibiotics or hormones. All the feed must also be from organic sources. The trick occurs when the seller labels the meat as organic but keeps the feedlot method of fattening a secret, thereby tricking the vast majority of the public who never suspect they have purchased feedlot beef. There is no official *organic* classification for beef, and using the term may be false advertising. However, the price of organic and grass-fed beef is extremely high, and the profit margins could be 300–500% greater than regular supermarket beef. This high profit margin provides extra funds for producers to promote their products with scare tactics and false information that claim supermarket feedlot beef is unhealthy. Many low-carbohydrate and Paleolithic diet gurus are jumping on the bandwagon and promoting organic and grass-fed beef because it sounds so pure and natural. We can be certain that a high percentage of the grass-fed beef sold is actually feedlot beef that has been mislabeled in order to reap the tremendous profits. The producer may have a pasture with grazing steers, but what percentage of the meat shipped is from steers raised in that pasture or the open range below?

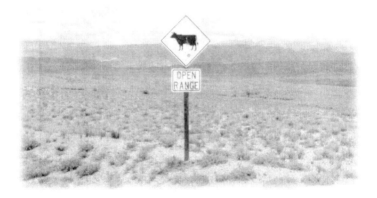

Does Beef Cause Cancer and Other Diseases?

Natural unprocessed fresh beef and other natural meats heal the body and prevent disease. Beef contains all of the essential nutrients needed to build a healthy body and the strong immune system needed to fight disease. All immune cells are made from polypeptides that are composed of amino acids derived from the digestion of meat. The following is a list of the major cells of the immune system.

- Lymphocytes are a category of adaptive cells that include B cells, T cells, and others that are made in the bone marrow from hematopoietic stem cells.

- Natural killer cells (or NK cells) are major cells that destroy cells that have been infected by viruses. NK cells also attack tumors. NK cells are cytotoxic lymphocytes of the innate immune system.

- Killer T cells, a T cell sub-group, destroy cells that have been damaged or infected with a virus or other pathogens.

- Helper T cells determine how the innate and adaptive immune systems should respond to pathogens.

- γδ T cells perform some of the same functions as helper T cells, cytotoxic T cells, and NK cells.

- B cells are lymphocytes that identify pathogens and mark them with antibodies that are bound to the surface. Antibodies and other immune system cells attack and destroy the identified pathogens.

Meat prevents cancer by building a strong immune system.

Chapter 8

Christian B. Allan, Ph.D., and Wolfgang Lutz, M.D., identified the connection between carbohydrate consumption and cancer in the following book:

Life Without Bread
by Christian B. Allan, Ph.D. and Wolfgang Lutz, M.D.

"After carbohydrates are consumed, the levels of sugar and glucose in the blood rise. The body responds by releasing insulin from the pancreas into the bloodstream. The carbohydrate theory of cancer is simple:

Too much insulin and glucose in the blood can cause cells to dedifferentiate, just as they do in cell lines, and thus can be a primary cause of dietary-related cancer." (Pages 169-170)

"There have been many studies done, in animals and people, that indicate that fat content in the diet is not responsible for breast cancer or any other cancer. We know there's a tendency to blame dietary fat for just about everything that goes wrong, but that's just a lazy way out. Time after time, the studies show it just isn't true." (Page 173)

"The Eskimos who ate only fat and protein never had any cancer in their population until a Western (high-carbohydrate) diet was introduced. Why don't we ever hear of cancer of the heart? Probably because the heart uses almost all fat for energy, thus cancer does not have a chance to develop in those cells. We hope that researchers will take the next step and start looking at what has been known for a long time. Dietary related cancer is a sugar metabolism disease just like all the others." (Page 177)

However, highly processed meats have been linked to colon cancer. Early results of a major new study suggest that eating lots of preserved meats, such as salami, bacon, cured ham, and hot dogs, could increase the risk for bowel cancer by 50%. Fresh red meats, including beef, lamb, pork, and veal, prevent cancer. Previous studies linking meat intake to colorectal cancer were fraudulent and produced distorted results because they grouped fresh and processed meats together.

Does Red Meat Cause Weak Bones?

Animal protein does not cause osteoporosis as falsely claimed. Amino acids from dietary protein are the building blocks for bone collagen that give bones strength to resist breakage. Weak hip joints are the result of a protein deficiency caused by the inadequate consumption of meat—not a calcium deficiency. Osteoporosis, low bone density, and hip fractures are common in elderly women because they are the group most likely to shun red meat and saturated fats. Collagen, not calcium, gives bones tensile strength. Magnesium is the supplement of choice for dense bone mineral deposits. I have never had a broken bone and do not take any calcium supplements, but I strongly recommend magnesium.

Does Eating Meat Cause Kidney Disease?

Eating large quantities of red meat will not give you kidney disease as often claimed. Dr. Richard K. Bernstein corrected the misunderstanding about kidney disease and dietary protein in his book.

Diabetes Solution - Chapter 9
by Dr. Richard K. Bernstein

"If you are a long-standing diabetic and are frustrated with the care you've received over the years, you have probably been conditioned to think that protein is more of a poison than sugar and is the cause of kidney disease. I was conditioned the same way—many years ago, as I mentioned,

I had laboratory evidence of advanced proteinuria, signifying potentially fatal kidney disease—but in this case, the conventional wisdom is just a myth."

"Non-diabetics who eat a lot of protein don't get diabetic kidney disease. Diabetics with normalized blood sugars don't get diabetic kidney disease. High levels of dietary protein do not cause kidney disease in diabetics or anyone else. There is no higher incidence of kidney disease in the cattle-growing states of the United States, where many people eat steak every day, than there is in the states where beef is more expensive and consumed to a much lesser degree. Similarly, the incidence of kidney disease in vegetarians is the same as the incidence of kidney disease in non-vegetarians. It is the high blood sugar levels that are unique to diabetes, and to a much lesser degree the high levels of insulin required to cover them (causing hypertension), that cause the complications associated with diabetes."

Are Confined Dairy Cows Unhealthy?

Dairy cows and special breeding stock are kept for several years until they are no longer productive. The dairyman or rancher must be concerned about the proper nutritional science for the animals in order to increase the health, productivity, and longevity.

Most dairy cows do not have a grass pasture in which to forage, especially in the larger operations. The basic controlled nutritional program for dairy cows is generally a combination of hay or straw, cereal grains, supplemental fats, vitamins, and minerals. The cows raised with a good controlled nutritional program are more productive and healthier than those with a grass pasture diet only contrary to the false statements made by the promoters of dairy products from grass-fed cows.

Barley is a preferred grain that gives the diary cow more condensed calories and increases body heat—a desirable effect to keep the cow warm. Barley has a good balance of protein, calories, and fiber. Remember, cows have a digestive system that processes the food by fermentation, including the complete digestion of fiber. This process is totally different from that in humans where fermentation results in inflammatory bowel diseases as I discussed in *Absolute Truth Exposed – Volume 1.*

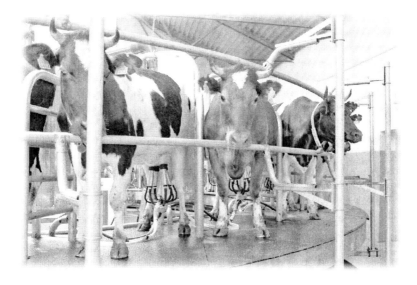

Mechanized Cow Milking Operation in Ukraine

Scientific studies have found that lactating dairy cows fed supplemental fats have a better conception rate and improved longevity. These fats can be a variety of animal and vegetable fats or a mixture of many different fatty acids. These fats are generally by-products of the food manufacturing industry.

Chapter 8

Is Premium High-Fat Kobe Beef Unhealthy?

The best beef in the world comes from Kobe cattle that have been raised in Japan since the second century. This high-fat beef comes from the black Tajima-ushi breed of Wagyu cattle raised in Hyōgo Prefecture, Japan, according to strict traditions. Herd isolation and strict breeding control have maintained the purity of the breed and high quality of the meat. The exceedingly high-fat Kobe beef has superior flavor and tenderness due to the uniformly marbled fat. The meat is served as a delicacy in expensive restaurants.

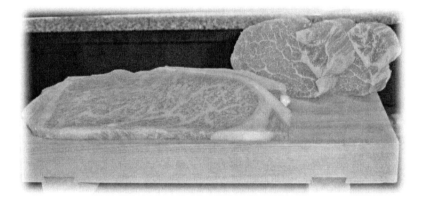

Premium Kobe Beef from Wagyu Cattle of Japan

The special treatment of the cattle, including hand massaging their hind quarters, makes the steaks and other cuts very expensive for the consumer. Recognizing the profit potential, cattlemen in other countries have also begun to raise and market the highly-prized meat from Wagyu cattle. Cattle ranchers in the United States have created a special beef by crossbreeding the Wagyu and Angus cattle to create a high-class meat called *Kobe-style* beef that has a darker color and bolder flavor. This special breed is fed grass and grain rather than the more expensive feed used in Japan. Most of the other Kobe and

Kobe-style beef producers also ignore the expensive hand massage.

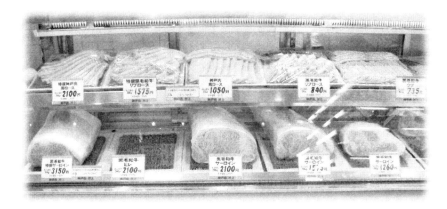

Japanese Market Selling Premium Kobe Beef

I am not suggesting you purchase Kobe beef unless cost is of no concern because it is very expensive. The high price proves that high-fat beef steaks are the most delicious and tender, and some people are willing to pay the price for this high-quality meat.

Why Is Beef an Awesome Health Food?

In summary, high-fat beef is an awesome health food that everyone should eat in generous amounts as often as desired. Scientific studies presented in previous chapters have shown that lowering the dietary intake of saturated fats will increase the risk factors for artery disease, diabetes, Syndrome X, and cancer, all of which have skyrocketed in recent years in concert with the dogma against red meat and saturated animal fats.

High-fat beef is an awesome health food.

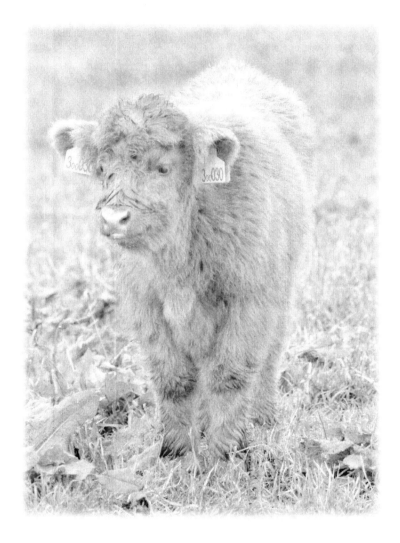

Scottish Highlands Calf

Reversing Heart Disease and Preventing Diabetes

Chapter 9

Paleolithic Diet Facts and Fiction

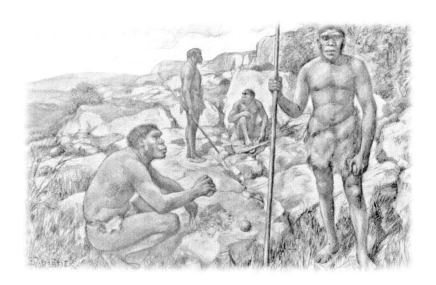

T he Paleolithic diet gets its name from theoretical ancient Paleolithic (hunter-gatherer) cavemen who are said to have been the forerunners to modern humans in the evolutionary tree. The diet derived from this philosophy arouses great emotion in devoted followers. The number of Paleolithic diet supporters may be equal to or greater than the number who favor the vegetarian diet, low-carbohydrate diet, or macrobiotic diet (a diet based on locally-grown whole grains, fruits, vegetables, and a limited amount of fish and other animal products). In this chapter, I will examine the Paleolithic diet by taking a fresh look at the archeological evidence, human physiology, and nutritional science. I will point out assumptions in the diet that I believe are pure conjecture. Although supporters may differ slightly, the Paleolithic diet was developed from the following typical assumptions:

- Paleolithic man evolved over several millions of years as a hunter-gatherer who hunted game animals for food and clothing and gathered vegetarian foods. He was neither hunter only nor gatherer only.

- Paleolithic man evolved on the diet as outlined below. Therefore, the assumption is made that this was the optimal diet for him and for us today.

- Paleolithic man did not cultivate grains or legumes and did not domesticate animals for milk and meat. Therefore, grains, legumes, milk, and milk products are not included in the Paleolithic diet.

- Paleolithic man ate the lean meat from game animals and discarded the fatty portions. He also discarded the pure fat layers found on many animals.

- Paleolithic man found bee hives from which he obtained honey.

Paleolithic Diet Facts and Fiction

Summary of the Paleolithic Diet

The foods listed in most Paleolithic diet books, websites, articles, and references must be unprocessed, organic, and free from genetically modified organisms. I list the typical groups and individual items below.

Caution!
I do not recommend the
Paleolithic diet outlined below!

- **Meat** – Beef, goat, lamb, pork, rabbit, fowl, fish, etc.

- **Game Meat** – Deer, elk, caribou, sheep, antelope, buffalo, bear, moose, turkey, duck, swan, goose, seal, pelican, kangaroo, and other wild game worldwide.

- **Fish** – Trout, bass, salmon, tuna, halibut, pike, cod, haddock, mackerel, herring, etc.

- **Shell Fish** – Lobster, shrimp, scallop, mussel, oyster, clam, crab, etc.

- **Poultry** – Chicken, turkey, goose, quail, dove, pigeon, etc.

- **Eggs** – Chicken, duck, quail, goose, etc.

- **Fats** – Natural animal fats, vegetable oils, etc.

- **Vegetables** – Brussels sprouts, eggplant, beet, celery, cauliflower, tomato, cucumber, asparagus, avocado, broccoli, cabbage, onion, pepper, etc.

- **Root vegetables** – Potato, sweet potato, carrot, yam, beet, turnip, parsnip, etc.

- **Squash** – Yellow, zucchini, butternut, acorn, pumpkin, etc.

- **Nuts** – Walnut, cashew, Brazil nut, pine nut, macadamia, chestnut, almond, hazelnut, pecan, etc.

- **Seeds** – Pumpkin, sunflower, sesame, etc.

- **Fruit** – Apple, pear, peach, grape, banana, orange, berries, grapefruit, plum, pineapple, mango, cantaloupe, watermelon, cherry, apricot, date, tangerine, etc.

- **Mushrooms** – Morel, button, Portobello, shiitake, etc.

- **Spices and herbs** – Ginger, pepper, garlic, onion, parsley, thyme, rosemary, mint, oregano, basil, chive, tarragon, dill, sage, etc.

- **Sweets** – Honey.

Caution!
I do not recommend the
Paleolithic diet outlined above!

I believe that many of the assumptions and conclusions used to formulate the Paleolithic diet are false, and the diet does not provide optimal health for people today as claimed.

Paleolithic Diet Mistake No. 1 - Evolution

Paleolithic diet mistake number one is the assumption that mankind evolved over several millions of years. Mankind has left behind the Great Pyramids of Egypt (4,500 years ago), the Great Wall of China extending 3,400 miles in length (started 2,700 years ago), Silbury Hill in England (4,600 years ago), and Stonehenge in England (5,000 years ago). These and other structures were made by man and date back approximately 4,500 years. Our complex languages like Greek date back 4,000 years with few changes in the modern languages. According to archaeological diggings, there are locations all over the Earth dating back 4,000 years where civilizations would typically choose to live, yet we cannot find any human settlements dating back 10,000 years. Where are the pictures of the structures they built 10,000 years ago? There aren't any because no structures existed. They simply do not exist because humans did not exist at that time. Ape-like creatures such as Home Erectus existed, but they are not human predecessors as claimed.

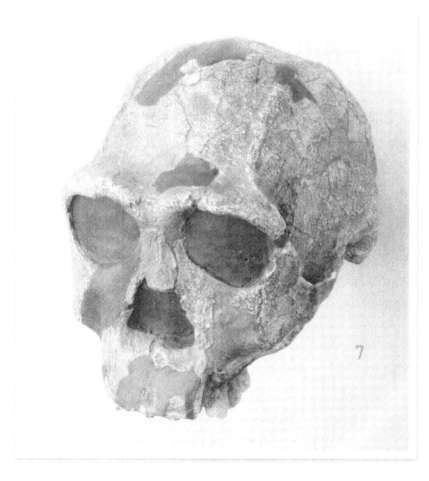

Homo Erectus Skull
Naturmuseum Freiburg, Breisgau, Germany

Create a timeline with 1,000,000 divisions representing years. Evolutionists tell us that humans have evolved very little over this timeline because evolution progresses very slowly. Based on the Theory of Evolution, we should easily find massive signs of civilization dating back a few hundreds of thousands of years, but the signs of civilization are not there. Humans have existed for the last six divisions only. The previous 994,000 divisions are completely empty. Evolutionists simply ignore the fact that intelligent humans suddenly appeared in the very recent past, certainly within the last 8,000 years. These humans were as smart as humans are today, maybe smarter. They completed awesome construction projects. Where are the cities that date back a mere 20,000 years? There are none. The foundations for many cities should exist if humans existed at that time, but not one city can be found. A simple settlement cannot be found that is 20,000 years old. The only crude tools and bones found are from ape-like creatures. Even these are questionable because the dating methods are not reliable.

The evolutionary theory is based on slow change over millions of years. If this were so, mankind 100,000 years ago should have been as smart as we are today. Why did they show absolutely no progress during the first 96,000 years of this period and explode with advancement in the most recent 4,000 years? The reason is the fact that intelligent humans did not exist 100,000 years ago.

My book, *Big Bang Theory,* provides detailed cosmological, geological, and archeological evidence which proves that life did not continue uninterrupted from the ancient ape-man periods to modern humans. The Earth experienced a violent destruction during the period that I call, *Chaotic Earth,* which was caused by a massive asteroid attack that totally annihilated the apes. This series of events is called *The Gap Theory.*

Paleolithic Diet Mistake No. 2 – Fruit Consumption

Paleolithic diet mistake number two is the assumption that the people consumed fruit on a regular basis. Cavemen did not have a constant supply of high-fructose fruits that are found in our modern supermarkets 365 days of the year. Paleolithic people certainly did not have a wide variety of fruit in any one location.

Paleolithic diet promoters open the "fruit door" to the raging fructose monster.

Most areas on Earth would have had a very few species of fruit available for the short ripening season only. Cavemen may have eaten a sour apple or two each year in some moderate climates.

Paleolithic people did not have access to all of the foods listed above as we have in our modern supermarkets. They had a very limited variety in any one area and different varieties a short distance away.

One author of a book about the diet of Paleolithic people suggests that we eat unlimited quantities of fruit. This is shocking because fruits are simply sugars with a scientific consistency no different from common table sugar. Paleolithic people did not have unlimited quantities of fruit available.

Paleolithic Diet Mistake No. 3 - Healthier

Paleolithic diet mistake number three is the assumption that eating a diet according to the above list will provide excellent health. We do not have sound scientific proof that Paleolithic people even existed, and we certainly have no idea whatsoever how their diet affected the health of the people. The assumption that Paleolithic people achieved optimal health on the diet available to them is only conjecture.

The ancient Eskimos and North American Plains Indians represent better examples of the true Paleolithic diet. Eskimos lived all winter on nothing but caribou meat from which they prepared a mixture of 80% fat and 20% lean protein. Other Eskimo tribes ate an all-meat and animal fat diet of seal, walrus, polar bear, moose, caribou, fox, wolf, whale, fish, and birds. During two expeditions between 1906 and 1912, explorers Vilhjalmur Stefansson and Karsten Anderson found their health to be excellent without eating fruits, nuts, seeds, vegetables, or honey.

The Paleolithic diet is neither scientific nor logical.

The North American Plains Indians lived almost entirely off the buffalo (bison) by preparing a mixture called *pemmican* made from dried lean meat mixed with rendered pure fat. The pemmican diet was 80% fat and 20% protein.

Scientific discoveries show that many groups of people primarily ate the flesh of only one animal species, such as bear, seal, salmon, deer, caribou, bison, or sheep, with very few other options. Many of these people had no fruits, vegetables, nuts, seeds, or honey.

Some references make the false claim that protein in corn fed to beef cattle is transferred to the protein in the meat. This claim is scientifically false. Fermentation in the cows' first stomach and further digestion in the other stomachs break the protein down into the individual amino acids that are then used to build new protein molecules in the cows' flesh. The protein molecules never go from the feed into the animals' flesh.

Paleolithic Diet Mistake No. 4 – Low-Fat Diet

Paleolithic diet mistake number four is the assumption that it was low in fat. Many references take the position that Paleolithic hunter-gatherers ate a lower fat diet because the flesh of wild game is much lower in fat than that of domestic beef. Indeed, wild game flesh is generally much lower in fat than supermarket feedlot beef, but Paleolithic people did not eat the meat only. In fact, studies have shown that ancient people like the North American Indians and Eskimos ate diets very high in animal fats. They preferred the fats and tended to waste the lean meat in times of plenty. Many references try to have it both ways. They say natural animal fat is healthy but go on to treat fat from farm animals as unhealthy, or they suggest that the fat in commercially raised animals is bad and fat from game animals is healthy. The assertions that domestic animal fats are unhealthy are scientifically wrong.

The Paleolithic people did not eat a low-fat diet.

One of the Paleolithic diet authors goes to great lengths to convince us that Paleolithic people ate a moderate to high-fat diet, but he suggests the modern supermarket shopper eat a low-fat diet by cutting off the skin from chicken and the fat from other meats. Obtaining a steady supply of food would have been a major effort for most Paleolithic cultures, and they would never have thrown away the fat from the kill except in rare periods of abundance. Neither would they have gathered low-calorie foods.

The incorrect assumption has been made that Paleolithic people preferred the lean meat and rejected the layers of fat on the animals. For example, lean venison does not taste good, and deer hunters routinely grind it with venison fat or beef fat to improve the flavor. The local supermarkets here in Colorado have a waiting list of hunters who want the suet (beef fat) trimmings to blend with the lean portions of the venison.

Some Paleolithic diet authors have stated that venison is 40% protein and 60% fat, but this figure excludes the layers of fat just under the hide. They suggest that Paleolithic people cut off the fat and threw it away, thereby making a deer roast only 19% fat. This presumption is utterly false. You can be certain that Paleolithic people, if they existed, never threw away animal fat. They would have preferred eating the fattiest meat first as evidenced in more recent but primitive cultures.

Paleolithic Diet Mistake No. 5 - Milk

Paleolithic diet mistake number five is the assumption that the fictitious Paleolithic people never consumed animal milk or milk products. We know that animal milk was consumed as far back as solid scientific information is available. Mammalian animals, such as cattle, goats, sheep, camels, and yak, could have provided milk. The Paleolithic diet supporters appear to have excluded animal milk based on modern diet preferences, not scientific facts or logic.

Paleolithic Diet Mistake No. 6 – Omega-6/Omega-3 Ratio

Paleolithic diet mistake number six is the claim that wild game meat has a much lower (better) omega-6/omega-3 fatty acid ratio than domestic beef. This assertion is put forth to give the impression that our current beef supply is unhealthy, which is false. The table in the previous chapter from her book, *Know Your Fats*, Dr. Mary G. Enig shows that omega-3 fatty acids are higher in supermarket beef and lamb roasts than in wild game. The Paleolithic diet supporters' claim that wild game has more omega-3 fatty acids is scientifically false.

Paleolithic Diet Mistake No. 7 – Same Diet for Millennia

Paleolithic diet mistake number seven is the false assumption that Paleolithic people evolved and adapted to the same diet over a period of tens of thousands of years or longer in accordance with the Theory of Evolution. Primitive people simply did not have access to the same diet for long periods of time. The conditions were too dynamic and the people were nomads. Promoters state that the diet will give us the best health because our Paleolithic ancestors adapted to these foods. The scientific evidence shows that the available foods would have been changing significantly in much shorter time periods.

The Paleolithic people were actually animals of the ape kingdom from which we are not descendants. The entire Paleolithic diet concept is wrong because the evolutionary theory is wrong.

Paleolithic Diet Mistake No. 8 – No Grains or Legumes

Paleolithic diet mistake number eight is the assumption that primitive people did not eat cereal grains and legumes. Ancient people were always frustrated with their inability to store fruits and vegetables. They ate and stored grains and legumes because these are the only two types of foods that can be stored for a long period of time.

Archeology has uncovered stored grains and legumes as old as the known existence of mankind. Egypt has many examples of stored grains and legumes that are thousands of years old—as old as the mummies. Ancient North American Indians left vessels containing grains, seeds, and legumes that have been stored for thousands of years, yet they are able to germinate and grow. Mankind has always eaten these foods whenever they were available because of the storage benefit. The exclusion of grains and legumes from the Paleolithic diet is not scientifically logical.

Chapter 9

It is also illogical to exclude grains but include seeds since cereal grains are essentially the same.

Paleolithic Diet Summary

The Paleolithic diet is pure conjecture without valid, confirmable scientific support. Paleolithic diet promoters take the liberty of fabricating the diet, the people, and their health because no science proves they existed, what they ate if they did exist, or the health outcome of the diet. The diet simply does not conform to reasonable assumptions about the diet and health of ancient Paleolithic people, if they existed at all.

A scientific analysis of the timeline for mankind proves that people could not have existed on Earth 50,000 years ago. Performing a reverse analysis of the progress of mankind raises grave questions about the existence of Paleolithic people. According to the Theory of Evolution, mankind 50,000 years ago would have been as smart as we are today, yet they achieved nothing, built nothing, left nothing, and made no progress. The science is clear. Mankind did not exist 50,000 years ago. The bones found in sediment are those for extinct species of ape-like creatures, not human predecessors.

The Paleolithic diet appears to be a compilation of unprocessed supermarket foods minus grains, legumes, and milk. The diet is composed of cascading false assumptions based on a non-existent premise as the foundation. The Paleolithic diet certainly will not allow you to reverse heart disease as I have done on my diet regimen.

Reversing Heart Disease
and
Preventing Diabetes

Chapter 10

Breaking Weight Loss Plateaus

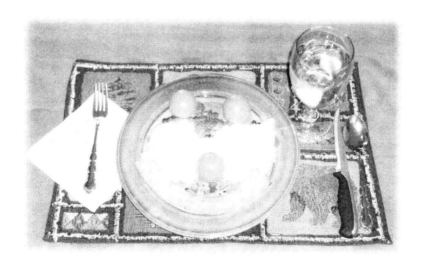

Fried Eggs, Bacon, and Tomatoes
Bacon is lower sodium cured without sugar.

Chapter 10

Stalls, plateaus, and low metabolism are common problems for people who are overweight or obese. Participants in most diet plans have good initial success, and the same can be said for the low-carbohydrate diet. People are highly motivated when they're convinced the diet plan they have chosen will be the one to solve their problem. The low-carbohydrate diet offers many initial advantages. Some of the early weight loss is body fluids, so the diet serves as an excellent diuretic. The high-carbohydrate, low-fat diet makes the body retain fluids and contributes to high blood pressure. This low-carbohydrate diet provides a natural normalization of blood pressure, and those on prescription blood pressure-lowering medications should be prepared to reduce their dosage. The low-carbohydrate diet also allows natural fats which curb the appetite and reduce carbohydrate cravings.

A friend started the low-carbohydrate diet and lost 14 pounds in the first 14 days. He was successful even though he was eating a tremendous number of calories. He hit his first stall and became discouraged when his weight loss completely stopped for the following two weeks. He didn't know what to expect, so he became impatient and returned to his old high-carbohydrate diet. By week six had regained all the weight. It's very important to understand stalls, plateaus, and low metabolism in order to stay on track and make the necessary adjustments to continue on a steady weight-loss curve.

A stall or plateau is a resting place for the body as it adjusts to the new reduced weight. Body weight will remain constant even though the participant is eating exactly the same diet that had provided his good weight loss in the past. This is very common and should be expected.

A reduced metabolism is normal on all diet programs as the body begins to lose weight. Diets which claim otherwise are simply wrong as many people who have experienced diet failures can testify. We often hear it said that a high metabolism is healthy, but that's a myth. A low metabolism is associated with longevity and anti-aging. Animal tests have proved time and time again that a low metabolism provides longer life. The metabolism will drop on the low-carbohydrate diet, which is a health improvement in itself. This low metabolism will require an adjustment in the diet in order to move off the stall or plateau and continue the downward trend. Reject all advice to raise your metabolism.

Other body reactions occur when making a sudden switch from a high-carbohydrate to a low-carbohydrate diet. Because people have rarely used fatty acids as their major energy source, the body is not accustomed to this and must make the adjustment. This period of adjustment can cause weakness or low energy, which will pass over time. During this period, the liver will produce ketones that can be measured in the urine and observed in the mouth. This symptom will pass within a few weeks. Do not think that weight loss has stopped simply because the ketone level has dropped.

General Guidelines
for a Stall and Plateau-Busting Diet

This plateau-busting diet is a low-carbohydrate diet with a little finessing to break a stall and proceed on the weight-loss curve. Knowing the general overall guidelines is important in order to avoid blindly following a strict meal program. You can eat the foods or recipes you desire as long as they comply with these guidelines.

Chapter 10

This stall and plateau-busting diet is more than that. It can be continued for the duration of your weight loss until you reach your goal even if it takes years. This diet plan can be used as a way of life for those who easily regain the weight. This plan is much different from other stall-busting diets that are limited in duration.

Don't be fooled by hype and claims of rapid weight loss that many programs promise. The weight loss of one pound (0.45 kg) per week should be considered normal for a person such as a large male with a high lean body mass. Others should expect less depending on their lean body mass. One half pound (0.23 kg) per week is normal for an average size female. Even so, mini-stalls will occur as weight is lost. Don't panic when a rare but small violation of the guidelines results in the uptick of several pounds. Simply return to the program and watch them fall away just as quickly.

Carbohydrates Must Be Severely Restricted

Carbohydrates are nonessential macronutrients for human health. Avoid carbohydrates because they contribute only calories in the form of sugars and cause many age-related degenerative diseases. Eat protein and fat on this plateau-busting diet because they are essential for human health. The total daily consumption of carbohydrates from the list of allowable non-starchy vegetables should be less than 20 gm., of which 3 gm. will most likely be classified as fiber. Breaking stalls requires strict adherence to a low-carbohydrate diet and the avoidance of fiber. Don't panic about a low-fiber diet. Fiber isn't the harmless indigestible food product that many claim. Bowel functions will become perfectly normal and natural without it. You can read a complete scientific analysis of dietary fiber in my book, *Absolute Truth Exposed – Volume 1.*

Eat Protein within Calorie Limits

Protein from red meat, fowl, fish, seafood, eggs, and cheese is allowed within the calorie limits. Protein is a very nutritionally dense food containing high levels of vitamins, minerals, and essential amino acids. The body can convert 58% of protein to glucose; therefore, high quantities of lean protein are not recommended. The protein should be from fresh or fresh-frozen animal products. Processed meats of any kind, such as deli meats, sausage, hotdogs, and ham, are strictly forbidden. Uncured bacon and bacon cured without maple sugar or other sugars are permitted. The ingredient list must not include sugar. Chicken and turkey that has been injected or coated with a solution of sugar, salt, or natural flavoring must be strictly avoided. However, salt that is applied externally to frozen poultry can be washed off with hot water immediately before cooking. Packaging labels for chicken and turkey should state that the poultry is minimally processed.

Soy protein is strictly forbidden. Whey protein and individual amino acids are permitted and particularly recommended for bodybuilders or those with intestinal or degenerative disc disease. Avoid protein powder until a weight goal has been reached. Grains, nuts, and seeds are unacceptable protein sources because they contain excessive amounts of carbohydrates.

Eat Fats Within Calorie Limits

In the following table, you will see that fat can comprise as much as 70% of the calories in this diet. Fats are vital for human life and contain nutritionally-dense, fat-soluble essential vitamins, such as A, D, E, and K. The percentage of dietary fat is increased by supplementing with omega-3 and omega-6 fatty acids, two critical elements for good health. Take Carlson's® Lemon Flavored Cod Liver Oil for EPA and DHA essential omega-3 fatty acids. Take borage oil with GLA omega-6 fatty acids, but strictly avoid all other omega-6 fatty acids from grains, vegetables, nuts, and seeds.

Substituting flax seeds or flax seed oil for omega-3 fatty acid is strongly discouraged because some people cannot break the fats down into the EPA and DHA omega-3 components, and flax seed oil is too high in inflammatory omega-6 fatty acids. Flax seed oil is promoted as a source for omega-3 fatty acids because it comes from a non animal source, but this diet is primarily animal protein and fats. Don't believe the hype about flax seed oil.

Fats from meat, fowl, fish, and seafood are permitted along with fats from eggs, coconut oil, butter, olive oil, and cheese. The cheese should be a hard type and never spreadable or liquid. Swiss cheese is preferred because of its lower salt content. Avoided cottage cheese because it contains carbohydrates, and scientific studies have proved it to be detrimental to bones.

Vegetables Are Moderately Restricted

Eat moderate amounts of non-starchy vegetables cooked any way you desire. Steam vegetables and add a small pat of butter or stir fry in a little coconut oil. Starchy vegetables, such as potatoes, yams, beets, turnips, pumpkins, and winter squash, are strictly forbidden. Limit moderately starchy vegetables such as carrots and peas. The best low-carbohydrate vegetables are green or yellow beans, cabbage, celery, peppers, spinach, cucumbers, tomatoes, zucchini, or yellow squash. Lettuce gives many people intestinal distress and is strictly forbidden for those with inflammatory bowel disease.

Strictly Avoid Table Salt

Salt causes water retention and high resistance to your weight loss. Use Morton's Salt Substitute® (potassium chloride) in a small, round, blue container that becomes its own shaker. Do not use other brands that contain monopotassium glutamate.

Strictly Control Calories

Restricting calories on the low-carbohydrate diet may not be necessary for those who lose weight easily. However, a stall, plateau, or stubborn metabolism requires total daily calorie intake to be strictly controlled. Consuming too many calories is the primary reason for failures on the low-carbohydrate diet. Simply eating an excessive amount of calories from protein and fat will result in weight gain. Calorie limitation is based on lean body mass, which is the total body weight minus the weight of body fat. A rough goal would be 20% body fat for males and 28% for females. You can guess your lean body mass goal by estimating your desired total weight goal for an ideal body shape. Example: A 5'- 6" (1676 mm) female should weigh about 133 pounds (60.3 kg), and a 6'-2" (1880 mm) male should weigh about 179 pounds (81.2 kg). You probably know your ideal weight based on your body type.

Example calculations for lean body mass (LBM) are as follows:

Female LBM = 133 x (1.00 - 0.28) = 96 pounds (43.5 kg)

Male LBM = 179 x (1.00 - 0.20) = 143 pounds (65 kg)

Total calories per day are according to the following table. The formula for calories is $(LBM/100)^{0.76}$ x 1400. This is a special mathematical formula that I developed because calories are not linear with weight. A smaller person requires more calories per lean body unit weight because heat loss is greater per unit weight for a smaller person. The table applies for both males and females. Do not use the following table to calculate calories based on total weight. Lean body mass is used to calculate calories because body fat does not burn calories. A very obese person is not allowed more calories simply because he weighs more than a slightly overweight person. Muscles, body organs, and heat loss account for the daily calorie requirement, not body fat. This table is a starting point only and may require adjustment up or down depending on the individual. Record your weight every day and compare the weekly change. The failure to lose weight over a two-week period requires a decrease in the daily calorie intake. Intermediate small plateaus can last as long as one week, so be patient. A two-week plateau should be cause for a reduction in calories.

Plateau-Busting Dietary Calorie Limits	
Lean Body Mass	**Calories per Day**
80	1100
90	1150
100	1200
110	1300
120	1400
130	1500
140	1600
150	1800
160	2000

Cheating - The Major Cause of Failure

Do not eat sweets or high-carbohydrate foods. A teaspoon of regular ice cream will block weight loss for at least two days. One third of a sugar cookie (one ounce) every other day will block the entire weight loss of one pound (0.45 kg) per week. You must be consistently diligent in your compliance with the food and calorie restrictions. Little slips render the diet worthless for those with a high-metabolic resistance to weight loss.

Typical Daily Food Guide

Start your stall-busting diet by strictly adhering to the following food table to prove to yourself that continued weight loss is indeed possible. Slowly switch to your favorite foods, but be sure to count every morsel of food and stay within the basic guidelines or calorie limit. The meat category can be any red meat, fowl, fish, or seafood. All meat weights are before cooking. Ground beef can be 80% lean. Canola mayonnaise in limited quantities can be used with lean meat, fish, or vegetables. Nuts will stop a good weight-loss trend dead in its tracks. Don't even think about eating nuts! Low-carbohydrate snacks and bars made with sugar alcohols are absolutely forbidden.

Do not consume any diet soft drinks or foods containing aspartame. The body converts aspartame to the amino acid phenylalanine that is the precursor for tyrosine. Tyrosine is the precursor for dopamine and the excitatory neurotransmitters, epinephrine and norepinephrine (commonly called *adrenalin* and *noradrenalin*). These neurotransmitters are powerful vasoconstrictors that raise blood pressure dramatically. Aspartame hypes the hormonal system and causes hunger, anxiety, and insomnia. Do not take phenylalanine and tyrosine supplements except as are naturally found in low-carb whey protein powder.

Example Foods Based on Body Size
Weight Shown Is Lean Body Mass (LBM)

Food Category	Small Female 80 pounds	Medium Female 100 pounds	Medium Male 140 pounds	Large Male 160 pounds
Breakfast				
Eggs	1	2	2	2
Bacon See Note 1	1 slice	1.5 slices	2 slices	2 slices
Stir-Fry Veggies	1/2 cup	3/4 cup	1 cup	1 cup
Cod Liver Oil See Note 2	1 tablespoon	1 tablespoon	1 tablespoon	1 tablespoon
Borage Oil	1 capsule	1 capsule	1 capsule	1 capsule
Snack				
Cheese	1 slice (1.1 oz)	1 slice (1.1 oz)	1 slice (1.1 oz)	2 slices (2.2 oz)
Lunch				
Meat	2 oz.	2 oz.	3 oz.	3 oz.
Veggies.	1 cup	1 cup	1.5 cup	2 cup

Snack				
Meat	1 oz.	1 oz.	1 oz.	1 oz.
Veggies	1/4 cup	1/4 cup	1/4 cup	1/4 cup
Dinner				
Meat	3 oz.	3 oz.	4 oz.	5 oz.
Veggies	3/4 cup	1 cup	1 cup	1 cup
Coconut Oil	1/2 tablespoon	3/4 tablespoon	1 tablespoon	1 tablespoon
Cod Liver Oil	---	---	1 tablespoon	1 tablespoon
Borage Oil	---	---	1 capsule	1 capsule
Snack				
Cheese	1 oz.	1 oz.	1.5 oz.	2 oz.

635

Total Calories	1116	1299	1770	1939
Total Fat, %	69	69	71	71
Sat. Fat, %	26	26	27	27
Poly. Fat, %	14	14	15	14
Mono. Fat, %	23	30	23	24
Protein, %	29	28	26	26
Carbs, %	3	3	3	3
Carbs, gm.	13	16	20	22
Fiber, gm.	5	6	8	9

Note 1 - The bacon must be uncured or cured without sugar. Fry the bacon over low heat. Add the eggs as soon as the bacon begins to sizzle. Stop cooking the bacon while it is still floppy with visible white fat. Pour off the excess fat. Do not cook the bacon until it is crisp as is common. High heat and over cooking oxidize the fats in crisp bacon and make it unhealthy.

Note 2 - Carlson's® Lemon Flavored Cod Liver Oil and borage oil with a high GLA fatty acid content are highly recommended.

Emergency Plateau Breaking Program

Too much protein can prevent weight loss and even cause weight gain on the low-carb diet in those with severe metabolic resistance. The body can convert 58% of the protein in meat to glucose. A higher-fat, lower-protein, low-carb diet can achieve an amazing drop in weight when the standard low-carb diet has failed. Try the following detailed eating suggestions. Drink regular coffee, black or herbal teas, or water. Avoid all fruit and vegetable juices and all diet or regular sodas.

Breakfast:

Eggs: Fry two large eggs in real butter or refined coconut oil for a large male or just one egg for a small female. A small amount of Swiss cheese on the eggs makes a tasty meal.

Tomato: One half of a large tomato or one small tomato for a large male. A small female should eat half that amount.

Pepper: One half of a medium-size red, yellow, or orange pepper is a nice addition.

Snack:

Cheese: One slice of Swiss cheese for a large male or half a slice for a small female.

Lunch:

Avocado: One avocado for a large male or half an avocado for a small female.

Tomato: One half of a large tomato or one small tomato for a large male. A small female should eat half that amount. Other low-carb vegetables can be eaten in reduced quantities.

Snack:

Candy: One piece of *Dove® Silky Smooth Dark Chocolate® Promises* for a large male or half a piece for a small female. Candy is not normally recommended on the low-carb diet. This is a rare exception to give the blood sugar a little boost and prevent the body from going into further metabolic resistance. Be careful. Having candy in the house can be very tempting. Let the chocolate melt in the mouth to enjoy the full flavor. Enjoy it with coffee or tea.

Dinner:

> **Meat, Fowl, or Fish:** Follow the above suggestions for a regular meal, but limit the quantity of meat. Select a high-fat choice such as roasted chicken thighs with the skin or high-fat beef burger without the bun, of course. Avoid a large serving of lean meat.

> **Green Beans:** Small serving of steamed or boiled green beans. Other low-carb vegetables can be eaten in reduced quantities.

Snack:

> **Cheese:** One slice of Swiss cheese for a large male or half a slice for a small female.

Addressing Muscle Loss on the Low-Carbohydrate Diet

A low-carbohydrate diet supporter posted on a message board that she was thrilled with her 100-pound weight loss, but she was certain that a good percentage of the loss was muscle. Actually, she was right. As people gain weight, they notice that their legs and hips become very muscular. The woman lost 100 pounds (45 kg) that caused her leg muscles to slim as well. Her legs were not carrying the extra load everywhere she went, so the muscles simply slimmed down. This has nothing whatsoever to do with the low-carbohydrate diet.

She could have kept the heavy muscles in her legs and hips if she had put on a weight suit and added the necessary weights in pockets to keep the total weight at her previous maximum. This technique would keep her leg and hip muscles in tact as if she were heavier. However, I don't think she would like the results because her upper body would be trim, but her lower body would look like that of a bodybuilder who only did leg exercises. Expect muscle mass to adjust in proportion to the total amount of body weight. Use bodybuilding techniques if you want heavier muscles.

Reversing Heart Disease and Preventing Diabetes

Chapter 11

Your Road to Reversing Heart Disease

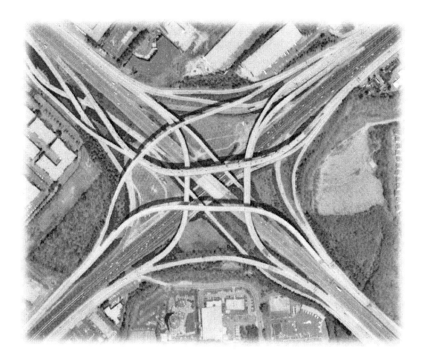

Your Road to *Success* Has Many Off-Ramps

Chapter 11

Congratulations! Because you are reading this book, you're one in a million who has the opportunity to enter the on-ramp to the Reversing Heart Disease Road on your way to **Success**. Reversing heart disease is like winning the jumbo lottery. Rarely does it happen, but you can begin to celebrate very soon. The road has more exits than alleys in Calcutta. You must work hard to avoid the slums.

I will try my best to get you on the road and keep you on the road until you reach Success, but you must put forth major personal efforts to make it happen. The first recommendation is to **erase your brain** of all nutritional, health, and dietary dogma that accumulated prior to reading this book. Yes, your brain, memory, prejudices, religion, education, and titles are major roadblocks to reversing heart disease. You have probably already encountered these obstacles if you disagreed with some of the information in previous chapters. If your mind is now clear from the fear of eating natural animal fats, you can enter the on-ramp to the Reversing Heart Disease Road. If not, you can only see it in the distance.

My regime reversed my heart disease.

Hopefully, you believe that heart disease can be reversed as I have done. Congratulations, if you do. You just maneuvered onto the on-ramp, and you are now on your way to Success. But don't relax too quickly. The road that leads to Success has many exits that will detour you to poor health and other unpleasant destinations. I will describe a few of the exits that you must avoid.

Now would be a good time to test the status of your mental condition. Proceed to the refrigerator, find the butter, slice off a

¼ x 1 inch (6 x 25 mm) chunk, pop it in your mouth, and enjoy the delicious fat. This is a very high-fat diet that will make it impossible for those with fat phobias to reach Success. I will never forget the comments on a low-carb forum when people listed their favorite fat treats. One woman said her favorite treat was ¼ pound (0.11 kg) of butter eaten in a couple of gulps. Obviously, she did not have a fat phobia. This should be your goal in order to stay on the road to Success.

Visualize six one-gallon (3.785 liter) milk jugs filled with thick saturated fat sitting on the table. You can't carry those six bottles of fat in your hands, but many people easily carry an identical 42 pounds (18.9 kg) of body fat. When I presented this visualization in a low-fat forum, the overweight members groaned. They were reducing dietary fat in the hope of losing weight. They did not understand that body fat comes from eating whole grains, fruits, and starchy vegetables that are all **Forbidden Foods** on my diet therapy program.

Beware of the exit sign labeled,
Dietary Fat Phobia → Exit

Look out! Bad advice is the next exit that will hit you in the face. Friends, family, and co-workers will insist that my diet therapy will surely kill you from *artery-clogging saturated fat.* They recommend zero-fat fruits, not knowing the liver turns fructose to blood fats faster than they can swallow. People with obsessive compulsive controlling disorder (OCCD) will be the most difficult to avoid.

They will get in your face, get mad, pout, argue, threaten, and as a last resort, shun you if you refuse to stuff your face with whole grains, fruits, and starchy vegetables. These people don't know that all carbohydrates enter the bloodstream as sugars after digestion. They drink low-fat milk not knowing that the liver quickly turns the lactose into blood fats, and insulin deposits it as slabs of body fat.

Beware of people with OCCD telling you what to do.
The exit sign says,
Dietary Advice from Friends → Exit

The next exit is the inability to endure a little discomfort. I often hear people admit that the food they are eating will cause long-term health problems, but they insist on eating it anyway. These people are addicted to carbohydrates and will not deny themselves.

The exit sign says,
Comfort Station → Exit

Others have a prescription drug phobia and strongly object to taking an antibiotic unless the infection is dripping puss. They insist that antibiotics are a health-damaging scam invented by pharmaceutical companies.

This exit is labeled,
Prescription Drugs will Kill You → Exit

Don't forget the purist who insists that all of his nutrition must come from the food he eats. He strictly avoids vitamins, minerals, and supplements based on the false claim that they are worthless or even worse, harmful. Actually, many physicians take this position.

This exit sign says,
Vitamins Are a Waste of Money → Exit

Those who insist on taking concentrated whole food supplements instead of pharmaceutical grade vitamins, minerals, and supplements will exit the road to Success.

This natural and appealing exit sign says,
Natural Whole Food Vitamins Only → Exit

Another exit from the road to Success tries to convince you that diet therapy will not improve your health because you are different. Those who take this exit believe the false theory that human physiology has wide variations among individuals. People respond differently to food and environmental conditions based on the diseases they may have, not on basic human physiology. For example, I can eat a big serving of ice cream and thoroughly enjoy it without any ill effects because I don't have diabetes or an inflammatory bowel disease. You may encounter several discomforts on my diet therapy program because of preexisting health conditions. These discomforts must be resolved by careful study, analysis, adjustments, and determination in order to stay on the Reversing Heart Disease Road. One exception is our genetic response to statin drugs as determined by the Genotype Tests performed by Berkeley HeartLab® as described in Chapter 4. There may be a few other scientific exceptions, but don't use these excuses for a quick exit.

Your health will suffer if you take the exit labeled,
You are Different → Exit

Many religions have taboos against certain foods and food groups. In fact, very few religions are devoid of such restrictions. Your religion could throw you over the guardrail, down the embankment, and off the road before you ever approach the first exit ramp. My diet therapy program restricts certain foods because they contain excessive amounts of unhealthy sugars.

Chapter 11

This is not a religious diet. Those with religious dietary taboos and vegetarians cannot stay on the road to Success. I can't help you resolve this conflict other than to recommend that you read my first book, *Absolute Truth Exposed – Volume 1*.

This exit sign will say,
Religious Taboos → You Just Crashed

It is possible to fully comply with the diet, supplement, and drug regimen that I have outlined in this book without the assistance of a physician, but I do not recommended this for most people. This brings us to the next exit from the road to Success. One person on my regimen wrote to say that his doctor threw him out of the office and told him to never come back. Others have written to explain the harsh threats they have received from their doctors. Go to a different doctor before he insists that you exit from the road to Success.

Don't take the exit labeled,
My Doctor Disagrees → Exit

Beware of the exit that will try to get you off the Reversing Heart Disease Road by suggesting or forcing you to lower dietary fat consumption. Health organizations in the United Kingdom and United States have recommended a high tax on high-fat foods to prevent us from eating them, but Denmark beat them to it in September 2011 by imposing a fat tax on foods with saturated fat above 2.5%. All English-speaking countries have an obesity epidemic because they meddle in the lives of the citizens with false health, diet, and exercise propaganda. Australia holds the record for obesity, having surpassed the United States last year. This is similar to the cigarette taxes that have been increasing at a steady rate over the past twenty years with the goal of improving people's health by financially forcing them to quit smoking. Yes, millions of people stopped smoking, but cancer in the United States has jumped to the leading cause of death due to the attack on dietary fats. Governments in several countries are threatening to restrict employment opportunities and medical benefits based on the person's weight as leverage to force people to eat carbohydrates. The government health departments falsely believe that dietary fat is a deadly poison that makes people obese and gives them diseases. Schools in the United States have begun to impose harsh restrictions on students by forcing them to choose a high-carbohydrate lunch, starvation, or expulsion; yet childhood obesity is ballooning above old records, and the kids are becoming juvenile Type 2 diabetics. The students will be forced to get a written statement from a physician in order to bring a healthy low-carbohydrate lunch from home. The governments could easily throw you off the road to Success by passing dietary laws against eating fat. Don't give in. Fight these obsessive compulsive controllers who are making obesity skyrocket.

Beware of the exit sign labeled,
Fat Tax → Exit or You Will Be Punished

Ostrich Syndrome is a mental dysfunction in which the sufferer has the tendency to dodge any personal responsibility by shifting every detail of his healthcare to a team of physicians. I have talked with many people with Ostrich Syndrome. They neither deny nor accept scientific information but simply respond by saying they intend to follow their physician's advice. This is well and good if you have my cardiologist as your physician, but most simply go along with the recommendations of their professional associations. I know two individuals with heart disease whose doctors are morbidly obese. (My cardiologist has an athletic physic, and he fully supports my diet, supplement, and drug regimen.) One of the physicians suggested that his patients eat the low-fat government diet. If you have Ostrich Syndrome, I hope you can overcome it, but what can an ostrich do except get eaten by the lions? Ostrich Syndrome is like a roadblock where you must exit.

This exit sign says,
Ostrich Syndrome → You Must Exit

A great many people will not accept the information I present despite my supporting documentation because contrary propaganda has been blasted into their minds since childhood. Those who simply cannot bring themselves to accept the scientific fats that red meat and saturated animal fats are healthy and heal the body will take the next exit ramp.

This exit sign says,
Brainwashed Syndrome → Exit

I wish you well on the Reversing Heart Disease Road. If you avoid the exit ramps, misleading signs, brainwashing, phobias, peer pressure, insults, threats, religious dogma, and government health organizations, you should arrive at Success in good health. Enjoy your trip.

Government intrusion into nutrition and healthcare in all English-speaking countries has caused obesity and many diseases to escalate in concert.

"I think that what you say is true."
Andrew, age 10

Luke 10:21 . . . "I thank thee, O Father, Lord of heaven and earth, that thou hast hid these things from the wise and prudent, and hast revealed them unto babes: even so, Father; for so it seemed good in thy sight."

Index

Index

651

Index

D

E

655

H

Index

Index

Index

Index

Index

Index

Index

Index

CPSIA information can be obtained
at www.ICGtesting.com
Printed in the USA
FSOW02n0434300615
8307FS